Sports Biomechanics

When working with sports men and women, the biomechanist is faced with two apparently incompatible goals: reducing injury risk and improving sports performance. Now in a fully updated and revised edition, *Sports Biomechanics* covers the fundamental principles that underpin our understanding of the biomechanics of both sports injury and performance, and explains how contemporary biomechanical science can be used to meet both of those goals simultaneously.

The first four chapters of this book look closely at sports injury, including topics such as the properties of biological materials, mechanisms of injury occurrence, risk reduction, and the estimation of forces in biological structures. The last four chapters concentrate on the biomechanical enhancement of sports performance, including analytical techniques, statistical and mathematical modelling of sports movements, and the use of feedback to enhance sports performance.

Drawing on the very latest empirical and epidemiological data, and including clear concise summaries, self-test questions and guides to further reading in every chapter, this book is essential reading for all advanced undergraduate and postgraduate students with an interest in biomechanics, sports injury, sports medicine, physical therapy or performance analysis.

Roger Bartlett is Professor of Sports Biomechanics in the School of Physical Education, University of Otago, New Zealand. He is an Invited Fellow of the International Society of Biomechanics in Sports and an Honorary Fellow of the British Association of Sport and Exercise Sciences, of which he was Chairman from 1991–4. Roger is a former editor-in-chief of the *Journal of Sports Sciences,* and *Sports Biomechanics.* He is the author of *Introduction to Sports Biomechanics: Analysing Human Movement Patterns* and co-editor of several other sports science books.

Melanie Bussey is a Senior Lecturer in Biomechanics and Sports Injuries in the School of Physical Education, University of Otago, New Zealand. She is a member of the International Society of Biomechanics, Sport Science New Zealand and Sports Medicine Association of Australia. She publishes in a broad spectrum of sport, clinical and biomechanical journals including the *Journal of Biomechanics, Clinical Biomechanics, Journal of Medicine and Science in Sport* and *Manual Therapy.*

Sports Biomechanics

Reducing injury risk and improving sports performance

Second edition

Roger Bartlett and Melanie Bussey

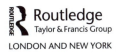

Routledge
Taylor & Francis Group

LONDON AND NEW YORK

First published 1999
by Routledge
2 Park Square, Milton Park, Abingdon, Oxon OX14 4RN
This second edition published 2012

Simultaneously published in the USA and Canada
by Routledge
711 Third Avenue, New York, NY 10017

Routledge is an imprint of the Taylor & Francis Group, an informa business

British Library Cataloguing in Publication Data
A catalogue record for this book is available from the British Library.

Library of Congress Cataloging in Publication Data
Bartlett, Roger
   Sports biomechanics: reducing injury risk and improving sports
   performance / Roger Bartlett, Melanie Bussey. – 2nd ed.
      p. cm.
   1. Sports – Physiological aspects.   2. Human mechanics.
   3. Sports injuries – Prevention.
   I. Bussey, Melanie. II. Title.
 ✓ RC1235. B372012
   617.1'027--dc23

                                        2011019516

ISBN: 978–0–415–55837–2 (hbk)
ISBN: 978–0–415–55838–9 (pbk)
ISBN: 978–0–203–86771–6 (ebk)

Typeset in Sabon
by RefineCatch Limited, Bungay, Suffolk

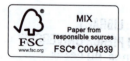

Contents

Figures

Tables

Preface

Sports biomechanics has two main concerns, on which this book focuses: the reduction of injury risk and the improvement of performance. It is a scientific discipline that is relevant to all students of the exercise and sport sciences, to those intending to become physical education teachers, and to all those interested in sports performance and injury. This book is intended as the companion volume to *Introduction to Sports Biomechanics: Analysing Human Movement Patterns*. Whereas that text mostly covers first and second year undergraduate material, this one focuses on third and fourth year undergraduate and postgraduate topics. The book is organised into two halves, which deal respectively with the two key issues of sports biomechanics: why injuries occur and how performance can be improved. Wherever possible, these topics are approached from a practical sport viewpoint. The mathematical element in biomechanics often deters students without a mathematical background. Where we consider that basic mathematical equations add to the clarity of the material, then these have been included, particularly in Chapter 4. However, we have otherwise avoided extensive mathematical development of the topics, so that the non-mathematical reader should find most of the material easily accessible.

The production of any textbook relies on the cooperation of many people other than the authors. We acknowledge the helpful contributions of several colleagues at our university, the University of Otago. In particular, the book could not have been produced without the backing of the Dean of the School of Physical Education, Professor Doug Booth. Neither would it have been possible without the inspiration provided by our many undergraduate and postgraduate students over the years. Roger Bartlett would like to thank his former honours student Anna Skelton for proof reading the drafts of his chapters and for suggesting the topics for the glossaries in those chapters, and to acknowledge the encouragement and psychological support provided by Jo Trezise and Jo Stuthridge during the gestation period of this book. Roger would also like to thank Professor Mike Hughes for permission to use and adapt some of the material from one of their joint chapters on performance analysis, and for inspiring much of his interest in that discipline. Melanie Bussey would like to thank graduate students Rhys Thorp and Neil Anderson for their aid in chasing down lost references and tedious file formatting. Most importantly, she would like to thank her family, husband Mike Sam and children Sophie and Jackson, for their patience, support and encouragement.

Roger Bartlett and Melanie Bussey

Introduction

Sports biomechanics has been described as having two aims that, at times, seem incompatible: the reduction of injury risk and the improvement of sports performance. The first four chapters of this book focus on the first of these aspects, the reduction of injury risk, while the last four chapters focus on the improvement of sports performance. At the end of the last chapter, the book comes full circle with a consideration of intervention strategies to reduce the risk of injury to fast bowlers in cricket.

The reduction of injury risk may involve a sequence of stages that begins with a description of the incidence and types of sports injury. The next stage is to identify the factors and mechanisms that affect the occurrence of sports injury. This relates to the properties of biological materials (Chapter 1), the mechanisms of injury occurrence (Chapter 2), the identifiable risk factors (Chapter 3) and the estimation of forces in biological structures (Chapter 4). Where deemed necessary, mathematical equations have been introduced, although extensive mathematical development of topics covered has been avoided.

Biomechanists use the principles and theories of physics and mechanical engineering to describe the forces and force-related factors that lead to injury. In a biomechanical model, it is the relationship between applied force and specific tissue tolerance to the applied force that determines the outcome of an inciting event.

In Chapter 1, we consider important mechanical concepts in the study of injury such as energy, external forces or load and the effects of loading on biological tissue along with an introduction to the important epidemiological concepts that support the biomechanical study of injury risk. The most important mechanical properties of biological and non-biological materials are explained. In particular, we outline the composition and biomechanical properties of bone, cartilage, ligament and tendon and their behaviour under various forms of loading. Muscle elasticity, contractility, the generation of maximal force in a muscle, muscle activation, muscle stiffness and the importance of the stretch–shortening cycle are all described.

To understand how sport participation may affect biological tissue and tissue tolerance to loads applied during sport participation, it is necessary to understand how biological tissue adapts to mechanical stress. In Chapter 2, we consider aspects of tissue adaptation and the effect of mechanical stress on bone, cartilage, muscle, ligament and tendons. Furthermore, we cover the biomechanical reasons why injuries occur in sport, and we distinguish between acute and overuse injury. An understanding is provided of the various injuries that occur to bone and soft tissues, including cartilage, ligaments and the muscle–tendon unit, and how these depend on the load characteristics. The sports injuries that affect the major joints of the lower and upper extremities, and the back and neck, are also covered.

Chapter 3 includes a consideration of some of the most general and common intrinsic and extrinsic risk factors in sport. Intrinsic risk factors are those factors that affect the load tolerance of the tissues within the athlete. Intrinsic factors considered in Chapter 3 are age, sex, anatomy, previous injury history, and movement technique. Extrinsic risk factors are those factors that influence the load characteristics applied to the tissues within the athlete while participating in sport. Under extrinsic risk factors, we consider the important characteristics of sports surfaces and how specific surfaces behave. The methods used to assess sports surfaces biomechanically and the injury aspects of sports surfaces are also covered. Attention is then given to the injury-moderating role of protective equipment. In addition to protective equipment, we consider various forms of athletic footwear, including running shoes, court shoes and field shoes, and important aspects of each in reducing injury and enhancing the relationship between the athlete and the surface on which they play. We look at various faults in movement technique across a range of individual and team sports and evaluate the effect of such faults on musculoskeletal injury.

In Chapter 4 the difficulties of calculating the forces in muscles and ligaments are considered, including typical simplifications made in inverse dynamics modelling. The equations for planar force and moment calculations from inverse dynamics for single segments and for a segment chain are explained, along with how the procedures can be extended to multi-link systems. The various approaches to overcoming the redundancy or indeterminacy problem are described. The method of inverse optimisation is covered, and attention is given to an evaluation of the various cost functions used. Finally, the uses and limitations of electromyography (EMG) in estimating muscle force are outlined.

The second aim of sports biomechanics, as we observed above, is the improvement of performance. This can involve certain aspects of sports equipment design and engineering, which can also help reduce the risk of injury; this is a major concern of the new discipline of Sports Engineering. In Chapter 5, we focus on Performance Analysis, a 'discipline' of sports science that has truly emerged and prospered since the first edition of this book. In the following two chapters, we look at the contribution sports biomechanics has made, and can make, to the improvement of sports performance – by improving the movement technique of the performer, through both qualitative (Chapter 6) and quantitative biomechanical modelling and analysis (Chapter 7). In Chapter 8, we conclude by looking at aspects of intervention strategies to improve performance.

Performance analysis can be considered to bring together various disciplines which are concerned with the analysis and improvement of sports performance. It is used extensively by sports movement analysts working 'in the field' with coaches and athletes. It can be seen, primarily, as an amalgam of sports biomechanics, notational analysis, and motor learning and control, with important contributions from sports technology and, when related to the analysis of performance, inputs from physiology, coaching science and, occasionally, psychology. In Chapter 5, we focus on the notational analysis and biomechanical analysis components of performance analysis, which are the aspects most directly involved with the analysis of sports performance, and we touch on the four-stage approach to structured performance analysis. The qualitative, semi-quantitative and quantitative approaches are outlined and contrasted. We then consider what notational analysis involves and how it is used to try to understand and improve performance of teams and individuals, and consider both hand notation systems and computerised notational analysis. We also outline some of the components of biomechanical analysis, such as analysis of phases of a sports technique, and movement principles as they relate to movement phase analysis and sports performance.

To improve sports performance, we effectively need some 'model' to which we can compare the current movement technique and performance of our athlete. In Chapter 6, we focus on the use of qualitative biomechanical analysis (in which we include semi-quantitative analysis) in the improvement of sports performance. Qualitative analysis is often used more directly than quantitative analysis in seeking to improve sports performance, as it is the approach most often used by coaches, teachers and performance analysts working with individual athletes and sports teams. We consider in more detail the four-stage structured analysis approach. A strong focus in this chapter is the use of deterministic models of sports performance to identify observable 'critical features' of the movement; we also look at alternative ways of identifying critical features. The use of qualitative biomechanical analysis software packages is overviewed. Qualitative analysis is not, however, only about observational analysis of video. It also involves the qualitative (and semi-quantitative) analysis of movement patterns and coordination patterns. We look at both of these types of pattern and see how they can enhance observational analysis of video footage. The coordination patterns we consider are angle–angle diagrams, phase planes and relative phase, and cross-correlation functions.

In Chapter 7, we consider the fundamentals underlying the quantitative biomechanical optimisation of sports movements, and focus on those approaches that have a strong emphasis on improving performance, albeit often more indirectly that the qualitative methods of the previous chapter. The relationships that can exist between a performance criterion and various performance variables are explained. The cross-sectional, longitudinal and contrast approaches to statistical modelling are described and the limitations of statistical modelling in sports biomechanics are evaluated. The advantages and limitations of computer simulation modelling, when seeking to evaluate and improve sports movements, are covered; brief explanations of modelling, simulation, simulation evaluation and optimisation are also provided. The differences between static and dynamic optimisation and global and local optimums are outlined. The interpretation and explanation of graphical representations of optimisation and the use of contour maps to identify likely ways to performance improvement are emphasised, in the context of studies of javelin throwing. We touch on models of human skeletal muscle and their use in both general computer simulation models of the sports performer and establishing optimal sports movements. The chapter concludes with the consideration of a more recent approach to modelling sports movements through the use of artificial intelligence, particularly artificial neural networks.

Chapter 8 considers how the results of performance analysis and of biomechanical studies of sports movements can be communicated and fed back to the athlete and coach to improve performance; this is the crucial intervention stage of the four-stage analysis process discussed in Chapter 6. The fundamental points that must be satisfied for feedback to the coach and athlete to be relevant are covered. The different forms of feedback that are now available are critically assessed. The strengths and weaknesses of the various models of performance covered in Chapters 6 and 7 and their limitations as intervention 'tools' are evaluated. The issues that must be addressed in seeking to optimise the provision of biomechanical information to the coach and athlete are discussed, with reference to some relevant motor learning literature. An overview and evaluation is provided of several forms of computer-based feedback. Finally, several intervention case studies are considered, mostly dealing with reducing injury risk in cricket fast bowlers.

1 Biomechanics of sports injury

Melanie Bussey

Knowledge assumed
Familiarity with human anatomy
Understanding of basic biomechanics

INTRODUCTION – THE SCIENCE OF STUDYING INJURY

BOX 1.1 LEARNING OUTCOMES

After reading this chapter you should be able to:

- recognise and use biomechanical terminology related to tissue function and injury
- describe the epidemiological and biomechanical perspectives of injury
- understand and explain the mechanical factors involved in tissue injury
- understand the basic material properties of human tissue
- explain the mechanical behaviours of human tissue
- understand the biomechanical functions of ligament, tendon, bone and cartilage.

For the purposes of this text we will use a simple working definition of sports injury, that is the disruption or failure of biological tissue in response to mechanical loading during sporting endeavours. To understand how injury to the musculoskeletal system occurs, it is necessary to know the loads and properties that cause specific tissues to fail. These relate to the material and structural properties of the various tissues of the musculoskeletal system: cortical and cancellous bone, cartilage, muscles, fascia, ligaments and tendons. The material properties that are important in this context are known as bulk mechanical properties. These are, for materials in general: density, elastic modulus, damping, yield strength, ultimate tensile strength, hardness, fracture resistance, fatigue strength and creep strength. It is important to understand not only how biological materials fail, but also how other materials can affect injury and how they can best be used in sport and exercise. The incidence of injury may be reduced or increased by, for example, shoes for sport and exercise, sports surfaces and protective equipment.

The study of sports injury is a multidisciplinary endeavour. Some examples of related disciplines include physiology, biomechanics, kinesiology, medicine, psychology, and epidemiology. Increasingly, the study of sports injury is also interdisciplinary, when researchers from differing disciplines combine their efforts to study injury with a new perspective. Each discipline comes with its own perspective on injury and its own specific vocabulary around injury. In this text we will be taking a distinctly biomechanical view of injury but we will also try to present data and knowledge from epidemiology and medicine to support and enrich the information given. Before undertaking any study of sports injury it is important to acknowledge the contribution of other disciplines and to understand how our biomechanical research may be informed by them.

Injury severity

From an epidemiology perspective the severity of an injury is defined by the amount of 'time lost'. Sports injuries are considered to be any injury resulting from participation in sport or exercise that causes either a reduction in that activity or a need for medical advice or treatment. Sports injuries are often classified in terms of the activity time lost: minor (one to seven days), moderately serious (eight to 21 days) or serious (21 or more days or permanent damage). The epidemiological model varies significantly from the clinical model. From a clinical perspective, injury severity is classified by the amount of structural involvement, physical signs, and extent of dysfunction. In the clinical model, the severity increases with the amount of damage experienced by the tissue; for example, ligament injury is graded first degree (mild damage to ligament), second (moderate ligament damage) and third degree (near or complete rupture of ligament). The need for both perspectives is clear. The epidemiological perspective is necessary to understand the link between injury and exposure time; this information is important to gain insight into injury incidence, injury reoccurrence and injury outcome. In contrast, the goal for the clinical model is finding and implementing the correct treatment protocol for that injury. Both perspectives are important to the biomechanist as both present information important to understanding the mechanical mechanisms related to the injury. For example, information about exposure times gives the biomechanist insight into the nature of the loading such as frequency, loading cycle, rest time, and potential cumulative effects of loading. Information about the amount of tissue damage is important to our understanding of specific tissue tolerance and the consequence of particular load characteristics.

Mechanism of injury

The mechanism of injury refers to the physical process responsible for given damage to a body system. Broadly, an injury mechanism should establish a cause and effect relationship. Because this term is loosely defined it has been open to interpretation by many different groups that research or treat injury. Thus, categorisation of mechanisms is quite variable, yet each system seems to work for the groups that use it and may be considered correct from that group's perspective. Categorisation of mechanisms is based on a combination of description of inciting event, description of mechanical factors and tissue responses to mechanical factors. Three of the most commonly used categorisations of mechanisms of injury are shown in Table 1.1. The reason we need a method of categorising injury mechanisms is so we can better understand the causes of injury so that we may design and implement appropriate injury prevention strategies.

Table 1.1 Three of the most commonly used categorisations of mechanisms of injury

SOURCE		
LEAD BETTER (2001)	COMMITTEE ON TRAUMA RESEARCH (1985)	BAHR AND KROSSHAUG (2005)
Contact	Crushing deformation	Description of inciting event including:
Dynamic overload	Impulsive impact	Playing situation
Overuse	Skeletal acceleration	Athlete–opponent behaviour
Structural vulnerability	Energy absorption	Whole body biomechanics
Inflexibility	Extent and rate of tissue deformation	Joint-tissue biomechanics
Impact		
Rapid growth		

Epidemiological perspective on injury

Epidemiology is the study of the incidence, distribution and determinants of disease and injury frequency within a given population (Woodward, 2005). Epidemiological studies can be descriptive or analytical. Descriptive studies examine the frequency, or incidence, and prevalence of injury occurrence. Incidence relates to the number of new cases that occur in a defined population during the time frame of the study, while prevalence refers to the total number of cases existing within a given population at a given time. Descriptive studies also look for patterns in injury occurrences by examining factors such as who gets injured, the location of injury, the time of occurrence and the type of injury. So, descriptive epidemiology provides the what, the who, the when and the where. Analytical studies examine the causal relationships for injury. So analytical epidemiologists ask the questions how and why injuries are taking place in order to establish relationships between injury occurrence and certain risk factors.

A risk factor is something that increases your chances of experiencing an injury. Sometimes, this risk comes from something you do such as not wearing a helmet while cycling. These risk factors we can manipulate to reduce our risk; they may be considered to be modifiable. At other times, there is nothing you can do; simply being of a certain age or cycling in certain weather conditions can increase your risk of injury. We cannot change our age, sex, climate etc., so these risk factors are non-modifiable.

Risk factors may also be categorised as intrinsic or extrinsic to the athlete. Intrinsic risk factors are those related to you, the athlete, specifically, such as age, sex, anatomical alignment, neuromuscular control and previous injury history. Extrinsic risk factors are those related to the sporting environment, such as use of protective equipment, climate, opponent skill or ability and rules of the game. Competing at a high standard increases the incidence of sports injuries, also contact sports have a greater injury risk than non-contact ones and in team sports more injuries occur during matches than in training, in contrast to individual sports.

Risk factors do not infer cause, which means that having one or more risk factors does not guarantee that you will experience a particular injury. What it means is that you are statistically more likely to experience an injury as compared to a person who does not have those risk factors. The cause of injury is multifactorial involving the inter-relationships between the intrinsic risks, extrinsic risks and mechanical factors present at the moment of the inciting event. There are many models that attempt to demonstrate the relationships between these factors. Perhaps the most cited is that of Meeuwisse (Meeuwisse, 1994; Meeuwisse *et al.*, 2007). Meeuwisse describes an athlete with intrinsic risks as predisposed to injury. Furthermore, according to the model, the factors that predispose the athlete may combine with the extrinsic factors related to the sport and environment to make an athlete susceptible to injury (Figure 1.1). However, the simple presence of these risk factors is not enough to produce injury. Rather, risk factors must combine with the appropriate mechanical factors during an inciting event to produce an injury. As an example, a female basketball player may be predisposed due to her sex (intrinsic non-modifiable risk) and weak hamstring muscles (intrinsic modifiable risk). This athlete might become susceptible to injury because of environmental causes, such as the need to get around a defender quickly (extrinsic modifiable risk). She might then experience an injury while performing a cutting manoeuvre (inciting event), which places excessive load (mechanical factor) on the anterior cruciate ligament (ACL), leading to disruption of the ligament fibres.

Figure 1.1 Model of relationship between risk factors for athletic injury, with examples of risk factors and inciting events and biomechanical knowledge gained (adapted from Meeuwisse, 1994).

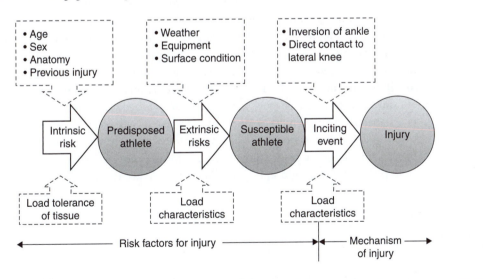

Biomechanical perspective on injury

From a very simplified viewpoint a biomechanist uses the principles and theories of the disciplines of physics and mechanical engineering to describe the forces and force-related (mechanical) factors that lead to injury. Arguably these factors are most closely related to the study of athletic injury as most athletic injuries can be related directly to mechanical causes (see the section below on energy). In the biomechanical model, the relationship between load applied and load tolerance determines the injury outcome of an inciting event. The critical feature for mechanical factors is that they must explain how the inciting event either resulted in a mechanical load in excess of that tolerated under normal circumstances or reduced the tolerance levels to a point at which a normal mechanical load cannot be tolerated (Fung, 1993). The mechanical factors may differ for each tissue and are dependent on the nature and type of load, its rate, the frequency of load repetition, the magnitude of energy transfer, and intrinsic factors such as age, sex and physical condition.

A biomechanical model will take tissue properties as well as load characteristics into account. As biomechanists we can use Meeuwisse's epidemiological model to emphasise the influence of load and load tolerance. For instance, intrinsic risk factors are seen in a biomechanical context, as those factors that affect the load tolerance of the tissues within the athlete, while extrinsic factors may be seen as those that influence the load characteristics (Figure 1.1). For example, if we look at age as an intrinsic factor, a masters standard athlete may have some devascularisation in the Achilles tendon, as can happen with increased age. The devascularisation causes a reduction in the elastic modulus and tendon resilience, thus decreasing the tendon's ability to tolerate large loads and increased load rates, making the tendon vulnerable to microtrauma. This athlete is predisposed to Achilles tendon injury. If we then look at an extrinsic factor such as the environment, say this athlete decides to switch from running on the beach to running on the road, he or she has changed the normal Achilles tendon load characteristics, increasing the magnitude of external repetitive loading to the Achilles tendon. Now this athlete is susceptible to Achilles tendon injury from either cumulative trauma, often seen in overuse injuries, or from some inciting event such as slipping on a wet road surface, which will increase the rate of loading to the Achilles tendon with a decreased load tolerance causing acute injury.

In the following sections we will cover some of the important mechanical concepts that are the foundation for studying injury from a biomechanical perspective. These concepts will form the grounding for Chapters 1 to 4 of this text.

ENERGY

Energy has been referred to as the primary agent of injury and, as such, is one of the most critical biomechanical concepts related to sports injury (Whiting and Zernicke, 2008). Energy is defined as the capacity to do work. It can assume many forms including chemical, electromagnetic, thermal and mechanical energy. Mechanical energy is the form most commonly related to sports injury and it is measured in joules (J).

The mechanical energy of a body can be classified according to the energy of its motion (kinetic energy, E_k) or the energy related to its position (potential energy, E_p). Linear kinetic energy is calculated as one half of the body's mass (m) multiplied by the square of its velocity (v) ($E_k = \frac{1}{2} m v^2$). Rotational kinetic energy is calculated using the mass moment of inertia (I) of the body in motion and its angular velocity (ω) ($E_k = \frac{1}{2} I \omega^2$). Potential energy can take two different forms. The first is gravitational potential energy, which is the potential of a body to do work as a function of height (h) with respect to a reference surface ($E_p = m g h$), where g is gravitational acceleration. So, a diver on a 10 m platform has a greater potential energy than a diver of the same mass standing on a 5 m platform. The second form of potential energy is deformation energy or strain energy, which is the energy stored in a body by virtue of its deformation. Simple examples of deformation energy are a stretched rubber band, a depressed spring board or a pole vaulter's bent pole. Deformation energy is particularly important in tissue biomechanics and is discussed further in the following sections.

The final concepts related to energy that every student studying injury should know are the principles of conservation of energy and transfer of energy. The principle of conservation of mechanical energy tells us that the net work done on a system is converted into kinetic and potential energy such that the total energy of the system remains constant throughout the motion (only when no external forces are acting on the system). Of course in sporting environments there is nearly always an external force acting on a system so mechanical energy is not entirely conserved. Don't panic, what this means is that some of the mechanical energy is converted to some other form, such as thermal or chemical energy. Also, in the case of an impact, some mechanical energy may be passed on from one system or body to another. Thus, conservation of energy indicates that energy is never destroyed rather it is transformed or transferred.

Transfer of energy is the mechanism by which energy is passed from one body to another. There are many sporting examples of transfer of energy. Energy transfer during a kicking motion can occur as energy moves from a proximal segment (e.g. the hip) to a distal segment (e.g. the foot). Another example is in a striking movement when a racquet makes contact with a ball in tennis. Energy transfer also occurs in collisions, as when a player tackles an opponent in rugby or American football. Transfer of energy can result in injury when the energy transferred exceeds the tolerance of the tissues involved.

LOAD, STRESS AND STRAIN

Load is referred to in this text as the sum of external forces applied to a material or tissue. When a load is applied to a body, that body may accelerate or the body may change in shape or configuration. This shape change is called deformation. There are three uni-directional load types. Compressive load occurs when equal and opposite loads are applied toward the surface of a body with a resulting deformation shortening and widening that body (Figure 1.2(a)). Tensile load occurs when equal and opposite loads are applied away from the surface of a body with a resulting deformation lengthening and narrowing of that body (Figure 1.2(b)). The third type of load is shear load where loads are applied parallel to the surface of the structure causing internal angular deformation (Figure 1.2(c)). Load deformation in some materials or tissues is obvious while in others it is unnoticeable. This is because the relationship between load and deformation is unique to the tissue or material type being loaded. Deformation is measured in absolute terms (e.g. mm) and we can depict the load–deformation relationship graphically in a load–deformation curve (Figure 1.3). The load deformation curve is useful for determining the mechanical properties of whole structures such as bone, an entire ligament or tendon, or an implant.

Figure 1.2 Uni-directional loads, with resulting deformation in wire-mesh outline: (a) compression; (b) tension; and (c) shear.

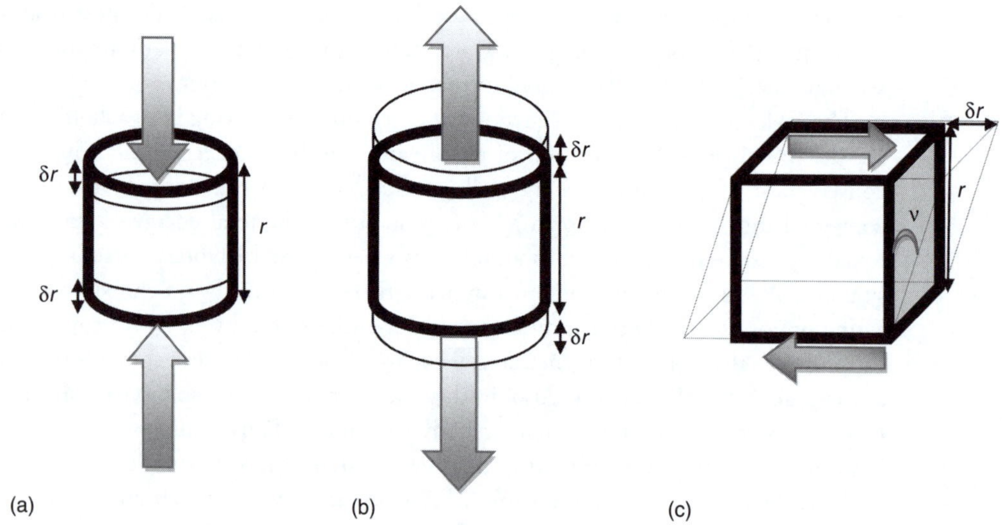

(a) (b) (c)

Figure 1.3 Load deformation curve for ligament.

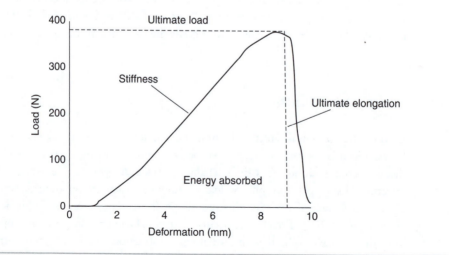

When a material is loaded, it undergoes deformation because the atomic bonds bend, stretch or compress. Because the bonds have been deformed, they try to restore themselves to their original positions, developing an internal resistance called stress. The standard (SI) unit of stress is the pascal (Pa), defined a 1 N distributed over 1 m^2. The stress (σ) is dependent upon the material properties of the tissue, the magnitude of the load and the cross-sectional area of tissue to which the load is applied ($\sigma = F/A$) where F is the normal force acting on the material and A is the area of an appropriate cross-sectional plane for the type of stress. The stresses in a material are known as the normal stresses when they are defined perpendicular to the relevant cross-section of the material (Figure 1.4). Normal stresses are categorised as compressive stresses (i.e. resistance to compressive loads) and tensile stresses (i.e. resistance to tensile loads). The third basic type of stress is shear stress. Shear stress is not a normal stress because it is applied tangential not perpendicular to the relevant cross-section of the material (Figure 1.2(c)). The shear stress (τ) and strain (v) (to be discussed a little further on) are calculated differently from normal stresses and strains: $\tau = F/A$ where A is the area over which the shear force acts and v is the angular deformation of the material in radians, or the angle of shear (Figure 1.2(c)). At every point in a stressed body there are at least three planes (Figure 1.4(a)), called principal planes, with normal vectors (Figure 1.4(b)). A principal plane is so called when the corresponding stress vector is perpendicular to the plane and where there are no shear stresses. The three stresses normal to these principal planes are called principal stresses (Figure 1.4(b)). For most loads experienced in sport, the stresses and strains developed in the tissues of the body, or in the materials making up sports equipment, are three-dimensional (Figure 1.4). Consequently, normal tension and compressive stresses are more commonly experienced in conjunction with bending or torsion (twisting) stresses, which were not mentioned in the opening paragraph. In such combined forms of loading, both the shape of the loaded structure and its material properties affect its ability to withstand loads.

Figure 1.4 Three-dimensional stresses in a material: (a) normal and shear stresses; (b) principal stresses (σ) and strains (ε). Dotted outline shows change in length of each side (δr) due to applied stress.

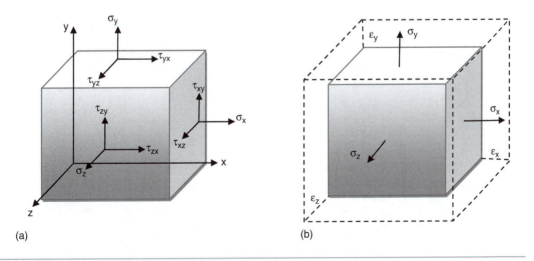

(a)

(b)

Structures that are relatively long and slim, such as human long bones, are likely to undergo bending. Bending is best illustrated in terms of a cantilever beam – a beam fixed at one end, for example a diving board of rectangular cross-section (Figure 1.5(a)). A force (F) exerted by the diver, acting perpendicular to the longitudinal axis of the beam, will tend to cause deflection or bending in the beam (Figure 1.5(b)). When bent, the material on the concave surface experiences compressive stress while the material on the convex surface experiences tensile stress (Figure 1.5(b)). These tensile and compressive stresses are a maximum at the outer surfaces of the beam and decrease toward the middle (Figure 1.5(c)). An axis somewhere between the two surfaces (it will be midway for a uniform rectangular cross section) experiences no deformation and hence no stress. This is known as the 'neutral axis'. The stress at any section of the beam increases with the distance, y, from the neutral axis (Figure 1.5(c)).

Figure 1.5 Bending of a beam: (a) cantilever beam represented as a diving board, with a rectangular cross section identified xs; (b) curved beam with top side under tension and bottom side under compression; (c) stress diagram representing stress distribution with respect to neutral axis; (d) transverse second moment of area.

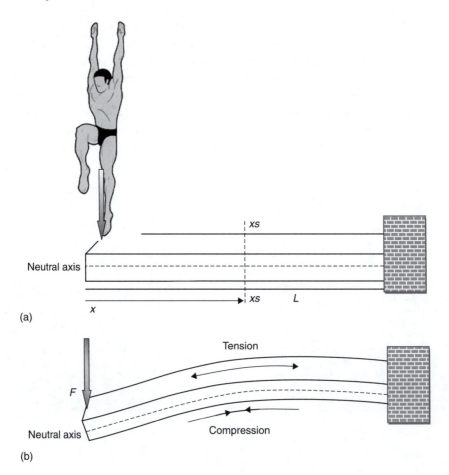

(a)

(b)

Figure 1.5 *Continued*

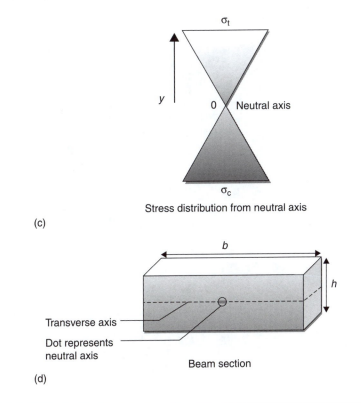

(c)

(d)

The forces acting on the beam create a moment on the beam, the bending moment (M_b). This moment generally varies along the beam, as for the example of a cantilever beam (Figure 1.5(a)). For such a beam, the bending moment at any section (e.g. *xs, xs*) is equal to the force applied to the beam (F) multiplied by the distance of its point of application from that section (x), which means the bending moment (M) will increase proportionally from zero at F to a value of FL at the base of the beam (Figure 1.5(a)). The stress can then be expressed as $\sigma = My/I_t$. Here y is the distance from the neutral axis and I_t is the second moment of area of the beam's cross section about the transverse axis that intersects the neutral axis (see Figure 1.5(d), where $I_t = bh^3/12$). The second moment of area sometimes known as the 'area moment of inertia' (I_t) is a property of a cross section that can be used to predict the resistance to bending and deflection about the neutral axis and its value depends upon the cross-sectional shape of the structure.

Torsion or 'twisting' is a common form of loading for biological tissues. It can be considered as similar to bending but with the maximum stresses being shear stresses. For a circular rod, the shear stress increases with radius (Figure 1.6(a)). The principal stresses – the normal compression and tension stresses – act at 45° to the long axis of the cylinder (Figure 1.6(b)). The shear stress caused by torsion is given by: $\tau = Tr/J_p$, where

Figure 1.6 Torsion stress applied to a cylinder: (a) the stress increases with radius – shear stress (τ) developed in response to torsional loading (T) where r is radius of the cylinder and J_p is the polar moment of inertia; (b) principal stresses (compressive (σ_c) and tension (σ_t)) act at 45° to long axis of cylinder.

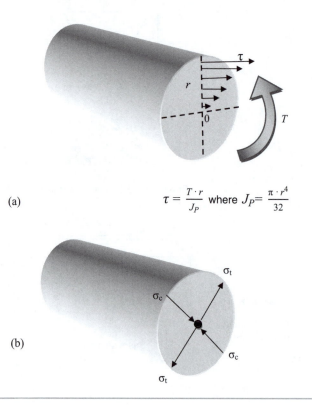

(a)

$$\tau = \frac{T \cdot r}{J_P} \text{ where } J_P = \frac{\pi \cdot r^4}{32}$$

(b)

r is the radial distance from the neutral axis, T is the applied torque about the neutral axis and J_p is the polar second moment of area. The polar second moment of area is the resistance to torsional load about the long axis of the cylinder. Torsional loading causes shear stresses in the material and results in the axes of principal stress being considerably different from the principal axes of inertia.

In both tension and bending, the resistance to an applied load depends on the moment of inertia of the loaded structure. Both the transverse moment of area (bending resistance) and the polar second moment of area (torsional resistance) are important. In structures designed to resist only one type of loading in one direction, the resistance to that type and direction of loading can be maximised, as in the vertical beam of Table 1.2. Biological tissues are often subject to combined loading from various directions. Bones, for example, are required to resist bending and torsional loads in sport. The strongest structure for resisting combined bending and torsion is the circular cylinder; to maximise the strength-to-weight ratio, the hollow circular cylinder is optimal. This shape provides reasonable values of both the transverse and polar moments of area (see Table 1.2), providing good load resistance and minimising mass.

Table 1.2 Relative resistance to bending and torsional loads.

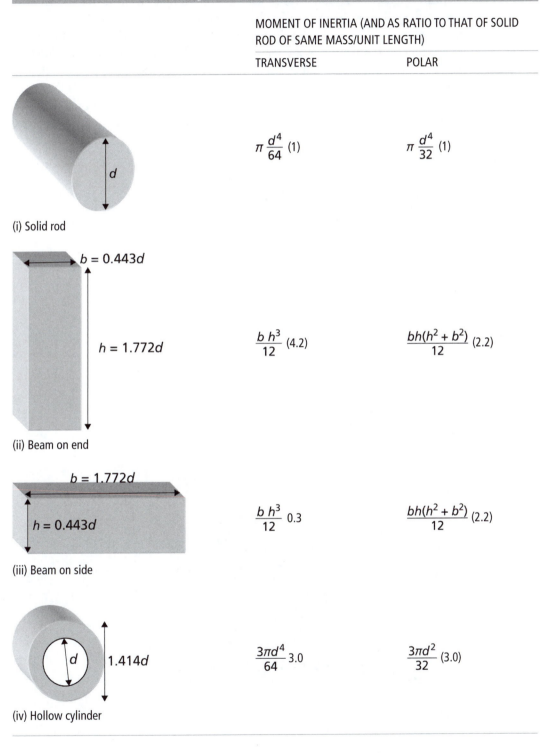

	MOMENT OF INERTIA (AND AS RATIO TO THAT OF SOLID ROD OF SAME MASS/UNIT LENGTH)	
	TRANSVERSE	POLAR
(i) Solid rod	$\pi \dfrac{d^4}{64}$ (1)	$\pi \dfrac{d^4}{32}$ (1)
(ii) Beam on end	$\dfrac{b\,h^3}{12}$ (4.2)	$\dfrac{bh(h^2 + b^2)}{12}$ (2.2)
(iii) Beam on side	$\dfrac{b\,h^3}{12}$ 0.3	$\dfrac{bh(h^2 + b^2)}{12}$ (2.2)
(iv) Hollow cylinder	$\dfrac{3\pi d^4}{64}$ 3.0	$\dfrac{3\pi d^2}{32}$ (3.0)

(i) Solid rod

b = 0.443d
h = 1.772d

(ii) Beam on end

b = 1.772d
h = 0.443d

(iii) Beam on side

d   1.414d

(iv) Hollow cylinder

Strain is a relative measure of deformation within a tissue or structure in response to externally applied loads. Strain (ε) is defined as $\varepsilon = \delta r/r$, where δr is the change in a specific dimension of the material, with an original value of r (Figure 1.4(b)). Linear strain (compressive or tensile strain) is measured as the amount of linear deformation (lengthening or shortening) of a sample divided by the sample's original length. This calculation results in mm/mm outcome and thus makes the expression of strain a non-dimensional parameter usually expressed as a percentage.

The relationship between stress and strain can be visualised by plotting stress as a function of strain (Figure 1.7). The stress–strain (σ–ε) ratio, the ratio of the stress

Figure 1.7 Stress–strain behaviour for a ligament: (a) stress–strain to failure; (b) viscoelastic behaviour of ligament energy loss represented in grey wavy shaded area while elastic energy represented in grey shaded area.

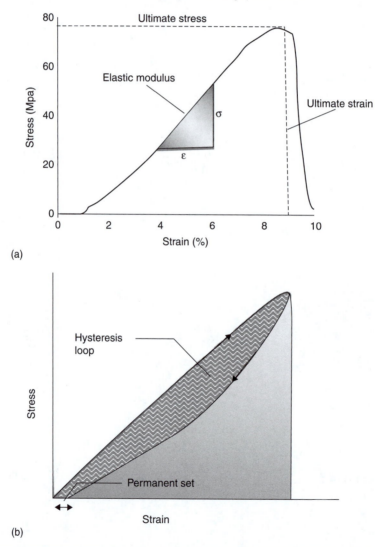

(a)

(b)

to the strain in that region for a particular load type, provides a numerical value of the material's stiffness called the modulus of elasticity or elastic modulus (E) or Young's modulus. It is important to note that, Young's modulus is only defined for the linear region of the stress–strain curve as in Figure 1.7. For tension or compression the modulus of elasticity (E) is defined as the ratio of tensile or compressive stress (σ) to tensile or compressive strain (ε). For shear, the shear modulus (G) is the ratio of shear stress (σ) to shear strain (ν).

So far we have only considered the linear relationships between load–deformation and stress–strain. Linear materials operate according to Hooke's Law, where stress and strain are linearly related such that the resulting strain is proportional to the developed stress ($\sigma = E\,\varepsilon$) (Figure 1.7(a)). The linear portion of the curve is referred to as elastic deformation. The term elastic is used because once the load is removed from the material or tissue it will return to its original shape, much like a rubber band. However, throughout their physiological range the mechanical response of most biological tissues is not entirely linear and, therefore, not entirely elastic. This is due to the non-linear characteristics created by the biological tissue's fluid component. If a material is strained beyond its elastic limit and the load is then removed, that part of the deformation that was elastic is recovered. However, a 'permanent set' remains, because the material has entered the region of plastic deformation, which represents an energy loss or hysteresis loop (Figure 1.7(b)). This energy loss is proportional to the grey shaded area under the stress–strain curve (Figure 1.7(b)). Hysteresis relates to differences in the load–deflection curve for loading and unloading and these can be particularly marked for viscoelastic materials (see next sub-section) (Figure 1.7(b)). Resilience is a measure of the energy absorbed by a material that is returned when the load is removed. It is related to the elastic and plastic behaviour of the material and to its hysteresis characteristics.

The area under the stress–strain curve up to any chosen strain is a measure of energy known as strain energy (Figure 1.7(a)). Strain energy is stored in any deformed material during deformation, as in a trampoline bed, vaulting pole, shoe sole, protective equipment, or compressed ball. Some of this energy will be recoverable elastic strain energy (grey shaded in Figure 1.7(b)) and some will be lost (i.e. converted to chemical or thermal energy) as plastic strain energy (grey wavy shaded area in Figure 1.7(b)). Plastic strain energy is useful when the material is required to dampen vibration or absorb energy, as in protective equipment. Elastic strain energy is useful when the material serves as a temporary energy store, as in a vaulting pole or trampoline bed or in a tendon during the stretch–shortening cycle.

Fatigue is the loss of strength and stiffness that occurs in materials when a load is cycled repetitively. The number of stress reversals that will be withstood without failure depends on the range of stress (maximum minus minimum) and the mean stress. The maximum range endured without failure for a mean stress of zero is called the fatigue limit; at this stress, the number of reversals that can be tolerated tends to infinity (Figure 1.8). Many overuse injuries can be considered, in effect, as fatigue failures of biological tissue (see Chapter 2).

Figure 1.8 Fatigue behaviour of a material.

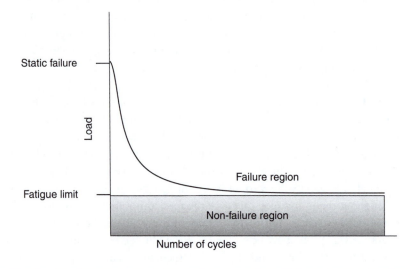

VISCOELASTICITY AND ANISOTROPY

Up to this point we have discussed mechanical properties without the influence of time. However, one of the major differences between biological materials and non-biological materials is how load affects them over time. The way a biological material responds to a load, the extent of deformation and energy lost, is dependent upon the rate at which the load is applied. This time dependent behaviour is called viscoelasticity. Viscoelasticity includes the terms viscosity (the resistance to fluid flow) and elasticity (a solid material property relating to a body's ability to return to its original bond formation). So, a viscoelastic material contains both fluid and solid material properties. For viscoelastic materials the stress (σ) is not only a function of strain (ε) but also of strain rate ($\dot{\varepsilon}= d\varepsilon/dt$). This time dependent behaviour suggests that a given material may display numerous different stress–strain curves depending on the strain rate, often offering a higher resistance when loaded faster (Figure 1.9).

Creep is an important mechanical characteristic of all viscoelastic materials. This phenomenon is observed in materials which deform as a function of time under a constant load; that is they continue to deform with time (e.g. Figure 1.10(a)). The measured strain is a function of stress, time and temperature. As the temperature of a material is increased, loads that cause no permanent deformation at room temperature can cause the material to creep. Putting theory into practice, this means that athletes should perform stretching activities after a warm-up; this will improve the creep response in connective tissue, reducing the stretch reflex and increasing the resting length of connective tissue. The creep response in biological tissue elicited from a static stretch may last from a few seconds up to several minutes. Another important

Figure 1.9 Example of rate dependent behaviour of cortical bone.

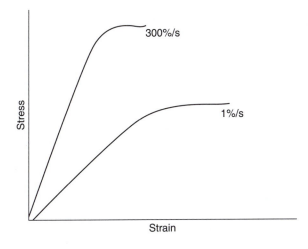

time dependent behaviour of viscoelastic materials is stress-relaxation. This means that a material undergoing a constant strain will began to relax, i.e. stress will be reduced (Figure 1.10(b)).

Anisotropy means the mechanical properties of a material are directionally dependent, as opposed to isotrophy, which implies homogeneity in mechanical properties in all directions. Biological materials (for example skin, bone and ligaments) are anisotropic, which means their mechanical properties depend on the direction in which they are loaded. For instance, the tibia is strongest when resisting compressive loads and weakest in resisting shear loads, while the Achilles tendon is strongest at resisting tensile loads. Further to direction dependence, the biomechanical properties of biological materials are also position dependent, such that some parts of the material behave differently from others. This is because most biological tissue is made of composite materials; that is they are non-homogeneous. For example, the type of bone, the region of the bone (e.g. the head versus the midshaft of the femur), and whether the bone is cancellous or compact, all affect its properties. What this means is that the same load may be applied in the same direction to different regions of the same tissue and yield different results.

Figure 1.10 (a) Creep behaviour – deformation of tissue under constant load; (b) stress-relaxation behaviour – stress will be reduced or material will 'relax' under a constant deformation.

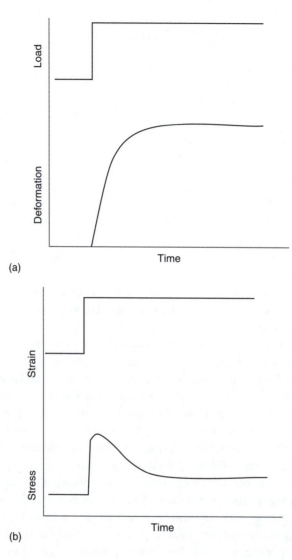

(a)

(b)

BONE

Structure and composition

There are two types of bone, cortical or compact bone and cancellous or trabecular bone. Cortical bone is dense and makes up 80% of the weight of the skeleton while cancellous bone is more porous. Cortical bone is a non-homogeneous, anisotropic, viscoelastic, brittle material which is weakest when loaded in tension. The major structural element of cortical bone is the osteon. These pack to form the matrix of the bone. The major structural element of cancellous bone is the trabeculae. The trabeculae have varying shapes and spatial orientations which give cancellous bone its airy, porous appearance. The orientation of the trabeculae corresponds to the direction of tensile and compressive stresses and is roughly orthogonal (Figure 1.11). This permits maximum economy of the structure as expressed by its strength-to-weight ratio. The trabeculae are more densely packed in those parts of the bone that have to transmit the greatest stress such as the head of the femur (Figure 1.11). The sponginess of cancellous bone helps to absorb energy but gives a lower strength than cortical bone does.

Figure 1.11 Bone composition of the femoral head.

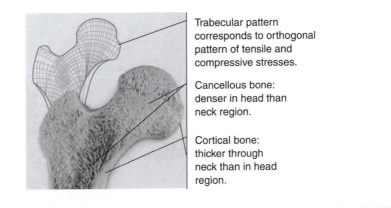

Trabecular pattern corresponds to orthogonal pattern of tensile and compressive stresses.

Cancellous bone: denser in head than neck region.

Cortical bone: thicker through neck than in head region.

The overall structure of long bones gives an optimal strength-to-weight ratio. This is made possible by the sandwich construction of a cortical shell with a cancellous core. In this type of non-homogeneous structure the soft component helps to prevent the stiff component from cracking while the stiff component helps prevent the soft one from yielding. The requirement for greatest stress resistance is at the periphery of the bone. A narrower middle section in long bones reduces bending stresses and minimises the chance of fracture. The cortical shell reduces in thickness at the epiphysis where cancellous bone becomes more prevalent. The shape of the epiphysis, being broader with a larger surface area, provides stability and reduces the stresses on the load-bearing surfaces.

Two fracture mechanisms occur in cortical bone. In the first of these, failure is ductile, which means extensive plastic deformation takes place before fracture as osteons and fibres are pulled apart. In the second, the failure is brittle owing to cracks running across the bone surface; a similar mode of failure occurs in cancellous bone, where cracks propagate along the length of the bone. Because of the anisotropy of bone (its properties depend on the direction of loading), the mechanisms of crack propagation depend on the orientation of the bone: cracks propagate more easily in the transverse than in the longitudinal direction. Bones that are more mineralised tend to experience brittle fracture whereas bones that are less mineralised tend to experience ductile fracture (Figure 1.12).

Figure 1.12 Load-deformation curves for different bone conditions. Ductile crack formation and propagation form of bone fracture.

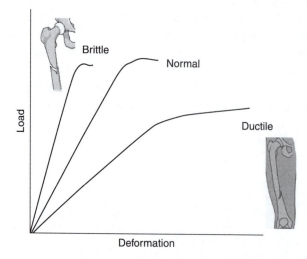

Loading and biomechanical properties

Because of its non-homogeneity, the type and distribution of load within the bone also affect its mechanical properties. These properties also vary with the direction in which the load is applied (anisotropy). For example, for cortical bone the elastic modulus is nearly twice as large along the long axis (17.9 GPa) as across it (10 GPa). The ultimate strength for human femoral cortical bone is 193 MPa when compressed longitudinally and is 133 MPa when loaded transversely. Thus, less energy is absorbed when bone is loaded transversely, which means that bone loaded transversely is more likely to experience brittle fracture with little yielding before breaking, as compared to bone that is loaded longitudinally. When reviewing the literature on material properties of bone it is notable that values for elastic modulus and ultimate strength are quite variable. This is due to the age and preparation of the bone as well as the rate of loading of the specimens, for example stiffness values for cancellous bone range from 1.4 MPa to 1.5 GPa. Studies have shown increased stiffness in older bone specimens as well as dry versus wet preparations and furthermore have shown stiffness and ultimate strength values to become more variable when loaded at rates exceeding the physiological range (Hansen *et al.*, 2008).

Bone is a viscoelastic material, thus rate of loading is important to its biomechanical behaviour. When bone is loaded as higher rates (within the physiological range) it becomes stiffer, having a greater elastic modulus, and sustains a higher load to failure (see Figure 1.9). The physiological range of strain rate varies only about 15% during activities of daily living, for example the strain rate in cortical bone during slow walking is 0.1%/s and about 3%/s during slow jogging and about 13%/s during fast running

(Hansen *et al.*, 2008). This rate dependent behaviour, characteristic of viscoelastic tissue, also tells us that the energy absorbed (proportional to the area under the stress–strain curve) increases with increasing strain rate. Strain rate is clinically important because it will influence the fracture pattern. Energy is absorbed by bone during loading and fractures forming in bone tissue allow energy to be released. Thus, a higher strain rate leads to greater energy, which leads to greater damage to the bone tissue.

CARTILAGE

Structure and composition

Of all types of connective tissue, articular (joint) cartilage is the most severely exposed to stress, leading to wear and tear. The main function of joint cartilage is to provide a smooth articular surface, helping to distribute the joint stress which varies with the amount of contact. For example, in the fully extended knee where probable weight-bearing is combined with ligamentous loading and muscle tension, the joint contact area is increased by the menisci. The increased area is maintained on initial flexion when weight-bearing is still likely, as during gait. In greater degrees of flexion, a gliding motion occurs over a reduced contact area; this reduced area is made possible by the reduction of load, as the collateral ligaments are relaxed and weight-bearing is no longer likely.

Articular cartilage is an avascular substance consisting of cells, collagen fibres and hyaline substance. Due to its lack of vascular, nerve and lymphatic supply, articular cartilage is dependent on exchange of synovial fluid for nutrients, oxygen and repair. Articular cartilage is structurally highly organised. Near the bone the collagenous fibres are perpendicular to the bone. The fibres then run through a transition zone before becoming parallel to the surface where an abundance of fibres allows them to move apart with no decrease in tensile strength. In the perpendicular zone, fibres weave around the cartilage cells, forming chondromes. Hyaline cartilage consists of between 20% and 40% chondroitin; this substance has a high sulphuric acid content and contains collagen and a polymer (chondromucoid) of acetylated disaccharide chondrosine. The concentration of chondroitin is lower in the surface zone because of the high content of collagen fibres, through adaptation to mechanical stresses.

Biomechanical properties

Cartilage has a high, but not uniform, elasticity. This is greatest in the direction of joint motion and where the joint pressure is greatest. Compressibility is about 50–60%. The deformation of cartilage helps to increase the joint contact area and range of motion. Normal cartilage has a typical viscoelastic behaviour. It has an elastic modulus in tension that decreases with increasing depth from the cartilage surface because of the collagen fibre orientation. The compressive modulus increases with load as the cartilage is compressed and the chondromes resist the load. The effect of load is to cause a rapid initial deformation followed by a more gradual increase (Figure 1.13). After the load is removed, cartilage returns to its initial elasticity within a relatively short time providing that the load was of short enough duration and low enough magnitude. A similar load held for a longer period, or a greater load, will cause more deformation and an increased impairment of elasticity, which may cause degeneration. Prolonged standing causes creep of the partly fibrocartilaginous intervertebral discs; this largely explains why people are tallest in the morning, losing 17 mm of height in the first two hours after rising. The ultimate compressive stress of cartilage has been reported as 5 MPa (Shrive and Frank, 1995). Its elastic limits are much lower for repeated than for single loading (Nigg, 1993).

Figure 1.13 Schematic representation of the effects of duration of loading on cartilage deformation.

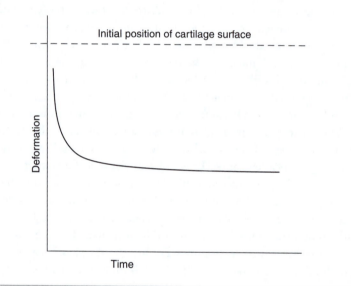

SKELETAL MUSCLE: MAXIMUM FORCE AND MUSCLE ACTIVATION

Two different forces can be distinguished for skeletal muscle. Active tension is the force produced by the contractile elements of a muscle as a result of voluntary muscle contraction. Passive tension is the force developed within the connective tissue of the muscle when the muscle surpasses its resting length. Total tension is dependent on the tension length characteristics of both the active and passive components of muscle (Figure 1.14). Total tension developed in a skeletal muscle is proportional to the number of cross-bridges in parallel. The number of cross-bridges between the filaments is maximal at resting length, therefore active tension is also at its maximum at resting

Figure 1.14 Length–tension relationship of skeletal muscle. Active tension derives from the interaction between myosin and actin. Passive tension can develop in the muscle's complex connective tissue, primarily in the tendons.

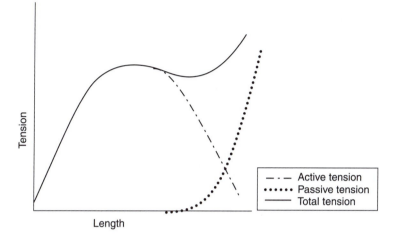

length. As the muscle is lengthened the filaments are pulled apart, thus the number of cross-bridges is reduced and so the active tension is decreased. As the muscle lengthens past resting length a passive tension begins to build in the connective tissue. As the muscle continues to lengthen there is an increase in the passive tension as well as an increase in the rate of development of passive tension.

The maximum force developed in each motor unit of a muscle is related to the number of fibres recruited, their firing (or stimulation) rate and synchrony, and the physiological cross-sectional area of the motor unit. The rate of active force production in a muscle is proportional to the number of sarcomeres in series. The factors affecting a muscle's ability to produce force include its length, velocity, fibre type, physiological cross-sectional area and activation. The force per unit physiological cross-sectional area is often known as the 'specific tension' of the muscle. A range of values for specific tension have been reported (e.g. Pierrynowski, 1995); a maximum value of 350 kPa is often used to estimate the maximum muscle force from its physiological cross-sectional area (pcsa). It should be noted that pcsa $= (m \cos\alpha)/(r_f/\rho)$, where m and ρ are the mass and density of the muscle, r_f is the muscle fibre length and α is the fibre pennation angle (Figure 1.15). The last two of these are defined when the muscle's sarcomeres are at the optimal length (2.8 mm) for force generation. The different values of specific tension cited in the literature may be caused by different fibre composition, determination of pcsa or neural factors.

Muscle activation is regulated through motor unit recruitment and the motor unit stimulation rate (or rate-coding). The former is an orderly sequence based on the size of the α-motoneuron. The smaller ones are recruited first; these are typically slow twitch with a low maximum tension and a long contraction time. The extent of rate-coding is muscle-dependent. If more motor units can be recruited, then this dominates. Smaller muscles have fewer motor units and depend more on increasing their stimulation rate.

Figure 1.15 Muscle fibre pennation angle α.

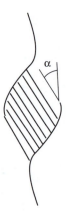

Mechanical stiffness

The mechanical stiffness of a muscle is the instantaneous rate of change of force with length, measured from the slope of the muscle tension–length curve (Figure 1.14). Unstimulated muscles possess low stiffness (or high compliance). Stiffness increases with time during tension and at high rates of change of force, particularly in eccentric contractions, in which stiffness values may be over 200 times greater than in concentric contractions. Stiffness is often considered to be under reflex control with regulation through both the length component of the muscle spindle receptors and the force-feedback component of the Golgi tendon organs. Some research, mostly on animals, has been carried out on the effects of blocking of reflex actions. The exact role of the various reflex components in stiffness regulation in fast human movements in sport remains to be fully established as do their effects in the stretch–shortening cycle (see below). It is clear, however, that the reflexes can almost double the stiffness of the muscles at some joints. Furthermore, muscle and reflex properties and the central nervous system interact in determining how stiffness affects the control of movement.

The stretch–shortening cycle

The natural state of muscle function may be more complex than partitioned descriptions of concentric, isometric and eccentric muscle contractions. In fact many of our everyday activities (e.g. walking, running, hopping) require more complex action of our muscles; this action is called the stretch–shortening cycle (SSC), in which muscle undergoes an eccentric phase quickly followed by a concentric phase (Figure 1.16(a)). An effective SSC requires three fundamental conditions: first, a well-timed preactivation of the muscles before the eccentric phase; second, a short and fast eccentric phase; third, an immediate transition between eccentric and concentric phases. This sequence of muscle action has been shown to vastly improve the force production during the concentric phase as compared with an isolated concentric muscle contraction (Figure 1.16(c)).

There have been alternative explanations for the phenomenon of the stretch–shortening cycle, particularly related to improved performance in countermovement

Figure 1.16 Idealised model muscle force–length curves: (a) stretch–shortening cycle – eccentric followed by concentric contraction – during the eccentric contraction energy is stored in the muscle tendon which results in a more powerful concentric contraction; (b) isometric followed by concentric contraction – shaded area represents the work done in the concentric phase.

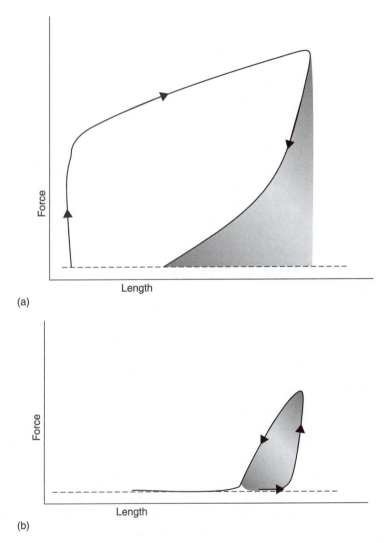

(a)

(b)

(Continued overleaf)

Figure 1.16 *continued* (c) three different muscle contraction conditions and associated force outputs.

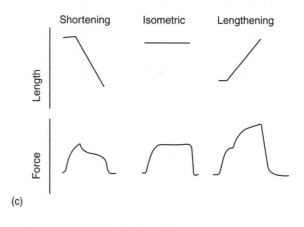

(c)

jumps; various theories have been proposed. First, the utilisation of stored elastic energy: the recoil of the tendinous structure would allow the velocity of shortening of the contractile element to proceed more slowly, thus enhancing force production owing to the force–velocity characteristics of muscle contraction. Second, rise time: the eccentric phase gives the muscle time to develop maximum tension. Third, the stretch reflex: the eccentric phase causes a stretch reflex which increases alpha stimulation to the muscles. Fourth, the effect of two-joint muscles: the stretch–shortening cycle optimises the transfer of energy from two joint muscles. Fifth, the effect of preload: if the muscle is preloaded to a high initial force, greater work will be produced in concentric contraction. For more information see Komi (2003).

Current evidence supports the following three mechanisms as being involved in SSC: elastic energy storage and release, preloading of the muscles involved, and reflex potentiation. Elastic energy is stored in the elastic elements of the muscle during the lengthening phase. We need to keep in mind that true eccentric contraction involves the lengthening of a muscle under active tension. If the muscle is not active then the lengthening is considered a stretch, not an eccentric contraction. Optimising elastic energy storage and release depends on the length of stretch, the velocity of the stretch, a short coupling time (transition between stretch to shorten), the force at the end of the stretch and the muscle stiffness. Preload of a muscle refers to the higher initial force at the start of the concentric phase of a stretch–shortening cycle than for a movement without a pre-stretch. This increased force in turn increases the work (measured from the area under the force–length curve) done in the concentric phase of the cycle (Figure 1.16(a and b)). Reflex potentiation involves the augmentation of the short and medium latency reflexes seen in the electromyogram from muscle fatiguing through repeated stretch–shortening cycles. This has been interpreted as regulation of muscle stiffness through the length-feedback component of the muscle spindles. There is still much work to be done in understanding the role of various reflex components and their effects on muscle stiffness regulation in the stretch–shortening cycle.

LIGAMENT AND TENDON PROPERTIES

Ligaments and tendons are soft collagenous tissues. Ligaments connect bone to bone and tendons connect muscles to bone. Both tendon and ligament are examples of organised dense fibrous connective tissue. This means that they have densely packed collagen fibres that run in parallel bundles (Figure 1.17). These types of tissues have great tensile strength primarily when tensile loads are applied parallel to the fibre lines. When unstressed, the fibres have a crimped pattern (Figure 1.17) owing to cross-linking of collagen fibres with elastic and reticular ones. This crimped pattern is crucial for normal joint mobility as it allows a limited range of almost unresisted movement.

Figure 1.17 Hierarchical ligament and tendon structure, showing crimp pattern of fibres (adapted from Towler and Gelberman, 2006).

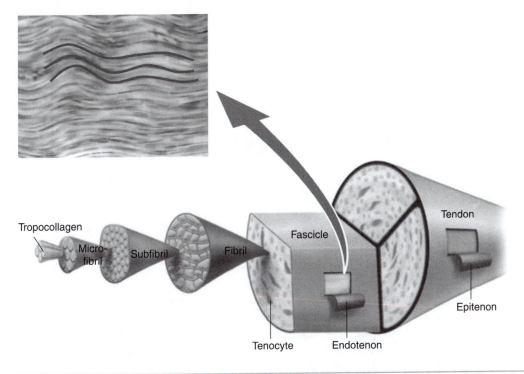

The stiffness of ligaments varies non-linearly with force. Because of their non-linear tensile properties (Figure 1.18), ligaments offer early and increasing resistance to tensile loading over a narrow range of joint motion. At higher forces, ligaments become stiffer and provide more resistance to developing deformations. This means that when the joint is displaced towards the outer limit of movement, collagen fibres are recruited from the crimped state to become straightened, which increases the resistance and stabilises the joint. Thus, daily activities, such as walking and jogging, are usually in the toe of the stress–strain curve (Figure 1.18) and strenuous activities such as landing, jumping

Figure 1.18 Model of anterior cruciate ligament loaded to failure (adapted from Lee and Hyman, 2002).

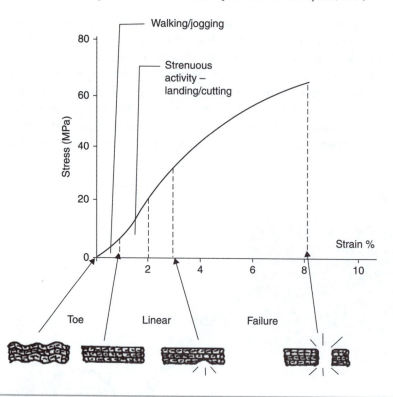

and cutting are normally in the early part of the linear region. The linear strain region may be as great as 20–40% and failure strains as high as 60–80%, much greater than for tendon.

All ligaments display viscoelastic properties: they creep – continue to deform under constant load; they experience stress-relaxation – under a fixed strain, the stress will decrease with time; they experience hysteresis – energy loss during loading and unloading, and they are strain-rate sensitive – stiffness increases with strain rate. For example Kennedy *et al.* (1976) found the ultimate failure load for the ACL to be 477 N at a strain rate of 40%/s but 678 N at a strain rate of 140%/s. The rate sensitive behaviour may be important in cyclic activities where ligament softening (the decrease in peak ligament force with successive cycles) may occur. Ligament stiffness, ultimate strength and energy to failure can be increased with training and exercise and reduced with immobilisation, inactivity and ageing.

Tendon tissue is similar to that of fascia, having large collagen content (70–80% dry weight). Collagen is a regular triple helix with cross-links, giving a material and associated structure of great tensile strength that resists stretching if the fibres are correctly aligned. Tendons are strong and, while no published consensus exists on the ultimate tensile stress of human tendon, values usually fall within the band of 45–125 MPa. Tendon is a relatively stiff material, having an elastic modulus of 800 MPa to 2 GPa (Fung *et al.*, 1986). Similar to ligament, the stiffness is smaller for low loads as the collagen crimping pattern causes a less steep gradient of the load–extension and stress–strain curves in the toe region (Figure 1.18). The toe region extends to about 3% strain, with the linear, reversible region up to 4% strain, and the ultimate (failure) strain around 8–10% (Nigg and Herzog, 2007). The compliance (elasticity) of tendon is important in how tendon interacts with the contraction of muscle tissue. When the tendon compliance is high, the change in muscle fibre length will be small compared to the length change of the whole muscle-tendon unit. As well as having a relatively high tensile strength and stiffness, tendon is resilient, having a relative hysteresis of only 2.5–10%. Within the physiological range, this represents limited viscoelastic behaviour for a biological material. Because of this, tendon is often considered the major site within the muscle-tendon unit for the storage of elastic energy. It should be noted that the energy storage is likely to be limited unless the tendon is subject to large forces, as in the eccentric phase of the stretch–shortening cycle.

SUMMARY

In this chapter we learned that the study of sports injury is a complex problem requiring a multidisciplinary approach to locate and implement effective solutions. The epidemiological approach offers us key information regarding the who, what, where and when of injury. The incidence, prevalence and risk factors are important aspects of the epidemiological study of injury. As biomechanists, we use the principles and theories of the disciplines of physics and mechanical engineering to describe the forces and force-related (mechanical) factors that lead to injury. However, it is important to acknowledge the contribution of other disciplines and to understand how our biomechanical research and understandings may be informed by them. For example, we can use Meeuwisse's epidemiological model to emphasise the influence of load and load tolerance such that intrinsic risk factors are seen as those factors that affect the load tolerance of the tissues within the athlete, while extrinsic factors may be seen as those that influence the load characteristics, which leads to a better understanding of the mechanism of injury. The remainder of the chapter looked at the most important mechanical properties of sports materials and biological tissues. Viscoelasticity, and its significance for biological materials, was explained. The composition and biomechanical properties of bone, cartilage, ligament and tendon, and their behaviour under various forms of loading, were considered. Muscle elasticity, contractility, the generation of maximal force in a muscle, muscle activation, muscle stiffness and the importance of the stretch–shortening cycle were all described.

STUDY TASKS

1 Compare and contrast the biomechanical and epidemiological perspectives on sports injury.
2 What mechanisms make a sequential motion of segments in high-speed activities, such as kicking a ball, the optimal coordination pattern?
3 Compare and contrast load–deformation and stress–strain curves.
4 Define stress and strain and provide clear diagrams of the different types of loading. Using a clearly labelled stress–strain diagram for a typical biological material, explain the material properties related to elasticity and plasticity.
5 Describe the anisotropic behaviour of biological tissue using stress–strain diagrams.
6 Using clearly labelled diagrams (such as stress–strain diagrams) where necessary, describe the differences between the behaviour of a material that is viscoelastic and one that is not.
7 Outline the most important material and mechanical properties of cartilage.
8 Draw a clearly labelled stress–strain diagram for a collagenous material, such as ligament or tendon. After consulting at least one of the items for further reading, describe fully the properties of collagenous materials.

GLOSSARY OF IMPORTANT TERMS

Cumulative trauma Caused by accumulated microtrauma resulting in acute or overuse type of injury. It is assumed that the acumulated microtrauma is caused by repeated overloading and inadequate rest of the tissues involved.

Degeneration A gradual deterioration of specific tissues changing them to a lower or less functionally active form.

Ductile To be drawn out, to become thinner or narrower before breaking.

Exposure A method of quantifying injury risk due to participation in sport. Injury rates are reported as per athlete-exposures (number of practices or games where the athlete might be exposed to injury risk) or time-exposures (amount of time spent practising or participating in risk activity). If an athlete participated in 100 practices per season lasting 60 minutes each, and sustains one injury during practice, the exposure risk is said to be 1 per 100 or 1 per 1000 hours.

Hooke's Law Within the elastic limit of a solid material, the deformation or strain produced by a stress of any kind is proportional to the force. If the elastic limit is not exceeded, the material returns to it original shape and size after the force is removed. If the elastic limit is exceeded, the material remains deformed or stretched. The force at which the material exceeds its elastic limit is called the 'limit of proportionality'.

Injury rate May be defined as case rates or athlete rates. Athlete rates are determined by dividing the total number of athletes injured by the total number of athletes participating. Case rates are determined by dividing the total number of reported cases occurring during the study period by the total number of population exposed to the possibility of injury.

Normal force The force component that is perpendicular to the surface of contact.

Orthogonal Two or more lines are said to be orthogonal if they are perpendicular or form right angles to each other.

Polar second moment of area Also known as the area moment of inertia, moment of inertia of plane area, or second moment of inertia, it is a property of a cross section that can be used to predict the resistance of beams to bending and deflection, around an axis that lies in the cross-sectional plane.

REFERENCES

Bahr, R. and Krosshaug, T. (2005) Understanding injury mechanisms: a key component of preventing injuries in sport. *British Journal of Sports Medicine, 39*, 324–329.

Committee on Trauma Research (1985) *Injury in America: A Continuing Public Health Problem*, Washington, D.C.: National Academy Press.

Fung, Y.C. (1993) *Biomechanics: Mechanical Properties of Living Tissues* (2nd edn), New York: Springer-Verlag.

Fung, Y.C., Schmid-Schonbein, G.W., Woo, S.L.Y. and Zweifach, B.W. (1986) *Frontiers in Biomechanics*, New York: Springer-Verlag.

Hansen, U., Zioupos, P., Simpson, R., Currey, J.D. and Hynd, D. (2008) The effect of strain rate on the mechanical properties of human cortical bone. *Journal of Biomechanical Engineering, 130*, 11–18.

Kennedy, J.C., Hawkins, R.J., Willis, R.B. and Danylchuk, K.D. (1976) Tension studies of human knee ligaments. Yield point, ultimate failure, and disruption of the cruciate and tibial collateral ligaments. *Journal of Bone and Joint Surgery – Series A, 58*, 350–355.

Leadbetter, W.B. (2001) 'Soft tissue athletic injury', in F.H. Fu and D.A. Stone (eds) *Sports Injuries: Mechanisms, Prevention, Treatment*, Philadelphia, PA: Lippincott Williams & Wilkins.

Lee, M. and Hyman, W. (2002) Modeling of failure mode in knee ligaments depending on the strain rate. *BMC Musculoskeletal Disorders, 3*, 3–8.

Meeuwisse, W.H. (1994) Assessing causation in sport injury: a multifactorial model. *Clinical Journal of Sport Medicine, 4*, 166–170.

Meeuwisse, W.H., Tyreman, H., Hagel, B. and Emery, C. (2007) A dynamic model of etiology in sport injury: the recursive nature of risk and causation. *Clinical Journal of Sport Medicine, 17*, 215–219.

Nigg, B.M. (1993) 'Excessive loads and sports-injury mechanisms', in P.A.F.H. Renström (ed.) *Sports Injuries: Basic Principles of Prevention and Care*, London: Blackwell Scientific, pp. 107–119.

Nigg, B.M. and Herzog, W. (2007) *Biomechanics of the Musculo-skeletal System* (3rd edn.), Hoboken, NJ: John Wiley & Sons.

Pierrynowski, M.R. (1995) 'Analytical representation of muscle line of action and geometry', in P. Allard, I.A.F. Stokes and J.-P. Blanchi (eds) *Three-Dimensional Analysis of Human Movement*, Champaign, IL: Human Kinetics, pp. 215–256.

Shrive, N.G. and Frank, C.B. (1995) 'Articular cartilage', in B.M. Nigg and W. Herzog (eds) *Biomechanics of the Musculo-skeletal System*, Hoboken, NJ: John Wiley & Sons, pp. 79–105.

Towler, D.A. and Gelberman, R.H. (2006) The alchemy of tendon repair: a primer for the sports mad scientist. *Journal of Clinical Investigation, 116*, 863–866.

Whiting, W.C. and Zernicke, R.F. (2008) *Biomechanics of Musculoskeletal Injury* (2nd edn), Champaign, IL: Human Kinetics.

Woodward, M. (2005) *Epidemiology: Study Design and Data Analysis* (2nd edn), Boca Raton, FL: Chapman & Hall/CRC.

FURTHER READING

Komi, P.V. (2003) *Strength and Power in Sport* (2nd edn), Oxford: Blackwell Science. Chapters 10 and 11, in particular, give a good explanation of what we understand about the stretch–shortening cycle.

Nigg, B.M. and Herzog, W. (2007) *Biomechanics of the Musculo-skeletal System* (3rd edn), Hoboken, NJ: John Wiley & Sons. Chapter 2, Biomaterials, provides a good summary of the biomechanics of bone, articular cartilage, ligament, tendon, muscle and joints, but is mathematically somewhat advanced in places.

Nordin, M. and Frankel, V.H. (eds) (1989) *Basic Biomechanics of the Musculoskeletal System*, Philadelphia, PA: Lea & Febiger. Chapters 1 to 3 and 5 provide a good and less mathematical summary of similar material to that in Nigg and Herzog (2007).

Özkaya, N. and Nordin, M. (1999) *Fundamentals of Biomechanics*, New York, Van Nostrand Reinhold. Chapters 13–17 contain detailed explanations of the mechanics of deformable bodies, including biological tissues. Many sport and exercise scientists may find the mathematics a little daunting in places, but the text is very clearly written.

2   Injuries in sport: how the body behaves under load

Melanie Bussey

Knowledge assumed
Familiarity with gross anatomy
Familiarity with basic human physiology
Basic knowledge of tissue mechanics from Chapter 1

INTRODUCTION – DEFINING MUSCULOSKELETAL INJURY

BOX 2.1 LEARNING OUTCOMES

After reading this chapter you should be able to:

- distinguish between overuse and acute injury
- understand the various injuries that occur to bone and how these depend on the load characteristics
- understand the effects of mechanical loading on growth and adaptation of human tissue
- describe and explain the injuries that occur to soft tissues, including cartilage, ligaments and the muscle-tendon unit
- understand the sports injuries that affect the major joints of the lower and upper extremities, the back and the neck.

Musculoskeletal injuries are often categorised according to their mechanisms of onset, termed either acute or overuse. Acute injury has a rapid onset and is often caused by a single external force or blow. Overuse injuries result from repetitive trauma preventing tissue from self-repair and may affect bone, tendons, bursae, cartilage and the muscle-tendon unit (Pecina and Bojanic, 1993); they occur because of microscopic trauma (or microtrauma). Overuse injuries are associated with cyclic loading of a joint or other structure, at loads below those that would cause traumatic injury. As discussed in Chapter 1, the failure strength decreases as the number of cyclic loadings increases, until the endurance limit is reached (Figure 1.8). The relationship between overuse injuries and the factors that predispose sports participants to them have been investigated for some sports.

This chapter is intended to provide an understanding of the causes and types of injury that occur in sport and exercise and some of the factors that influence their occurrence. In Chapter 1, we noted that injury occurs when a body tissue is loaded beyond its failure tolerance. In this chapter, we will focus on sport and exercise injuries that affect the different tissues and parts of the body.

BONE

In Chapter 1 we introduced the gross structural components of bone: cortical and trabecular. When discussing bone growth, modelling, remodelling and adaptation it is also important to familiarise yourself with the bone structures at the tissue level; these are primary, secondary and woven bone. You should also become familiar with bone structures at the cellular level including osteoblasts, osteocytes, bone-lining cells and osteoclasts.

- **Primary bone** refers to bone tissue that is laid down where no bone tissue has existed before, and comprises several types of bone that differ morphologically, physiologically and in their mechanical properties. It cannot be deposited without pre-existing structure such as cartilaginous substrate or woven bone. Forms of primary bone are primary osteons, plexiform and primary lamellar bone. Primary osteons are the principal structures of compact bone and plexiform bone. Plexiform bone is highly oriented cancellous bone with trabecular plates thickening due to endosteal or periosteal surface apposition, sometimes seen in children undergoing growth spurts (further information about primary bone formation in children is available in Chapter 3). Primary lamellar bone is arranged in circular rings around the endosteal and periosteal bone and the trabeculae in the epiphyses of long bones.
- **Secondary bone** is mature bone tissue that has an organised appearance with collagen fibres that are arranged in lamellae. There are primarily three types of bone cells responsible for bone remodelling. Osteoclasts are multinuclear bone cells of hematogenous origin that reabsorb bone which releases calcium into the serum. Osteoblasts are mononuclear bone forming cells, they synthesise collagen matrix and deposit bone material within it, which produces mineralised bone. Once the osteoblast surrounds itself with mineralised bone tissue it is referred to as an osteocyte.
- **Woven bone** is bone tissue laid down during fracture healing and callous formation. It is laid down rapidly and thus has a more disorganised arrangement of collagen fibres and osteocytes. Further, woven bone may be laid from new, which makes a unique type of bone tissue. Typically woven bone has a lower mechanical strength compared to primary or secondary bone, possibly due to the disorganised pattern and lower proportion of non-collagenous proteins. Because of its rapid growth and its high cell-to-bone volume ratio, it is believed that the purpose of woven bone is to provide a mechanical support to a fractured bone by way of splint.

Modelling, remodelling and adaptation

The processes of modelling (bone growth) and remodelling (replacing of old or damaged bone) are not very different at the cellular level. Modelling and remodelling of bone results from the action of osteoblasts and osteoclasts in response to mechanical and hormonal stimulus. If these processes occur at different locations within the bone, and the bone morphology is altered, then the bone is considered to have undergone the process of modelling (Frost, 1990). In homeostatic equilibrium, bone resorption and formation are balanced, meaning they are occurring at the same location within the bone and the bone morphology is not changing. In this instance the bone is considered to have undergone the process of remodelling (Frost, 1990). During the process of remodelling, old bone is replaced and defects such as microfractures are repaired by coupling the action of these cells such that old bone is continuously replaced by new tissue so that it adapts to mechanical load and strain. The remodelling cycle consists of three consecutive phases: resorption, reversal and formation. Resorption begins with the migration of partially differentiated preosteoclasts to the bone surface where they form osteoclasts. After the completion of osteoclastic resorption, there is a reversal phase when mononuclear cells appear on the bone surface. These cells prepare the surface for new osteoblasts to begin bone formation and provide signals for osteoblast differentiation and migration. The formation phase follows with osteoblasts laying down bone until the resorbed bone is completely replaced with new. Upon completion, the surface is covered with bone-lining cells and a rest period begins until a new remodelling cycle is initiated. The stages of the remodelling cycle have different lengths. Resorption probably continues for about two weeks, the reversal phase may last up to four or five weeks, while formation can continue for four months until the new bone structural unit is completely created. The overall integrity of bone appears to be controlled by hormones and many other proteins secreted by both hemopoietic bone marrow cells and bone cells.

Bone adaptation requires bone cells to detect mechanical signals and integrate these signals into appropriate changes in the bone architecture (Turner, 1998). The initial concept of bone adaptation was presented by two scientists, Wolff and Roux, in the late 1800s; their findings were that bone architecture is determined by mechanical stresses (particularly tension and compression) placed on bone. The concept that bone adapts to the mechanical loads placed on it is commonly referred to as Wolff's law. Today, the term Wolff's law is seen as rather outdated because the rules that are accepted to govern bone adaptation to mechanical load are not compatible with Wolff's original findings. There are three fundamental rules of bone adaptation. First, bone adaptation is driven by dynamic rather than static loading. Second, only a short duration of mechanical loading is necessary to initiate an adaptive response in bone cells. The third rule is that bone cells accommodate to the everyday mechanical loading environment making them less responsive to routine loading signals (Turner, 1998). What is meant by the last rule is that bone appears to maintain its current structure unless exposed to overload or underload. Overload causes bone modelling or bone growth, while underload causes remodelling or resorption of bone material. We know that increasing exercise intensity will cause overload to our system and lead to increased bone mineral density. Reducing activity, from bed rest or immobilisation, will cause underloading to the system and lead to bone resorption and decreased bone mineral density.

Fracture of bone

A fracture is a serious injury that causes damage to the bone material and may also cause damage to surrounding soft tissue (e.g. muscle, ligaments, nerves, blood vessels). In the sporting environment, fractures may be the result of direct trauma, as in a direct impact or collision, or the result of indirect trauma, for example when a limb becomes trapped and causes the athlete to fall awkwardly. From a mechanical perspective bone fails secondary to shear, tension, compression, bending, torsion, or combined loading and the fracture morphology reflects the failure mode. Some common fracture morphologies are as follows.

Diaphyseal impaction fractures

Diaphyseal impaction fractures are usually caused by an axial compressive load offset from the longitudinal axis of the bone. The diaphyseal bone is driven into the thin metaphyseal bone producing the fracture pattern most common from axial loading, examples of which include the Y type supracondylar fracture of the femur or humerus (Table 2.1). This is a common injury to the phalanges in ball sports such as cricket and basketball, which occurs when the ball impacts the tip of the finger.

Transverse fracture

A transverse fracture is characterised by a fracture line that is perpendicular to the long axis of the bone (Table 2.1). Transverse fractures can occur from failure under tensile loading, which is an unlikely mechanism in any sport, or from bending loads. As discussed in Chapter 1, a long bone may be viewed as a cantilevered beam; during bending, the portion of bone on the concave side will experience compressive stresses while the portion of bone on the convex side will experience tensile stresses. Because cortical bone is weaker in tension than compression, bone failure begins on the tensile side (Figure 2.1). The failure mechanism is crack propagation at right angles to the bone's long axis from the surface layer inwards (Figure 2.1). The diaphysis of any long bone subjected to a bending load can be affected. The forces may be delivered directly to the bone, as when the leg or arm is directly struck with an object (e.g. a tackling body). Forces may also be delivered indirectly to the diaphyseal region, for example from a fall from a significant height.

Table 2.1 Basic fracture patterns		
FRACTURE PATTERN	**LOAD**	**APPEARANCE**
Diaphyseal impaction	Axial compression	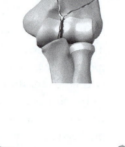
Transverse	Bending	
Spiral	Torsion	
Oblique transverse and butterfly	Axial compression and bending	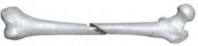
Oblique	Axial compression, bending and torsion	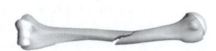

Figure 2.1 Transverse fracture propagation: (a) bending load applied to bone causes tension stress on one side of the neutral axis and compression stress on the other; (b) the fracture propagates from the side of bone under tension stress and the crack continues at right angles to the bone surface.

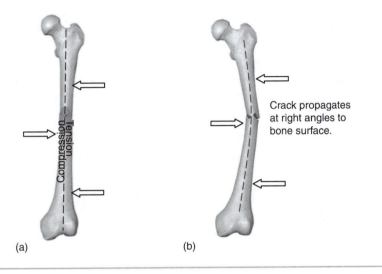

(a)   (b)

Spiral fractures

Spiral fractures (Table 2.1) are relatively common in sport. They are caused by torsional loading, usually in combination with other loads. Torsion creates a state of pure shear between parallel transverse planes. In other planes (at other angles with respect to the longitudinal axis) tensile and compressive stresses are present, and they become a maximum at a 45° angle to the longitudinal axis. The spiral propagates at an angle of about 40–45° to the bone's longitudinal axis, causing the bone under tension to open up. In experimental testing of human cadaver long bones, spiral fractures were only produced from torsional loading (Kress *et al.*, 1995). Typical examples occur in skiing, from the tip of the ski catching in the snow and producing large lateral torques in the calf, in overarm throwing movements, where the implement's inertia creates a large torque in the humerus, and in contact sports when the foot becomes trapped and the player turns or is tackled.

Oblique, oblique transverse and butterfly fractures

An oblique fracture is characterised by failure of bone at a 30–45° angle to the longitudinal axis. These fractures (Table 2.1) are caused by a combination of axial compression and bending loads with a less important torsional contribution. The fracture morphology reflects the dominant loading type. As in Figure 2.1(a), on one side of the bone's neutral axis the bending stress is compressive (Figure 2.2) and is cumulative with the axial compressive stress. On the other side of the bone's neutral axis the bending stress is tensile; this can partially cancel the axial compressive stress. If the axial and bending stresses are of similar magnitude, the resultant oblique transverse fracture is a

Figure 2.2 A compressive load applied to a bone will tend to cause an oblique fracture pattern whereas a bending load applied to a bone tends to cause a transverse fracture pattern. When the two types of loading are combined, the resulting fracture pattern is a combination of the two and may appear as an oblique transverse or butterfly fracture.

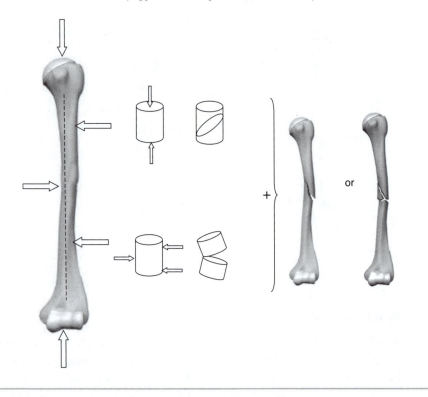

combination of the two; it is part oblique, failure in compression, and part transverse, failure in tension due to bending. The combined effect is an oblique transverse or butterfly fracture as shown in Figure 2.2. A long oblique fracture line is common when torsion is the predominant force. However, please note that a long oblique and a spiral fracture may be indistinguishable from a two-dimensional X-ray. A shorter line of fracture propagation commonly occurs when the predominant force is bending or compression that results in a more transverse orientation and a 'shorter' oblique fracture (e.g. Levine, 2002, p. 505). The butterfly fracture is a special case, caused by the bending load impacting the oblique 'beak' against the other bone fragment. These fractures can occur when the thigh or calf receives a lateral impact when bearing weight, as in tackles or in children with greater elasticity.

Alternatively, transverse loading of the shafts of long bones can result in an oblique fracture pattern as well as fragmentations. This pattern of bone failure is most likely due to the bone's intrinsic response to tensile stresses (Kress *et al.*, 1995).

There are two mechanical reasons for fracture to occur in bone: first is excessive stress and the second is weakened bone material leading to reduced load tolerance. The mechanical reasons for excessive stress in a bone material are as follows.

- **Excessive loading** If the magnitude of the load exceeds the strength of a particular structure, that structure will fail. The greater the magnitude of the load, the greater the amount of energy associated with its application. This energy is dissipated in deforming the bone, breaking the intermolecular bonds (fracturing), and in the soft tissues around the bone. Greater energy causes more tissue to be destroyed and a more complex fracture, as in oblique, oblique transverse, butterfly and comminuted fractures. Comminuted fractures are typically only seen in very high energy impacts, as in car accidents and are very uncommon in the sporting environment.

- **Excessive load rate** As discussed in Chapter 1, bone, along with other biological materials, is viscoelastic; its mechanical properties vary with the rate of loading. It requires more energy to break bone in a short time (such as an impact) than in a relatively long time, for example in a prolonged force application. However, in such a short time, the energy is not uniformly dissipated. The bone can literally explode, because of the formation of numerous secondary fracture lines, with an appearance resembling a comminuted fracture.

- **The dimensions of the structure are small for the magnitude of load** The geometry of bone greatly affects its mechanical behaviour. Bones with a larger cross sectional area are generally stronger and stiffer. In bending, the cross sectional area and distribution of bone about the neutral axis affect the bone's mechanical behaviour. For instance long bones tend to have more and heavier bone tissue distributed at a distance from the neutral axis (Figure 2.3). This configuration gives the long bone a larger area moment of inertia, or resistance to bending moments. The same relationship exists for resistance to torsional loading. Bones with more bony material distributed away from the neutral axis have an increased polar moment of inertia and, therefore, increased resistance to torsion loads. Studies have shown that the smallest cross sectional area is the most vulnerable point for bone fracture. Thus, more fractures occur in the tibia than in the femur because the tibia has a smaller area moment of inertia than the femur. Furthermore, torsional loading of the tibia or femur is more likely to cause fractures within the distal portion or middle third of the shaft as opposed to a third of the femur shaft which is approximately twice the shear stress in the proximal section because the proximal section has a larger polar moment of inertia (Figure 2.3).

- **Geometry of acting forces is unfavourable to the material** Forces acting on a bony structure have a line of action and a direction that produce moments with respect to joints. The magnitude of these moments determines the internal loading of the material within the structure or bone. Forces that have moment arms that are large with respect to the relevant joints may cause excessive stresses within the bone material (Nigg and Herzog, 2007).

- **Excessive frequency of load application** Bone failure due to repeated loading is called fatigue fracture or stress fracture. Fatigue fractures may be produced by a few repetitions of a high load, approaching the yield strength of bone or by many repetitions of a lower load, within the elastic limit of bone. The development of fatigue fractures is not solely dependent upon the number of applications of a load but is more reliant upon the frequency of the load application, meaning the number of repetitions of a load within a given time. Frequency of load is important

Figure 2.3 Femur with cross sections from just above the adductor tubercle and middle third of shaft. Note the distance from the neutral axis (grey dot in cross section) to heavier bone mass; as you can see, the proximal section (A) has a higher polar moment of inertia than the middle section (B) due to bone mass distribution.

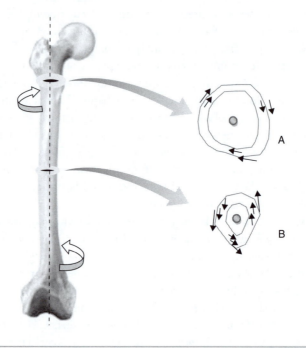

because bone as a living tissue has the ability to remodel and repair with time, thus fractures only occur when the rate of the remodelling process is surpassed by the fatigue process. Three theories have been proposed for the etiology of stress fractures. First, muscle fatigue theory; muscles become fatigued through the course of physical activity, which reduces their ability to contract. If muscles cannot contract they are ineffective in storing energy and reducing the stresses imposed on bone. The result is increased loads imparted to bone from normal physiological loads. The second is increased muscle strength (overload) theory; this is underpinned by the fact that muscle responds to training more quickly than bone. The corresponding increase in muscle tension generated from stronger muscle places larger bending loads on bones. This imbalance may increase the risk for fatigue fractures in bone before the bone has the opportunity to adapt to the increased bending load. The third theory is the remodelling theory, which explains that repetitive stress overload causes accelerated remodelling, which causes imbalance between bone resorption and replacement leading to a decrease in bone density and strength. Once bone density is diminished, further stress applied to the weakened bone may lead to fatigue fractures.

Two reasons have been proposed for weakened bone material leading to reduced load tolerance.

- **Reduced bone mineral density** Bone density has a direct relation to a bone's material properties and ultimate breaking strength. Bones with a lower bone density will potentially fracture at lower forces. Athletes with a reduced bone mineral density are at risk of an insufficiency fracture. An insufficiency fracture is a type of stress fracture that occurs during normal stress on a bone of abnormally decreased density. Stress fractures account for approximately 5–15% of all sports injuries in different populations, with a higher incidence among runners. The tibia is the most commonly reported stress fracture site, particularly in runners, followed by the fibula, metatarsal and pelvis.
- **Surgical intervention** Surgical screws or drill holes inserted in bone tend to create stress risers that can weaken bone and lead to fractures under normal physiological loading. The bone strength is reduced because the defect prevents the stresses imposed during normal loading from being distributed evenly throughout the bone (Nordin and Frankel, 1989) (Figure 2.4). Instead the stress riser acts to concentrate stress at the defect site. For this reason, athletes who have had a surgical correction of a fracture using plates or pins held in place with screws are at high risk of re-fracture. Depending upon specific fracture and surgical circumstances, remodelling of these deficits may take from one month to a year after removal of plates or pins.

Figure 2.4 Exaggerated example of the effect of bone defect on stress distribution in bone: (a) when load applied to bone stress is distributed evenly through the bone; (b) defect in bone causes stress to be concentrated around this point deflecting normal stress lines and creating shearing stress around the defect.

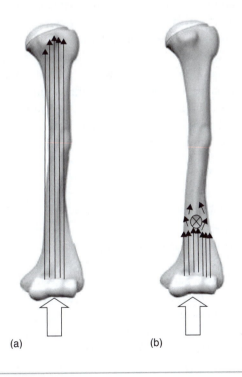

(a)   (b)

ARTICULAR CARTILAGE

Much of the relevant anatomical and mechanical properties of articular cartilage were covered in Chapter 1. Functionally articular cartilage is responsible for control of motion, transmission of load and maintenance of stability. Articular cartilage is plastic and capable of deformation, decreasing the stress concentration by increasing the load-bearing area. It is an avascular substance consisting of cells, collagen fibres and hyaline substance. Due to its lack of vascular, nerve and lymphatic supply, articular cartilage is dependent on exchange of synovial fluid for nutrients, oxygen and repair. Thus, cartilage has poor healing qualities and the lack of nerve supply means many injuries go unnoticed until they invade the surrounding tissues, such as the subchondral bone, synovial lining or periosteum.

Adaptation of articular cartilage

Articular cartilage, similarly to bone, appears to respond to mechanical loading. Mechanical forces have great influence on the synthesis and rate of turnover of articular cartilage molecules, particularly proteoglycans. The articular cartilage appears to react to both load frequency as well as magnitude of load. Regular cyclic loading of the joint (within the normal physiological range) from physical exercise causes the cartilage to swell, enhances the synthesis of proteoglycans, increases the pericellular matrix and increases the number of cells per unit of cartilage which, in turn, increase the cartilage stiffness. However, continuous compression of the cartilage diminishes the synthesis of proteoglycans and may cause damage to the tissue through necrosis. Excessive loading can cause decrease synthesis and increased degradation in cartilage tissue while underloading, caused by prolonged bed rest or joint immobilisation, can lead to significant cartilage atrophy. The atrophy is characterised by a reduction in the synthesis of proteoglycans and the total amount of proteoglycans, along with an increase in fibrillation of the surface cartilage and a decrease in the size and amount of the aggregated proteoglycans (Whiting and Zernicke, 2008).

Injury to articular cartilage

Cartilage injuries may be acute, from single impacts, often occurring at the time of other significant joint injury. For example it has been estimated that 40–70% of anterior cruciate ligament (ACL) injuries are accompanied by some articular cartilage damage which will lead to chronic joint disease such as osteoarthritis. There are several grading systems available to classify articular cartilage damage, which typically grade damage according to depth of tissue involvement. These systems tend to be joint and even site specific, for example the Outerbridge classification system commonly used for the damage to the femoral articular cartilage of the knee (Cameron et al., 2003) (Figure 2.5).

Figure 2.5 Articular cartilage injuries may be graded according to the Outerbridge classification which grades the surface carti- lage from 0 to IV according to damage and appearance. Grade 0 would appear normal and healthy. Grade I cartilage injury has some softening and swelling. Grade II injury has a partial thickness defect with fissures on the surface that do not reach subchon- dral bone or exceed 1.5 cm in diameter. In Grade III injury the fissure has extended to the level of subchondral bone in an area with a diameter greater than 1.5 cm. Finally, we see a Grade IV injury with a deep fissure that exposes the subchondral bone.

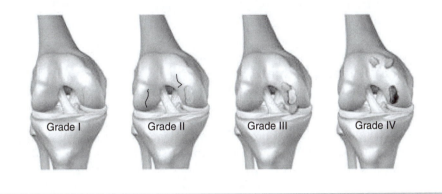

Other than acute injury the most common issue with articular cartilage in athletes is excessive wear leading to degenerative joint disease. Wear is defined as 'the removal of material from solid surfaces by mechanical action' (Nordin and Frankel, 1989). Excessive wear of the cartilage may arise from several mechanical triggers, such as abrasion, fatigue wear or poor fluid redistribution. Abrasion is caused by loose particles within the joint abrading the cartilage surface. Whereas fatigue wear occurs from an accumulation of microscopic damage of the cartilage due to repetitive stressing. Poor fluid redistribution may cause excessive wear particularly with rapid repetitive loading. When rapid loads are applied to cartilage, fluid is redistributed to the compacted area to relieve stress in the tissue; if this response is delayed or if loading is so rapid that there is not enough time for the redistribution response then damage to the tissue is likely to occur.

Osteoarthritis is a common joint condition in athletes. It is a progressive disorder of the joints caused by gradual wearing of cartilage with eventual exposure of subchondral bone which leads to the development of bony spurs and cysts at the margins of the joints. There are two prevailing thoughts on the cause of osteoarthritis. The first is that it is initiated from surface wear, through the depletion and fibrillation of superficial collagen network. The second is that it is initiated from subchondral bone; when the joint is exposed to impact loading, structural changes occur to the subchondral bone that alter the stress pattern on the joint surface leading to mechanical failure of the carti- lage and structural damage of the cartilage surface.

LIGAMENTS AND TENDONS

While structurally and mechanically very similar, ligaments and tendons have different roles in the musculoskeletal movement system. The ligament is a bone-to-bone connector and its role is to enhance mechanical stability of joints, guide movement within the physiological range and limit excessive motion at joints. Tendon is a muscle-to-bone connector and its role is to transmit tensile loads from muscle to bone and to improve the mechanical efficiency of muscles by optimising the distance of the muscle belly from its insertion.

Adaptation of tendon and ligament

Age

Generally the mechanical properties and composition of tendons and ligaments are greatly influenced by age and ageing. In the skeletally immature child, tendons and ligaments are more viscous so they are more compliant. As the child grows there is a consistent increase in the stiffness and modulus of elasticity until skeletal maturity is reached, at which time there is a plateau in the rate of change in mechanical properties until middle age. During middle age and beyond, the collagen within the ligaments and tendons becomes more cross-linked, which causes a decrease in collagen compliance; there is a decrease in viscosity and an increase in the elastin component. The net effect of these changes appears to increase tendon compliance. Furthermore, there is a weakening at the attachment and insertion sites increasing the risk of avulsion injury in ageing athletes.

Mechanical loading

As with other tissues we have discussed, ligaments and tendons respond to mechanical loading. However, our knowledge of how mechanical loading mediates structural changes within the tissue is weak, as there has been far less research conducted on ligament and tendon than on bone. Nonetheless, from our knowledge gained mostly through animal models, we can make several observations. First, increase in tensile loading from resistance training appears to increase the ultimate tensile strength and may also increase the cross-sectional area of tendons and ligaments. Second, positive adaptations in ligaments and tendons occur more slowly than adaptations in bone, possibly owing to a poorer vascular supply compared to bone. Third, disuse during immobilisation will lead to atrophy and a reduction in ultimate strength (Figure 2.6). Finally, immobilisation has a more rapid and sizeable affect on the mechanical properties of ligaments and tendons than increased loading from exercise.

Remodelling after injury

After the inflammatory phase begins to wind down (one to four days) the tissue enters the proliferation phase (day three to six weeks) where scar tissue is developed. During the proliferation phase granulation tissue is formed consisting of fibroblasts, collagen

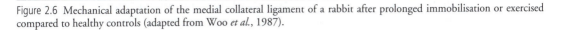

Figure 2.6 Mechanical adaptation of the medial collateral ligament of a rabbit after prolonged immobilisation or exercised compared to healthy controls (adapted from Woo *et al.*, 1987).

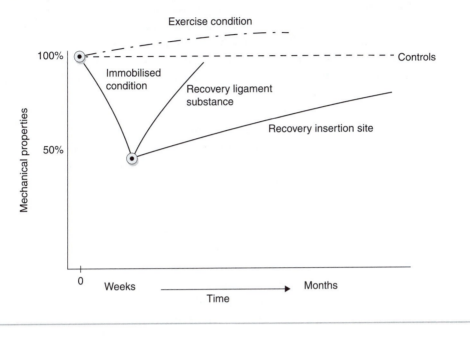

and capillary buds. By the sixth day fibroblasts begin producing collagen fibres that are laid in a random fashion, forming scar tissue. The tensile strength of the scar tissue rapidly increases in proportion to the rate of collagen synthesis. As the tensile strength increases the number of fibroblasts diminishes to signal the beginning of the maturation phase. The maturation phase lasts from six weeks to one year. During this phase collagen fibres that make up scar tissue are remodelling according to tensile forces and strains in the tissue.

Injury to ligament

Ligaments function to stabilise joints and transmit loads; however, they also contain important mechanoreceptors. This means that ligaments are also important to the sense of position within our joints (proprioception). Therefore, when a ligament is injured we tend to suffer a loss of stability, potential joint misalignment, abnormal contact pressure and a loss of position sense or proprioception. When a joint loses its stability or alignment there is an increased stress on the articular cartilage, which has been related to the amount of secondary osteoarthritis found in athletic populations. Athletes most at risk are those with excessive ligament laxity, previous ligament injury or poor muscle strength.

Injury to ligaments is almost always acute and can be the result of either direct or indirect mechanisms. Ligament failure is often caused by bending and twisting loads applied distally to a limb as, for example, landing on uneven ground or in a rugby tackle. Failure depends on the load rate and is normally one of three types. First, bundles of ligament fibres can fail through shear and tension at fast load rates; this mid-substance tear is the most common mechanism of ligament injury. Second, bony avulsion failure can occur through cancellous bone beneath the insertion site at low loading rates; this occurs mostly in young athletes, whose ligaments are stronger than their bones or in older athletes with underlying pathologies. Finally, cleavage of the ligament–bone interface is possible, although rare because of the strength of the interface.

Ligament injuries are clinically categorised according to the amount of tissue injury. In Grade I injuries, some micro-failure of collagen fibres may have occurred but clinical symptoms (pain, function and discolouration) are negligible. Grade II produces progressive failure of the collagen fibres which results in partial ligament rupture. There is a decrease in strength and stiffness by up to 50% and an increase in clinical symptoms (more pain, increased joint instability, loss of natural gait pattern, increased swelling and discolouration). A Grade III injury is defined by macro-failure of collagen fibres, with complete or near complete rupture of the ligament structure. A Grade III injury produces the greatest clinical symptoms: loss of stability, loss of function (unable to sustain body weight), palpable deformation, increased swelling and discolouration. Notably, people who experience a Grade III ligament injury report greater pain during the trauma and less pain after initial trauma than for a Grade II injury. This is probably due to disrupted pain receptors within the ligament.

Some studies have shown that, mechanically, the healed ligament does not recover its cyclic behaviour or stress relaxation characteristics; its strength after recovery is, at most, 70% of its original strength. Protective equipment, such as taping, knee and ankle braces, and wrist guards, can help to reduce the incidence of ligament sprains; such equipment is highly recommended in athletes who have suffered recurrent sprains.

Injury to tendon

Tendons transmit the contraction force of muscles to bone causing motion at our joints. Although tendons have a variety of shapes, such as the broad, flat, sheet-like aponeurosis of the latissimus dorsi or the long, thin pen-like structure of the biceps brachii, regardless of shape all tendons have high tensile strength. Injuries to tendons can be acute or from overuse trauma. Acute tendon injury often involves a mid-substance rupture at high strain rates. However, this type of injury is uncommon in athletes without underlying tendon pathology (see below). In a true acute tendon injury, that is failure without the existence of underlying pathologies, failure occurs either at the musculotendinous junction (e.g. strain of gastrocnemius at the musculotendinous junction in 'tennis leg') or at the bony attachment, called an avulsion injury. Avulsion injuries are most common where a large muscle attaches to a relatively small bony protrusion, for example the attachment of the hamstring muscles at their origin.

There are several common tendinopathies caused by overuse trauma. The most common is tendinosis, which refers to a non-inflammatory condition of the tendon at the cellular level caused by a breakdown in the collagen matrix, cells, and the vascular components of the tendon. In a tendon affected by tendinosis some collagen fibrils may not assume the correct parallel orientation or may not be uniform in length or diameter, in addition to other cell abnormalities and the ingrowth of blood vessels. Tendinosis is believed to be the most common cause of spontaneous tendon rupture. Two other common overuse tendinopathies are peritendinitis and tendinitis. Peritendinitis is defined as an inflammation of the paratendon, which is the loose connective tissue filling the interstices of the fascial compartment around the tendon. The term tendinitis is now used to describe a symptomatic degeneration of the tendon with vascular disruption and inflammatory repair response. The American Academy of Orthopaedic Surgeons recommends using three sub-groupings of tendinitis: first, purely inflammation with acute haemorrhage and tear; second, inflammation superimposed upon pre-existing degeneration; and third, calcification and tendinosis changes in chronic conditions.

MUSCLE

Skeletal muscles have been termed the 'basic elements of movement mechanics' because the force production within a muscle powers human movement. Of course it is not only the force production that is important to movement but also the transmission of the load produced by the force from muscle to bone that creates movement at joints. To that end the muscle-tendon unit is a crucial component, as it stabilises and absorbs energy in load transmission and is a key element linking the force-generating muscle fibres and the force-transmitting collagen fibres of the tendon.

Adaptation

The ability of muscle to adapt to mechanical load is obvious, and we can easily see the effect if we contrast the physique of a power lifter with that of a cross-country skier. From this example we may note that not only the amount but also the type of training (specificity) appears to have an influence on human muscle. Endurance training increases the oxygen carrying potential of muscle and tends to have a less significant effect on size of the total muscle. Resistance training, on the other hand, will increase the total size of a muscle's myofibrillar cross section in turn increasing the muscle's size and mass. In addition to the changes in the contractile component, exercise training also increases the stiffness in the non-contractile components allowing the passive force production to be more efficient. As with other human tissues, muscle tends to atrophy in response to disuse and hypertrophy when subjected to overload.

Immobilisation and disuse

Immobilisation and disuse tend to cause significant atrophy (as determined by cross-sectional area) in the slow twitch fibres as well as a reduction in aerobic capacity. Specifically, the loss of muscle mass has been linked to a decreased muscle fibre size, and a decrease in the number of myofibrillar proteins, phosphocreatine, glycogen, potassium and enzymes necessary for glycolysis and oxiditative phosphorylation. Additionally, there is a thinning of the sarcolemma and weakening of connective tissue resulting in a decrease in the elastic modulus and resilience of the muscle-tendon unit. The extent of the atrophy is proportional to the time of immobilisation or disuse and the rate of atrophy is rapid for the first two to four weeks, then progresses more slowly as the immobilisation period continues.

Age

Our muscle strength tends to peak between ages 20 and 30 then plateaus until around age 50 where strength begins to decline. The strength loss between ages 20 and 70 has been estimated to be around 30%. Although the mechanisms are not entirely clear, the reasons for decreased force production with ageing are linked to a total reduction in muscle mass, a decrease in the total number of muscle fibres, decrease in cross-sectional area of fast twitch fibres and a decrease in the total number of motor-neurons. Resistance training programmes have been shown to slow the rate of decline and improve muscle mass in ageing populations.

Injury

Muscle trauma accounts for 10–30% of all reported sporting injuries. Injury to muscles is most commonly due to acute trauma. Acute trauma may result from direct impacts or muscular tears called strains. When there is a direct impact to a muscle, that muscle experiences a large compression force as it is compressed between the impacting object and the underlying bone. This type of direct impact injury is called a contusion and may cause tearing of the muscle fibres and bleeding within the muscle compartment. Sport-related contusions tend to be worse because of the magnitude of blood flow through the muscle tissue at the time of the injury. During exercise the amount of blood flow in the muscles may increase from approximately 0.8 l/min to 18 l/min. Generally, the rule of thumb is that the amount of tissue damage caused by the impact is associated with the amount of blood flow in the muscle at the time of injury; the greater the blood flow, the greater the tissue damage.

A muscular strain occurs when the load applied to a muscle exceeds the tissue tolerance and is most often associated with eccentric muscle activity. It is believed that high eccentric forces create high shear stresses between the myofibrils and the endomysium, which may cause injury to the sarcolemma, basal lamina and the dystrophin-associated glycoprotein complex (Gao et al., 2008). The amount of fibre damage is related to the number of muscle fibres that are being contracted while under passive stretch and the rate of loading of the eccentric force. The fibre damage may be very mild, such as that experienced after a strenuous workout. This type of damage is referred to as delayed-onset muscle soreness (DOMS). Alternatively, the fibre damage can be extensive causing complete or near complete rupture of the muscle. Strains are graded similarly to ligament sprains. First degree strains are mild with less than 5% of muscle fibres involved with no significant associated loss in strength or range of motion. There will, however, be pain with active or passive movement. Second degree strains are more moderate, involving 25% and possibly up to 75% of the fibres within the muscle. There is a more significant loss in function and greater pain. With a second degree tear the deformity caused by the torn muscle fibres will be palpable, maybe even obvious to the naked eye. A third degree strain typically involves a complete disruption or rupture of the muscle.

Most common sporting activities that result in muscle strains are activities that involve acceleration, deceleration, landing, jumping and cutting. In these activities the muscles must function eccentrically until the energy in the moving limb is absorbed and concentric muscle action can begin. Biarticular muscles, such as the hamstrings, gastrocnemius and rectus femoris, are at high risk because they can be stretched by two joints to the point that the passive tension within the muscle limits the joint motion. Furthermore, strains commonly occur near the end of an activity or when the athlete has not had sufficient rest, because fatigued muscle is more susceptible to strain injuries. A fatigued muscle is susceptible to strain injuries because it has a reduced capacity for load and energy absorption before failure. More specifically it has been noted that a fatigued muscle has a reduced capacity for energy absorption during the early stages of muscle stretching, as compared to non-fatigued muscle (Mair et al., 1996). Thus, to absorb the same amount of energy, the fatigued muscle must undergo greater lengthening (Figure 2.7). This increase in muscle length is where injury may result.

The muscle-tendon unit is subject to strains induced by stretch. Such strains are often cited as the most frequent sports injuries, and are usually caused by stretch of the muscle-tendon unit, with or without the muscle contracting. They occur most commonly in eccentric contractions, when the active muscle force is greater than in other contractions and more force is produced by the passive connective tissue. Multi-joint muscles are particularly vulnerable as they are stretched at more than one joint. These muscles also often contract eccentrically in sport, as when the hamstrings act to decelerate knee extension in running. Sports involving rapid limb accelerations, and muscles with a high type II fibre content, are frequently associated with strain injuries. Injuries may be to the muscle belly, the tendon, the muscle–tendon junction or the tendon–bone junction, with the last two sites being the most frequently injured. The increased stiffness of the sarcomeres near the muscle–tendon junction has been proposed as one explanation for strain injury at that site. The muscle–tendon junction can be extensive; that of the semimembranosus, for example, extends over half the muscle length.

Figure 2.7 Vertical and horizontal shaded areas relate to equivalent energy absorption for fatigued and non-fatigued states of muscle (adapted from Mair *et al.*, 1996). According to Mair *et al.*, to absorb the same amount of energy as non-fatigued muscle a fatigued muscle must lengthen to 70% of its rupture length. Therefore, when faced with the same amount of energy to absorb, the fatigued muscle may become injured whereas the non-fatigued muscle will not.

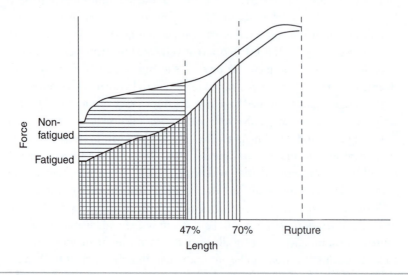

The following sections provide some examples of injuries to the joints and tissues of the body that occur in sport. These are only a few of many examples; they have been chosen to provide an insight into the biomechanics of sports injury. For an epidemiological approach to sports injuries, refer to Caine *et al.* (1996; 2010).

THE HIP, GROIN AND THIGH

Injuries to the groin are common in sport accounting for 3–11% of all injuries in sports such as ice hockey, soccer, speed skating, swimming and athletics. Sports such as soccer and ice hockey have the highest incidences of groin injuries ranging between two and five injuries per 1000 hours of participation. Most commonly groin injuries result from overuse mechanisms although acute trauma injuries do occur.

The most common acute injuries to the groin area are muscle strains to the adductor longus, iliopsoas or abdominal muscles. Injuries to the muscle-tendon units are the most common, particularly to the rectus femoris, adductor longus and iliopsoas, with the first of these the most susceptible (Renström, 1994). Muscle tears and strains, particularly to the two-joint muscles, can be caused by sudden strain on an incompletely relaxed muscle, either by a direct blow or indirectly as in sprinting. Tackling or checking is a common mechanism of injury to the conjunct tendon of the transverse abdominis and internal oblique muscles. Injury may occur when an athlete has become unbalanced and is trying to recover from a tackle (either as the tackler or the tackled) (Figure 2.8).

Figure 2.8 In an attempt to recover from a tackle the groin and lower abdominal muscles are at risk from attempting to contract forcefully a lengthened muscle. This figure depicts the mechanism of injury for both tackler and ball carrier in soccer. The tackler overextends the hip and trunk in an attempt to get a better reach to the ball; she loses her balance and must recover the overextended limb and trunk with a quick, forceful contraction. The ball carrier is also at risk of a groin injury here, as her foot is hung up on the tackler's foot, thereby adding an unexpected eccentric load to the hip and groin as the athlete tries to kick the ball.

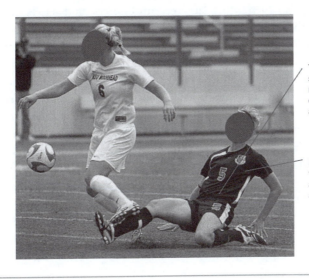

Tackle attempt causes spine extension and right rotation, with left hip extension, external rotation and abduction.

Recovery–flex trunk with left rotation. While attempting to flex, adduct and internally rotate left hip.

Most common injuries to the thigh are quadriceps contusions and hamstring strains. Contusion to the quadriceps, often referred to as a 'charley horse', is one of the most common injuries in contact sports and may account for 8–23% of all injuries in sports such as soccer, hockey, ice hockey, American football and rugby. The most common injury mechanism is thought to be passive failure of the muscle tissue from non-penetrating, blunt, compression force probably delivered from an opponent's knee, elbow or helmet. The type and amount of muscle damage may be related to the mass, velocity, size and shape of the impacting object (Crisco *et al.*, 1994). There are two kinds of contusion; intramuscular, when muscle fibres are torn within the perimysium, or intermuscular, when both the muscle fibres and perimysium are torn. An intramuscular contusion is most problematic because the build-up of fluid within the muscle sheath can lead to increased pressure within the muscle, known as compartment syndrome. The increased pressure may cause further damage and necrosis within the muscle and delay the healing. A further complication of intramuscular contusions is the risk of calcification of the hematoma called 'myositis ossificans'. Very little is known about the mechanism of myositis ossificans but the predominant theory is that the condition results from ossification of proliferating fascial connective tissue (Hait *et al.*, 1970) and is highly dependent upon an individual's predisposition to the condition.

Hamstring strain is common in sprinting and in sports that require fast running or sprinting as a major component such as rugby, American football, soccer and Australian

Rules football. It has been hypothesised that the hamstrings are most susceptible to injury during the terminal swing phase of running (Chumanov *et al.*, 2007; Schache *et al.*, 2009). While running at high speeds there is a large inertial force acting about the knee during terminal swing and it is proposed that this force must be transmitted to the hamstrings. Thus, terminal swing has been implicated because at this point the hamstring is experiencing large eccentric forces, and has been shown to undergo active lengthening in an attempt to decelerate the swinging thigh and shank and absorb some of the imparted inertial force. Other theories include motor control deficits that lead to poor coordination, for instance between the two heads of biceps femoris, and that may make this muscle more prone to injury. Athletes who have had hamstring strain are more likely to experience recurrent strains. It is thought that one-third of athletes who experience a hamstring strain will face a recurrent strain within the first year after their return to sport. Furthermore, subsequent injuries are more severe than the original. Thus, there is still much we do not understand about the mechanism of hamstring strain, which is crucial in developing proper rehabilitation techniques.

Overuse injury

Hamstring tendinitis commonly affects biceps femoris at its insertion. Other injuries include osteitis pubis, a painful inflammation of the symphysis pubis, which is common in soccer players and also affects runners and walkers. In walking, the hip joint has forces of three to five times body weight (BW) to transmit. The hip joint forces that result from ground impact, such as those experienced in running, are obviously much greater. The most common fracture is to the femur when subject to a combination of axial compression, torsion, shear and bending loads. The force transmitted from the hip joint to the femur has shear, compressive and bending components, which can cause fracture at various sites. Stress fractures to the femur neck and shaft have increased and are associated with repetitive loading in long- and middle-distance runners and joggers (Renström, 1994).

'Snapping hip' is a condition where a snapping is felt on the outside of the hip around the greater trochanter and may be caused by the muscles of the tensor fascia lata or gluteus maximus translating back and forth over the greater trochanter. This condition is common in dancers and can result in abrasion wear and inflammation to the muscle fibres, tendons and bursae. Acetabular labral tear is a common repetitive stress injury experienced by golfers, cyclists, horseback riders, soccer players and martial artists. Generally it is accepted that the mechanism is repetitive external hip rotation or forceful twisting, although up to 74% of labrum tears have unknown causes (Lewis and Sahrmann, 2006). Joint incongruity or decreased joint surface area have been documented as strong risk factors for labral tears. Poor joint congruency places increased stress on the acetabulum and the labrum and is associated with further joint disease and articular cartilage degeneration.

THE KNEE

The knee is a major weight-bearing joint and it is located between two of the body's longest bones. These two facts make the knee highly susceptible to soft tissue injury due to shear and torsion loads. In fact, some research reports that up to 32.6% of all sports injuries involve the knee and that the activities leading to most injuries were soccer (35%) and skiing (26%). The most common acute injuries in the knee involve damage to the anterior cruciate ligament (ACL), the medial collateral ligament (MCL) and either meniscus. The knee is also a common site for overuse injury in athletes, the most of which are tendinopathy and wear to the articular cartilage of the tibia, femur or patella.

The most common knee ligament injuries in sport are to the ACL and the MCL. The ACL prevents excessive anterior translation of the tibia and helps to control the gliding of the tibia on the femur during extension and flexion. It also plays an important rotational role in the 'screw home' mechanism of the knee. As the knee reaches full extension the tibia externally rotates to lock the knee into the meniscus, the ACL acts to resist hyper-extension and becomes taught. The MCL protects the knee against valgus directed forces and consists of three layers: superficial, deep, and posterior. The largest and most crucial of the three layers is the superficial layer. It has about twice the tensile strength of the ACL and is a flat, triangular band of collagen that runs from the medial femoral condyle to the medial aspect of the tibia. These ligaments are commonly damaged (70%) during activities involving sudden acceleration or deceleration, such as a sudden change in direction when cutting or landing from a jump. Cutting and landing manoeuvres combine axial loading with abduction and external rotation, which place large rotational moments and shear forces on the knee structures (Figure 2.9). Female athletes are at much higher

Figure 2.9 Non-contact mechanisms for anterior cruciate ligament injury.

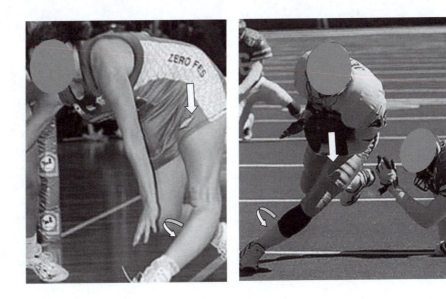

risk for non-contact ACL injury, up to eight times more likely than their male counter-parts (more on this topic follows in Chapter 3). If the magnitude of loading is excessive it may result in tearing of the MCL, ACL and the medial meniscus. This type of injury is often referred to as the 'terrible triad' or the 'unhappy triad'. The unhappy triad is most likely (95%) to occur when the mechanism of injury creates a loading that leads to a Grade III tear of the MCL. The other 30% of ACL and MCL injuries occur from direct contact mechanisms that put excessive load on the joint, for example in a rugby or American football tackle (Figure 2.10).

Because of the MCL's location and attachments to the joint capsule it can withstand greater loads without complete rupture and has better healing ability than the ACL. The ACL is the knee ligament that suffers the most frequent total disruption. Once ruptured 70–80% of patients lose the rotational stability at the knee and, because the ACL is a more isolated ligament without the physiological support of the joint capsule such as the MCL, it has poor healing abilities; thus, surgical repair is highly recommended. Because the mechanical properties of tendon closely resemble those of ligament, the repair of the

Figure 2.10 Direct contact mechanisms for anterior cruciate ligament injury.

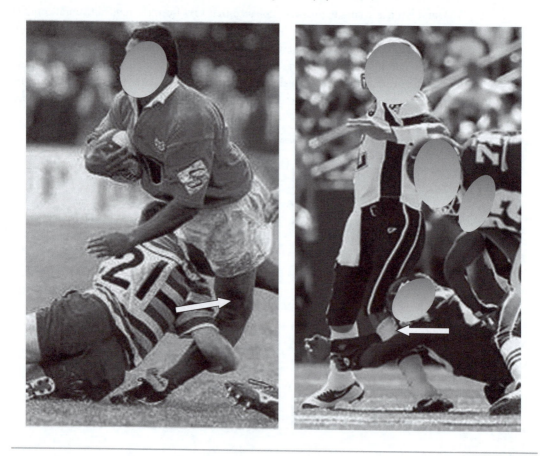

ACL involves replacement of the damaged ligament with tendon tissue. The tendon tissue that is usually chosen for the repair will come from the surrounding area, either from the patellar tendon, or from the semitendinosus tendon or the combined tendon of the semitendinosus and gracilis (hamstring grafts). When the tissue selected for the repair comes from the patient's own tendon it is called an autograft. In some countries surgeons also give patients the option to have a graft from a cadaveric donor; this is called an allograft. The difference between the patellar or hamstring grafts is in the insertion points. Grafts from the patellar tendon include small pieces of bone taken from the patella and tibial tuberosity (the graft is called a bone-patellar tendon-bone graft), Figure 2.11, while the hamstring grafts do not contain bone plugs. The mechanical advantage of the bone-patellar tendon-bone graft is that the resulting ligament-bone attachment is physiologically and mechanically more reminiscent of the original ligament attachment. The area where tendon attaches to bone is more mineralised and has increased stiffness compared to the rest of the tendon tissue. The bone-patellar tendon-bone graft has been shown to provide a greater reduction in joint laxity over the straight tendon graft, most probably because of the increased stiffness. Thus, the

Figure 2.11 Bone-patellar tendon–bone autograft taken during reconstruction surgery of an anterior cruciate ligament. The bone plugs are clearly visible.

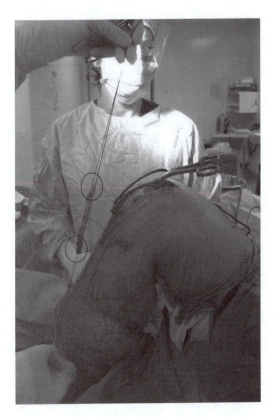

bone-patellar tendon-bone graft has been recommended over the hamstring graft for those with excessive general joint laxity (Kim *et al.*, 2008). The drawback of bone-patellar tendon-bone graft is greater pain associated with the surgery and long term (>one year) pain associated with kneeling (Biau *et al.*, 2006). The pure tendon graft has been shown to have quicker recovery and less long term pain symptoms and is recommended to those with normal joint laxity.

With injury mechanisms that damage the ACL or MCL there is a great risk of also damaging the meniscus within the knee. The menisci are 'C' shaped pieces of cartilage that act as shock absorbers and provide anteroposterior and mediolateral stabilisation between the tibia and femur owing to their shape. Because the MCL is physically attached to the medial meniscus, a load that is great enough to stretch the MCL may also damage the medial meniscus. In fact the medial meniscus is injured ten times as frequently as the lateral meniscus. Current research shows that if meniscus injury and repair accompany ACL injury and repair there is a much greater risk of degenerative joint disease, like osteoarthritis, long term (Neuman *et al.*, 2008).

Overuse injury

Patellar tendinosis also called 'jumper's knee' is an overuse injury of the patellar tendon. High demands on the extensor mechanism result in disruption of tendon fibres, chronic overload of the tendon leading to degenerative changes within the tendon structure. Prevalence of patellar tendinosis is greatest in sports such as volleyball, basketball, figure skating and tennis, in which the forces at the patellofemoral joint are large. Mechanisms are still under debate but some anatomical anomalies may act as contributing factors. For example, reduced flexibility in the quadriceps, patella alta (high riding knee cap) or weak hamstring muscles could increase the strain on the patellar tendon during repeated jumping.

Iliotibial band syndrome is a common overuse injury in runners (12% of running injuries) and cyclists or other athletes who use running to train for, or as a major component in, their sports. Iliotibial band syndrome is characterised by localised pain on the lateral aspect of the knee. Typically, pain presents just after activity; however, as the condition worsens the pain may occur during activity. The mechanism of injury in runners is impingement of the posterior edge of the iliotibial band against the lateral epicondyle of the femur just after foot strike in the gait cycle. The friction force between the iliotibial band and epicondyle is greatest as the athlete flexes the knee to, or slightly below, 30°. Thus, downhill running and running at slower speeds may exacerbate iliotibial band syndrome as the knee tends to be less flexed at foot strike. In cyclists, the iliotibial band is pulled anteriorly on the down-stroke and posteriorly on the up-stroke; this repetitive movement leads to irritation and microtrauma. There are several anatomical abnormalities that may contribute to iliotibial band friction injury. In runners, anomalies such as excessive foot pronation, leg length discrepancy, lateral pelvic tilt, genu valgus, and reduced flexibility in the gluteal or quadriceps muscles will increase the strain on the iliotibial band. In cyclists, excessive external tibial rotation

(>20°), genu varus, and exaggerated knee extension will place excessive strain on the iliotibial band and increase the likelihood of lateral knee pain.

There are two kinds of joint wear associated with the knee; the first is chondromalacia, which refers to softening and deterioration of the underside of the kneecap. This condition is common in young athletes and the mechanism may be related to a direct trauma to the patella, overuse, poor alignment of the knee joint, or muscle imbalance. Any of these mechanisms may lead to friction and rubbing under the kneecap resulting in abrasion damage to the surface of the cartilage. The sensation is a dull pain around or under the kneecap that worsens when compression load is increased to the kneecap, for example when walking downstairs or downhill, climbing stairs, doing squats, or sitting with knees bent for a long period of time. The second common knee condition associated with joint wear is osteoarthritis, which is the most common type of arthritis in athletes. It is a degenerative disease that results in a gradual wearing away of the joint cartilage. The mechanisms related to osteoarthritis were discussed in the section on articular cartilage above. Typical symptoms of osteoarthritis are pain, inflammation, a loss of the range of motion of the knee, and morning stiffness that decreases with motion.

THE ANKLE

The ankle is the most commonly injured joint in sport, accounting for around 10–15% of total injuries. Both acute and overuse injuries are common in the ankle and few sports are immune. The most common acute injuries are ligament sprain and fractures. About 13.9–17% of traumatic sports injuries involve sprain of the ankle ligaments, and 85% of these involve the lateral ligaments. A small moment in the frontal plane (up to 0.16 BW in walkers) transmits load to the lateral malleolus. The medial malleolus, with the deltoid ligaments, prevents talar eversion. The stress concentration within the joint is high owing to the small load-bearing area but, within the physiological range of 10° dorsiflexion to 20° plantar flexion, the load transmitted to the ligaments remains low. When ranges exceed these or loads are directed to invert or evert the foot the ligament loads increase significantly. Sprains to the lateral ligaments caused by plantar flexion and inversion will damage only the anterior talofibular ligament in 75% of cases. Furthermore, in 20–25% of lateral sprains, the damage to the anterior talofibular ligament is combined with damage to the calcaneofibular ligament as well. Medial ankle sprain of the deltoid ligament is caused by an eversion mechanism and is quite rare (<3%), while injury to the tibiofibular ligament by forced dorsiflexion also accounts for only 3% of ankle ligament injuries.

The occurrence of lateral ankle sprain is highly associated with increased susceptibility to repeat ankle sprains. In fact between 20 and 75% of athletes will suffer recurrent ankle sprains and a further 25% report 'frequent sprains' (i.e. more than two per season). An athlete who suffers recurrent or frequent ankle sprains may have a chronic instability. Chronic instability may be characterised as functional or mechanical. A mechanical instability is characterised by joint mobility beyond the physiological range, which may be associated with changes in either flexibility or compliance. This means that ligament structures may have increased in length due to stretching, leading to increased flexibility at the joint, or the ligaments have reduced stiffness or increased compliance leading to greater mobility for a given load. A functional instability is characterised by a 'giving way' and is linked to impaired proprioception, neuromuscular control, strength deficits and possibly impaired postural control. If an athlete's instability is seen as functional then it is possible to retrain the ankle and improve function. However, if the athlete has a mechanical instability he or she should consider bracing if their sport allows such devices, if not he or she should consider surgery to correct the joint laxity.

The ankle is a common fracture site in sport, the mechanism is supination combined with internal rotation of the foot often occurring when the foot adheres to the surface while the inertial force carries the rest of the leg and body forward, creating a shearing mechanism across the ankle joint (Figure 2.12). The result may be fracture of the fibula at the level of the joint, fracture of the medial malleolus or dislocation of the talus with significant disruption to the ligaments and other soft tissue (Figure 2.12).

Figure 2.12 Examples of fracture of the fibula with dislocation of talus. In both examples ((a) and (b); (c) to (e)) the athlete attempts to brake or change direction by planting the foot slightly supinated. In (c) the athlete lands with foot slightly supinated and internally rotated; (d) the foot appears to adhere to the surface while the rest of the athlete's body continues on its path creating a shearing mechanism at the ankle joint; (e) resulting in fracture of the fibula and dislocation of the talus.

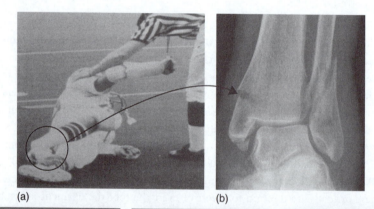

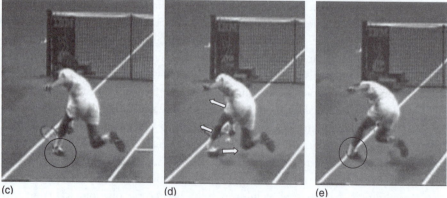

Overuse injury

Overuse pathologies in the tendons of the ankle are common in runners and running-related sports. The most common tendinopathies for runners are tendinosis and peritendinitis in the tibialis posterior tendon or the peroneal tendons. The Achilles tendon is one of the largest and strongest tendons in the body and is responsible for transmitting large loads; for example, everyday loads on the Achilles tendon may range from 850 N for walking (Pourcelot *et al.*, 2005) to 2233 N in jumping and 3786 N in single leg hopping (Fukashiro *et al.*, 1995). The Achilles tendon is one of the most common sites for tendon rupture in sport; the incidence of rupture is 18 per 100,000. The most affected group are males (averaging six males for every female) aged 35 to 50 years. Injuries occur in many sports that involve running and jumping particularly American football, team handball, volleyball, basketball, tennis, squash, badminton and long distance running. The main sporting mechanisms are: landing and cutting manoeuvres (e.g. gymnast landing Figure 2.13(a)); sudden dorsiflexion of a plantar flexed foot (e.g. badminton backing up to take a shot, Figure 2.13(b)); and a taut tendon struck by a

Figure 2.13 Examples of sporting mechanisms of Achilles tendon injury. (a) Sudden dorsiflexion of a plantar flexed foot; (b) Landing mechanism: in this photo there is a noticeable deformity in the line of the calf due to the tendon rupture; (c) Depicts the surgery for repairing a ruptured Achilles tendon.

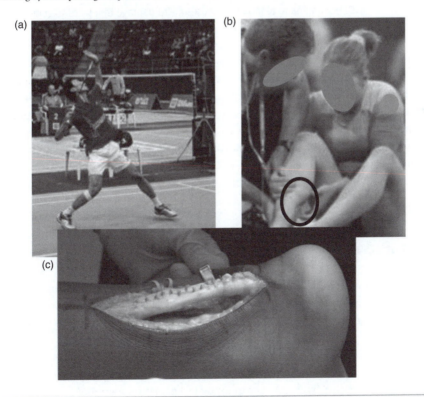

Table 2.2 Factors associated with Achilles tendinosis in athletes

FACTOR	MECHANISM
Training errors	Sudden increase in running mileage
	Sudden increase in running intensity
	Hill running
	Resumption of intense training after a period of inactivity
Surface	Repetitive jumping and landing on hard surfaces
	Running on uneven terrain
Equipment	Shoes with inadequate shock absorption
	Shoes with heel wedge less than 38 mm
	Loose fitting heel counter
	Excessively narrow or flared heel base
Anatomical	Poor tendon blood supply
	Thin heel pad
	Rear foot valgus in a flexible foot
	Rear foot varus in a rigid foot
	Tibial varum
	Proximal limb and pelvic malalignments
	Gastrocnemius-soleus strength-to-tendon-size imbalance
Other	Age and tendon collagen changes that may be associated with age
	Direct trauma to tendon that causes micro-damage that leads to cumulative trauma.

blunt object (e.g. baseball bat, squash racquet, or tennis racquet). When the Achilles tendon is ruptured there is a significant loss in strength and function at the ankle joint, which can be restored through surgical repair (Figure 2.13(c)). Contributing factors to Achilles tendinopathies are multifactorial including training errors, equipment faults and anatomical factors (Table 2.2). Research suggests that Achilles tendon rupture is most often secondary to a degenerative process rather than a primary injury. Often the mechanical structure of the tendon is compromised through pre-existing tendinosis, systemic disease, steroids, or fluoroquinone antibiotics.

THE WRIST AND HAND

Hand and wrist injuries are common in virtually all sporting endeavours. In fact, 3–9% of all sport related injuries involve the hand and wrist. In contact sports, such as rugby or American football, hand and wrist injuries account for 15% of all injuries, while in gymnastics the percentage is even higher at 46–87%. Injuries may be classified as acute or overuse.

The most common acute injuries to the wrist are a scaphoid fracture, a Colles fracture (distal radius fracture), a scapholunate ligament sprain and injuries to the distal radioulnar joint and triangular fibrocartilage complex. The most common inciting incident for these types of acute injuries is falling on an outstretched hand. Thus, injuries such as these are often referred to as FOOSH (Falling On An OutStretched Hand) injuries. The mechanical mechanism underlying FOOSH starts with the load applied to the outstretched hand which is transmitted along the whole upper extremity as an axial compression force and a bending moment. Of course, FOOSH is not all there is to know; the angle of the hand to the ground and the flexion angle of the wrist dictate the magnitude of the bending moment on the radius and the compression and shear forces applied to the scaphoid. Studies have shown an increased risk to the schaphoid in falls with the wrist hyperextended 90° or more combined with 10° or more of radial deviation. In falls with less than 90° wrist hyperextension a Colles fracture of the distal radius is more likely. Sports where the FOOSH mechanism is common are roller-skating or roller blading, skateboarding, snowboarding, skiing, and cycling. Injuries to the triangular fibrocartilage complex may also be seen in sports that place excessive tensile load on the wrist, such as the pole vault, waterskiing, golf, and racquet sports.

The most common joint injuries in the hand involve the proximal interphalangeal joint, the distal interphalangeal joint and the metacarpophalangeal joint of the thumb. The proximal interphalangeal joint is one of the most commonly injured joints in sports. Collateral ligament injuries of the proximal interphalangeal joint are quite common due to axial loading and flexion forces, mechanisms commonly seen in ball sports such as basketball, netball, cricket, softball, rugby and American football. Common distal interphalangeal injuries are 'mallet finger', disruption of the extensor mechanism, and 'jersey finger', disruption of the flexor mechanism. Mallet finger is usually caused by an object (e.g. a ball) striking the finger, creating a forceful flexion of an extended distal interphalangeal joint. The extensor tendon may be stretched, partially torn, or completely ruptured, or separated by a distal phalanx avulsion fracture. Disruption of the flexor digitorum profundus tendon, also known as jersey finger, commonly occurs when an athlete's finger catches on another player's clothing, often seen in tackling sports such as American football or rugby. The ring finger accounts for 75% of jersey finger cases. Common injuries to the metacarpophalangeal joint of the thumb are dorsal dislocations and collateral ligament injuries. Collateral ligament injury called 'gamekeeper's' or 'skier's' thumb is typically caused by a radially directed force on an abducted thumb.

Overuse injury

Tendinopathy is relatively common in the wrist tendons, particularly in sports involving repetitive movements, such as tennis, squash, badminton and canoeing. De Quervain's syndrome, stenosing tenosynovitis of the first dorsal compartment, is the most common tendinitis of the wrist in athletes. Activities requiring repetitive forceful grasping along with ulnar deviation place excessive pressure and friction on the abductor pollicis longus and extensor pollicis brevis as they glide over the radial styloid process. This syndrome is common in activities such as golf, squash, racquet ball, badminton and fly fishing. The second most common tendonitis is found in the extensor carpi ulnaris tendons often found in rowing and racquet sports that use excessive ulnar deviation. Oddly enough this injury is common in the non-dominant hand in tennis players who use a two-handed stroke. Dorsal impingement syndrome is common in sports requiring repetitive wrist flexion accompanied by high axial loading, such as gymnastics. Dorsal impingement may cause dorsal capsulitis, inflammation of the joint capsule or synovitis, or inflammation of the synovial membrane.

THE ELBOW

Elbow injuries account for about 2–5% of all sport related injuries. Anatomically, the elbow is a stable joint. Accordingly, acute single-event injuries such as fracture or dislocation require high energy mechanisms and are not overly common in sport. Repetitive and low energy overuse problems, such as tennis elbow and chondromalacia of the olecranon compartment, are the most common type of elbow injury. Yet a third type of injury in the elbow is the acute single-event injury overlaid on tissue made vulnerable by an overuse injury mechanism.

The most common acute single-event mechanism is FOOSH. Sports where acute elbow injury is common are those where there is a likelihood of high energy transfer as in sports where the athlete is travelling at high speeds, such as cycling, skiing and speed skating, or sports performed at a height, such as the pole vault, gymnastics, ski jumping and ski aerials. If the elbow is somewhat flexed, posterolateral dislocation may occur. If the elbow is fully extended, transmission of force up the radius may produce a fracture of the radial head or capitellum. Varus or valgus shear forces at the time of impact may cause fracture of the condylar and supracondylar structures. These injuries are more common in children whose bones are incompletely formed; ligament injuries and joint dislocation are more common in the mature skeleton. If the elbow is abducted with hyperextension, loading causes an axial force plus a bending moment equal to the product of the force's moment arm from the elbow and the magnitude of the force. This loading causes tension in the medial collateral ligament and lateral compression of the articular surfaces and can lead to fracture of the radial neck or head and, after medial ligament rupture, joint dislocation or subluxation. A direct blow on a flexed elbow axially loads the humeral shaft, which may fracture the olecranon or cause Y- or T-shaped fractures to the humerus articular surface.

Overuse injuries

Overuse injuries are more frequent in the elbow when there is a repetitive passive elongation of a muscle undergoing active contraction. The tensile forces in an eccentric contraction are high and may cause tearing in the muscle-tendon units, the myotendinous junction or the tendon origin. 'Tennis elbow', an inflammation of the lateral epicondyle (lateral epicondylitis), is the most common overuse injury of the elbow, and is often seen in athletes with a poorly executed backhand, that causes the wrist to flex involuntarily while the extensor carpi radialis brevis is contracting to stabilise the wrist and racket. 'Golfer's elbow', inflammation of the medial epicondyle (medial epicondylitis) affects the common flexor tendon origin and is seen when tension is applied to the wrist and digital flexor tendons and pronators while they are being contracted.

Combined injuries

Tear or rupture of the ulnar collateral ligament usually occurs in a ligament previously weakened by overuse and is often seen in repetitive throwing mechanisms. Repeated throwing exposes the medial side of the elbow to valgus shear forces which cause strain in the ulnar collateral ligament during the late cocking and early acceleration phases. In adolescents, tension from the strained ulnar collateral ligament and the flexor and pronator muscle groups can cause an avulsion fracture of the medial epicondylar apophysis, called 'little leaguer's elbow'. 'Thrower's elbow' is a whiplash injury caused by hyperextension, leading to fracture or epiphysitis of the olecranon process. 'Javelin thrower's elbow' is a strain of the medial ligament caused by failure to achieve the classic 'elbow-lead' position, as in roundarm throwing.

THE SHOULDER

The shoulder is one of the most complex and mobile joints in the human body owing to its five separate articulations (sternoclavicular, acromioclavicular, coracoclavicular, glenohumeral and scapulothoracic joints). Injuries to the shoulder joint are common in sports, particularly overhead throwing events where the incidence of injury may range from 3 to 57% of all reported injuries. Common acute injuries to the shoulder include acromioclavicular sprain, glenohumeral dislocation, and fracture of the acromion, clavicle or humerus.

Because the articulations of the shoulder girdle are interconnected, they function much as a unit in bearing loads and absorbing shock, thus a single mechanism may cause various injuries to one or more structures around the shoulder complex. A common mechanism of shoulder injury in sport is falling onto the shoulder of an adducted arm, common in contact sports (rugby, American football and ice hockey), cycling, horse riding, skiing and wrestling (Figure 2.14(a and c)). In these sports, force is transmitted along an adducted arm that compresses the head of the humerus against the coracoacromial arch resulting in separation of the acromioclavicular joint, injury to the rotator cuff muscles or fracture of the acromion or glenoid neck. If the arm is partially abducted, fracture of the clavicle is likely (Figure 2.14(c)). The glenohumeral

Figure 2.14 Common sporting mechanisms of shoulder injury: (a) and (c) falling on to the shoulder of an adducted arm, which is common in contact sports; (b) direct contact mechanism may cause posterior dislocation of shoulder or fracture of clavicle; and (d) common mechanism of glenohumeral dislocation in rugby, tackling with abducted and externally rotated arm.

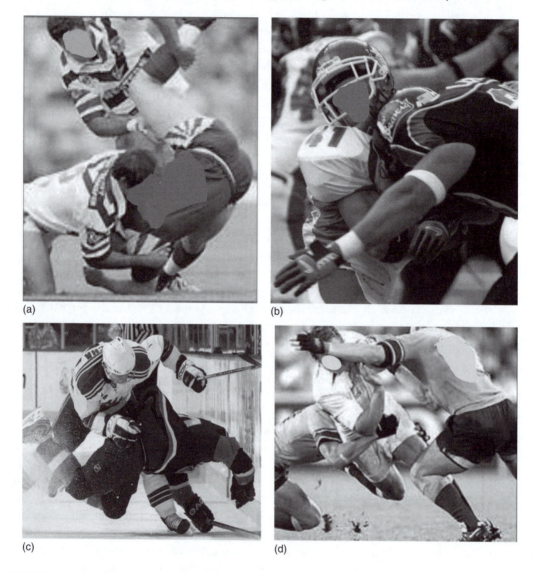

(a)

(b)

(c)

(d)

joint is the most commonly dislocated joint in the body. Anterior glenohumeral dislocation is most likely, particularly in young athletes, when the arm is fully abducted and externally rotated (Figure 2.14 (d)). Posterior dislocation, which is far less common, can occur from a heavy frontal shoulder charge in field games (Figure 2.14(b)) or by a fall in which the head of the humerus is forced backwards while the humerus is inwardly rotated.

In overhead sports movements, such as javelin throwing, baseball pitching and serving in tennis, the joints of the shoulder region often experience large ranges of motion at high angular velocities, often with many repetitions. A range of injuries have been associated with an overhead throwing mechanism termed rotational injuries. Typically rotational injuries include tears of the labrum, and strain or rupture of the rotator cuff and the biceps brachii. Two phases of the throwing action have been associated with labrum injury. During the cocking phase the shoulder externally rotates and the humeral head translates anteriorly; as the thrower's body moves forward, the inertial force on the arm creates further external rotation. In a forceful or high speed throw (or throw-like action) the inertial force is greater, therefore, there is greater external rotation force placed on the shoulder. During this over-rotation the posterior rotator cuff may become impinged between the glenoid labrum and the humeral head; long term this can cause degeneration of the superior labrum and the rotator cuff tendons. The second most problematic phase is the deceleration phase. During deceleration the rotator cuff muscles are active to resist the distraction force at the shoulder placing a large tensile force on these muscles. Tensile failure is common in the supraspinatus tendon or the long head biceps tendon while these muscles are actively trying to decelerate the arm and elbow. Injuries to the tendon or associated muscle range from micro- to macro-damage and ruptures. The supraspinatus is vulnerable near the insertion where there is a region of low vascularity. It is thought that the reduced vascularity may be responsible for the high incidence of tendinosis and ruptures at this site. Superior labral tears, otherwise known as SLAP lesions, have also been found in repetitive throwing athletes. The mechanism is thought to be related to the large force in the biceps muscle acting to decelerate elbow extension. The force of the long head of the biceps pulls the labrum away from the glenoid creating the SLAP lesion.

Overuse injury

Dynamic stabilisation of the glenohumeral joint is achieved by the coupling of the forces of the supraspinatus, infraspinatus, teres minor and subscapularis (collectively known as the rotator cuff) and the three heads of the deltoid muscle. Abduction of the arm requires the deltoid and rotator cuff to work in tandem, while the movement is mostly powered by the deltoid, the force couple in the rotator cuff is required to maintain glenohumeral congruence to provide a stable fulcrum for humeral rotation. Thus, injury or damage to the rotator cuff muscles, which cause weakness or laxity within that muscle group, can lead to long term degenerative damage to articular surfaces or the labrum owing to improper congruence of the humeral head and glenoid fossa.

Overuse injuries to the rotator cuff are common in sports with a repetitive overhead action, such as volleyball, swimming, throwing and tennis. The most common cause of shoulder pain in these sports is thought to be impingement. Impingement is the compression and mechanical abrasion of the rotator cuff structures as they pass beneath the coracoacromial arch during elevation of the arm. Many tendons pass through the limited subacromial space, such as the long head of biceps brachii, the supraspinatus, the infraspinatus, teres minor and subscapularis, as well as the subacromial bursa. Several popular theories exist as to the etiology leading to impingement, including anatomic abnormalities of the coracoacromial arch (Zuckerman *et al.*, 1992); tension overload; ischemia, or degeneration of the rotator cuff tendons; and shoulder kinematic abnormalities (Ludewig and Cook, 2000). This topic will be discussed further in Chapter 3.

THE HEAD, NECK AND BACK

Head and neck injuries account for around 11% of the sports injuries that require hospital treatment. Traumatic head injuries in sport are most commonly caused by falls or collisions during which the brain moves violently within the skull. Injury to the brain may be classed as primary or secondary. A primary brain injury is the result of tissue deformation caused at the time of impact from the mechanical force acting on the brain. It is believed that the tissue deformation causes specific biochemical changes at the level of the cell membrane, which is responsible for the observed effects of the trauma. Secondary damage may occur as a complication to the primary injury and results from hypoxic and ischemic damage which may cause swelling and or infection. Impact injuries depend on the site, duration and magnitude of the impact and the magnitude of the acceleration of the head. Recent research also suggests that a genetic factor may be involved in the outcome of head trauma (Hang *et al.*, 2006). Damage from head impact is cumulative so each injury makes the athlete more susceptible to further injury and carries long term risk for neurological and cognitive defects. Chronic head injuries have been associated with repeated sub-threshold blows that can lead to a loss of psycho-intellectual and motor performance. Most closely connected with boxing, such injuries have also been reported from repeated heading of fast-travelling soccer balls (Figure 2.15).

Flexion, extension and lateral flexion cause a bending load on the spine, rotation causes a torsional load and axial loading leads to compression. A shear load is caused by any tendency of one part of the spine to move linearly with respect to the other parts (Evans, 1982). The vertebral bodies, intervertebral discs and the posterior longitudinal ligament resist compression; the neural arches, capsule and interspinous ligaments resist tension (Figure 2.16).

Injury to the cervical spine has been associated with axial loading, such as by head-first impact with an opposing player, when slight flexion has removed the natural cervical lordosis. The high elastic content of the ligamentum flavum pre-stresses the discs to about 15 N, with an associated interdisc pressure of 70 kPa. In compression, bulging of the vertebral endplate can occur, which can then crack at loads above 2.5 kN, displacing nuclear material into the body of the vertebra as the disc disintegrates. Axial loading combined with bending or shear is a common mechanism of injury to the cervical spine in rugby front row forwards during scrummaging. A rugby union scrum consists of two packs of eight players divided into the three front row, second back row

Figure 2.15 High speed soccer ball or fist may transmit considerable force to the head.

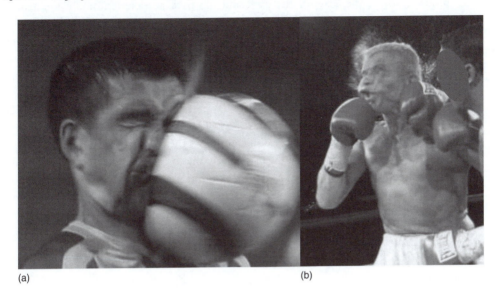

(a)   (b)

Figure 2.16 The spinal ligaments under loading of a motion segment.

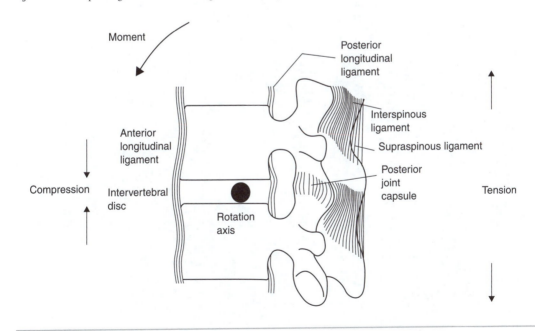

and three back row. The magnitude of force applied by one pack upon the other is proportional to the mass of the pack and the pack acceleration at the moment of impact (engagement). Therefore, the compression forces are particularly high during engagement, for example the pack force has been measured at 8 kN in professional players (Milburn, 1990). At this moment if players act to collapse the scrum, the shear and bending stresses placed on the cervical vertebra may exceed tissue tolerance (Figure 2.17). Although, front row forwards have the highest frequency of catastrophic spine injuries during scrummaging, there has been an increasing frequency of cervical spine injuries sustained during the tackle (MacQueen and Dexter, 2010).

The bending load caused by flexion compresses the vertebral body and increases the tension in the posterior ligaments, particularly the interspinous ligament, which has a breaking force of around 2 kN. Such loads result in fracture of the vertebral body before any ligament failure, as the load on the anterior part of the vertebral body is three to four times greater than the tension in the ligament.

The spine, particularly its cervical and thoracolumbar regions, is highly vulnerable to torsion, with discs, joints and ligament all being susceptible to injury. Although a single

Figure 2.17 Top figure shows scrum engagement and bottom one shows that scrum collapse can place excessive compression and torsion stress on the cervical spine of a front row player.

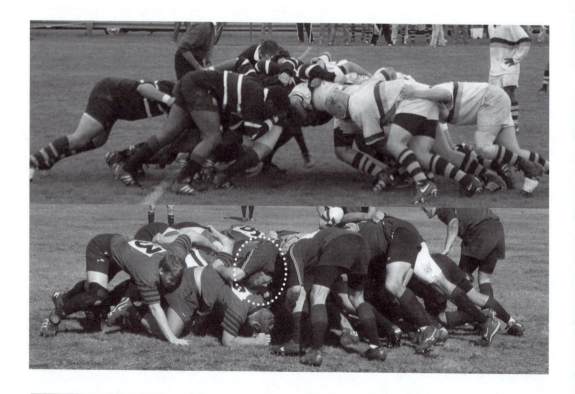

type of loading can cause injury, the spine is more likely to be damaged by combined loading. Rotation of the flexed spine can lead to tearing of the posterior ligament, the joint capsule and the posterior longitudinal ligament. Rotation of the extended spine can lead to rupture of the anterior longitudinal ligament.

Tensile loads on the spine can occur through decelerative loading in the abdominal region, for example in gymnastic bar exercises. This can result in failure of the posterior ligaments or in bone damage. Limited extension at between the fifth and sixth cervical vertebrae (C5–6) and linked flexion at C6–7 and C7–T1 (the first thoracic vertebra) causes those regions to be particularly vulnerable to extension and flexion injury respectively. Overall the cervical spine is most prone to such injury. In the thoracic spine, sudden torsion can injure the tenth to twelfth thoracic vertebrae, which are between two regions of high torsional stiffness.

The probability of injury from a load of brief duration depends on both the peak acceleration and the maximum rate of change of acceleration (jerk) that occur (Troup, 1992). Injury is more likely either when prolonged static loading occurs or in the presence of vibratory stress. Resistance to injury depends on the size and physical characteristics of the spine, muscular strength, skill and spinal abnormalities. High disc pressures, which might lead to herniation, have been associated with twisting and other asymmetric movements because of high antagonistic muscle activity. Lateral bending or rotation combined with compression is usually responsible; participants in sports such as tennis, javelin throwing, volleyball and skiing may be particularly vulnerable (Pope and Beynnon, 1993).

Low-back pain affects, at some time, 80–85% of a given population; as such it is difficult to link the occurrence of non-specific pain to particular sport involvement. However, the literature tends to focus on three mechanical issues: weight-loading, forceful rotations and forceful hyperextension. Weight-loading involves high or repetitive spinal compression which may be exacerbated by any imbalance in the strength of the abdominal and back muscles. This mechanism has been implicated as a risk for low back pain in sports such as weight-lifting, running and horse-riding. Rotation-causing activities involve forceful twisting of the trunk, as in racket sports, golf, discus throwing, and aerial movements in gymnastics and diving. Forceful hyperextension has been implicated in sports such as volleyball, rowing and swimming. Obviously, activities involving all three of these are more hazardous. An example is the 'mixed technique' used by many fast bowlers in cricket (see also Chapter 8). Here the bowler counter-rotates the shoulders with respect to the hips from a more front-on position, at back foot strike in the delivery stride, to a more side-on position at front foot strike. At front foot strike, the impact forces on the foot typically reach over six times body weight. This counter-rotation, or twisting, is also associated with hyperextension of the lumbar spine. The result is the common occurrence of spondylolysis (a stress fracture of the neural arch, usually of the fifth lumbar vertebra, L5) in fast bowlers with such a technique (Elliott et al., 1996). Spondylolysis is present in around 6% of individuals (Pecina and Bojanic, 1993); it is far more common in, for example, gymnasts. Although it is often symptomless, it can be a debilitating injury for gymnasts, fast bowlers in cricket and other athletes.

SUMMARY

In this chapter, the load and tissue characteristics involved in injury were considered along with the terminology used to describe injuries to the human musculoskeletal system. The distinction between overuse and traumatic injury was made clear. An understanding was provided of the various injuries that occur to bone and soft tissues, including cartilage, ligaments and the muscle-tendon unit, and how these depend on the load characteristics. The causes and relative importance of the sports injuries that affect the major joints of the lower and upper extremities, and the back and neck were also covered.

STUDY TASKS

1   For each main type of tissue (bone, cartilage, ligament, muscle, tendon) explain which load types are most closely associated with injury.
2   Distinguish between acute and overuse injuries and provide examples of the latter for each of the tissue types in Study Task 1.
3   For each of the tissue types outlined in Study Task 1, outline the effects of immobilisation.
4   Describe the most likely scenario for acute injury of the Achilles tendon.
5   How does exercise affect tissue adaptation in muscle and ligament?
6   Prepare a synopsis of throwing injuries associated with the shoulder and elbow.
7   Define the three activities that are considered to relate most closely to lumbar spine injuries and outline their relative importance in at least two sporting activities of your choice.
8   What are the mechanical reasons for excessive stress in a bone material leading to fracture? For each reason, identify a sport scenario that might lead to excessive stress causing fracture in an athlete.

GLOSSARY OF IMPORTANT TERMS

Abrasion (graze) Skin surface broken without a complete tear through the skin.
Adhesion Bands of fibrous tissue, usually caused by inflammation.
Avulsion fracture Fracture where the two halves of the bone are pulled apart.
Bursitis Inflammation of a bursa.
Calcification Deposit of insoluble mineral salts in tissue.
Callus Material that first joins broken bones, consisting largely of connective tissue and cartilage, which later calcifies.
Cancellous bone Internal material of long bone; appears trellis-like.
Capsulitis Inflammation of the joint capsule.

Collateral ligament An accessory ligament that is not part of the joint capsule.

Comminuted fracture One in which the bone is broken into more than two pieces.

Contusion Bruise, usually caused by an escape of blood from ruptured vessels after injury.

Cortical bone Outer layer (cortex) of bone having a compact structure.

Diaphysis The central ossification region of long bones (adjective: diaphyseal).

Dislocation Complete separation of articulating bones consequent on forcing of joint beyond its maximum passive range.

Epiphysis The separately ossified ends of growing bones separated from the shaft by a cartilaginous (epiphyseal) plate.

Epiphysitis Inflammation of the epiphysis.

Fracture A disruption to tissue (normally bone) integrity. In traumatic fracture a break will occur, whereas in a stress fracture the disruption is microscopic.

Haemarthrosis Effusion of blood into a joint cavity.

Inflammation Defensive response of tissue to injury indicated by redness, swelling, pain, loss of function and warmth.

Laceration An open wound or cut.

Metaphysis Region of long bone between the epiphysis and diaphysis.

Osteitis Inflammation of bone.

Peritendinitis Inflammation of the tissues around a tendon (the peritendon).

Rupture or tear Complete break in continuity of a soft tissue structure.

Sprain Damage to a joint and associated ligaments. The three degrees of sprain involve around 25%, 50% and 75% of the tissues, respectively. Grade I sprains are mild and involve no clinical instability; grade II are moderate with some instability; and grade III are severe with easily detectable instability. There may be effusion into the joint.

Strain Damage to muscle fibres. A grade I strain involves only a few fibres, and strong but painful contractions are possible. A grade II strain involves more fibres and a localised haematoma, and contractions are weak; as with grade I, no fascia is damaged. Grade III strains involve a great many, or all, fibres, partial or complete fascia tearing, diffuse bleeding and disability.

Subluxation Partial dislocation.

Tendinitis Painful tendon with histological signs of inflammation within the tendon.

Tendinopathy Disease of the tendon including tendinitis, tendinosis and tenosynovitis.

Tendinosis Degenerative condition of a tendon.

Tenosynovitis Inflammation of the synovial sheath surrounding a tendon.

Valgus Abduction of the distal segment relative to the proximal one (as in genu valgum, knock-knees).

Varus Adduction of the distal segment relative to the proximal one (as in genu varum, bow-legs).

REFERENCES

Biau, D.J., Tournoux, C., Katsahian, S., Schranz, P.J. and Nizard, R.M.S. (2006) Bone-patellar tendon-bone autografts versus hamstring autografts for reconstruction of anterior cruciate ligament: meta-analysis. *British Medical Journal, 332,* 995–1001.

Caine, D.J., Caine, C.G and Lindner, K.J. (eds) (1996) *Epidemiology of Sports Injuries,* Champaign, Il: Human Kinetics.

Caine, D.J., Harmer, P. and Schiff, M. (eds) (2010) *Epidemiology of Injury in Olympic Sports,* Chichester, Wiley-Blackwell.

Cameron, M.L., Briggs, K.K. and Steadman, J.R. (2003) Reproducibility and reliability of the outerbridge classification for grading chondral lesions of the knee arthroscopically. *The American Journal of Sports Medicine, 31,* 83–86.

Chumanov, E.S., Heiderscheit, B.C. and Thelen, D.G. (2007) The effect of speed and influence of individual muscles on hamstring mechanics during the swing phase of sprinting. *Journal of Biomechanics, 40,* 3555–3562.

Crisco, J.J., Jokl, P., Heinen, G.T., Connell, M.D. and Panjabi, M.M. (1994) A muscle contusion injury model. *The American Journal of Sports Medicine, 22,* 702–710.

Elliott, B.C., Burnett, A.F., Stockill, N.P. and Bartlett, R.M. (1996) The fast bowler in cricket: a sports medicine perspective. *Sports Exercise and Injury, 1,* 201–206.

Evans, D.C. (1982) 'Biomechanics of spinal injury', in E.R. Gozna and I.J. Harrington (eds) *Biomechanics of Musculoskeletal Injury,* Baltimore, MD: Williams & Wilkins, pp. 163–228.

Frost, H.M. (1990) Skeletal structural adaptations to mechanical usage (SATMU): 1. Redefining Wolff's law: The bone modeling problem. *The Anatomical Record, 226,* 403–413.

Fukashiro, S., Rob, M., Ichinose, Y., Kawakami, Y. and Fukunaga, T. (1995) Ultrasonography gives directly but noninvasively elastic characteristic of human tendon in vivo. *European Journal of Applied Physiology and Occupational Physiology, 71,* 555–557.

Gao, Y., Wineman, A. and Waas, A. (2008) Mechanics of muscle injury induced by lengthening contraction. *Annals of Biomedical Engineering, 36,* 1615–1623.

Hait, G., Boswick, J.A. and Stone, J.J. (1970) Heterotopic bone formation secondary to trauma (myositis ossificans traumatica). *Journal of Trauma, 8,* 405–411.

Hang, C.H., Chen, G., Shi, J.X., Zhang, X. and Li, J.S. (2006) Cortical expression of nuclear factor kappa after human brain contusion. *Brain Research, 1109,* 14–21.

Kim, S.J., Kim, T.E., Lee, D.H. and Oh, K.S. (2008) Anterior cruciate ligament reconstruction in patients who have excessive joint laxity. *Journal of Bone and Joint Surgery, 90,* 735–741.

Kress, T.A., Porta, D.J., Snider, J.N., Fuller, P.M., Psihogios, J.P., Heck, W.L., Frick, S.J. and Wasserman, J.F. (1995) 'Fracture patterns of human cadaver long bones', in *International Research Counsel on the Biomechanics of Impact,* Brunnen: IRCOBI, pp. 155–169.

Levine, R.S. (2002) 'Injury to the extremities', in A.M. Nahum and J.W. Melvin (eds) *Accidental Injury,* New York: Springer-Verlag, pp. 491–522.

Lewis, C.L. and Sahrmann, S.A. (2006) Acetabular labral tears. *Physical Therapy, 86,* 110–121.

Ludewig, P.M. and Cook, T.M. (2000) Alterations in shoulder kinematics and associated muscle activity in people with symptoms of shoulder impingement. *Physical Therapy, 80,* 276–291.

MacQueen, A.E. and Dexter, W.W. (2010) Injury trends and prevention in rugby union football. *Current Sports Medicine Reports, 9,* 139–143.

Mair, S.D., Seaber, A.V., Glisson, R.R. and Garrett, W.E. (1996) The role of fatigue in susceptibility to acute muscle strain injury. *The American Journal of Sports Medicine, 24,* 137–143.

Milburn, P.D. (1990) The kinetics of rugby union scrummaging. *Journal of Sports Sciences, 8,* 47–60.

Neuman, P., Englund, M., Kostogiannis, I., Fridéon, T., Roos, H. and Dahlberg, L.E. (2008) Prevalence of tibiofemoral osteoarthritis 15 years after nonoperative treatment of anterior cruciate ligament injury. *The American Journal of Sports Medicine, 36,* 1717–1725.

Nigg, B.M. and Herzog, W. (2007) *Biomechanics of the Musculo-skeletal System* (3rd edn), Hoboken, NJ: John Wiley & Sons.

Nordin, M. and Frankel, V.H. (1989) *Basic Biomechanics of the Musculoskeletal System* (2nd edn), Baltimore, MD: Williams & Wilkins.

Pecina, M.M. and Bojanic, I. (1993) *Overuse Injuries of the Musculoskeletal System,* Boca Raton, FL: CRC Press.

Pope, M.H. and Beynnon, B.D. (1993) 'Biomechanical response of body tissue to impact and overuse', in P.A.F.H. Renström (ed.) *Sports Injuries: Basic Principles of Prevention and Care,* London: Blackwell Scientific, pp. 120–134.

Pourcelot, P., Defontaine, M., Ravary, B., Lemâtre, M. and Crevier-Denoix, N. (2005) A non-invasive method of tendon force measurement. *Journal of Biomechanics, 38,* 2124–2129.

Renström, P.A.F.H. (1994) 'Groin and hip injuries', in Renström, P.A.F.H. (ed) *Clinical Practice of Sports Injury: Prevention and Care,* London: Blackwell Scientific, pp. 97–114.

Schache, A.G., Wrigley, T.V., Baker, R. and Pandy, M.G. (2009) Biomechanical response to hamstring muscle strain injury. *Gait & Posture, 29,* 332–338.

Troup, J.D.G. (1992) 'Back and neck injuries', in T. Reilly (ed) *Sports Fitness and Sports Injuries,* London: Wolfe, pp. 199–209.

Turner, C.H. (1998) Three rules for bone adaptation to mechanical stimuli. *Bone, 23,* 399–407.

Whiting, W.C. and Zernicke, R.F. (2008) *Biomechanics of Musculoskeletal Injury* (2nd edn), Champaign, IL: Human Kinetics.

Woo, S.L., Gomez, M.A., Sites, T.J., Newton, P.O., Orlando, C.A. and Akeson, W.H. (1987) The biomechanical and morphological changes in the medial collateral ligament of the rabbit after immobilization and remobilization. *Journal of Bone Joint Surgery, American Volume, 69,* 1200–1211.

Zuckerman, J.D., Kummer, F.J., Cuomo, F., Simon, J., Rosenblum, S. and Katz, N. (1992) The influence of coracoacromial arch anatomy on rotator cuff tears. *Journal of Shoulder and Elbow Surgery, 1,* 4–14.

FURTHER READING

The three IOC Medical Commission publications below are of the Encyclopaedia of Sports Medicine series. They contain much useful and interesting material on sports injury from many international experts.

Caine, D.J., Harmer, P. and Schiff, M. (eds) (2010) *Epidemiology of Injury in Olympic Sports,* Chichester, Wiley-Blackwell.

Frontera, W.R. (ed) (2003). *Rehabilitation of Sports Injuries: Scientific Basis,* Malden, MA: Blackwell Science.

Zatsiorsky, V.M. (ed) (2000) *Biomechanics in Sport: Performance Improvement and Injury Prevention,* Malden, MA: Blackwell Science.

3 Risk factors for sports injury

Melanie Bussey

Knowledge assumed
Familiarity with basic
biomechanical concepts
(Chapter 1)

INTRODUCTION – UNDERSTANDING INJURY RISK FOR INJURY PREVENTION

BOX 3.1 LEARNING OUTCOMES

After reading this chapter you should be able to:

- identify common intrinsic and extrinsic risks in sport
- differentiate between modifiable and non-modifiable risk factors
- identify most common injuries associated with specific risk factors
- identify the specific risks to paediatric and masters athletes
- identify the risks to the female athlete that differ from risks to the male athlete
- identify the most common movement technique faults and associated injury risks in various individual and team sports
- understand the mechanical behaviour of sports surfaces and the associated risks to the athlete
- understand how workload may influence injury risk to the throwing athlete
- understand how to reduce injury risk by using the appropriate footwear and protective equipment.

Prevention of sports injuries is particularly important for clinicians and researchers involved in improving sports performance and caring for athletes. Van Mechelen (1992) outlined a sequence to be used in conducting injury prevention research. According to this model one must first examine the magnitude of the problem, which is usually identified using epidemiological data. Specifically we are looking for information about the incidence, prevalence and severity of the injury in question. The second step involves identifying the risk factors and mechanisms for injury, which requires systematic steps to examine athletes, their training regimens, their competitive schedules and sporting environments. The third and fourth steps are associated with implementing injury prevention strategies and assessing their effectiveness. Prevention and intervention have become crucial points for researchers and clinicians. However, before these types of studies can be used, the risk factors for injury must be clearly established.

As discussed in Chapter 1, intrinsic risk factors (relating to the athlete) are seen in a biomechanical context, as those factors that affect the load tolerance of the tissues within the athlete, while extrinsic factors (relating to the environment) may be seen as those that influence the load characteristics (Figure 1.1). Assessment of risk is complex because most factors do not act in isolation. To produce a model of a particular injury to a particular athlete we may need to examine how multiple risk factors interact to create an environment favourable to that injury. And yet, there may be just one specific factor that is required and without it no injury would occur (Meeuwisse *et al.*, 2007). In this chapter, we will examine known risk factors associated with various sports and athlete groups. Specifically, we will focus on intrinsic and extrinsic risks and present, where possible, the supporting epidemiological and mechanical data and information.

INTRINSIC RISK FACTORS RELATED TO INJURY

Intrinsic risk factors are those factors that affect the load tolerance of the tissues within the athlete. These include age, sex, previous injury history, body size, local anatomy, movement technique, aerobic fitness, muscle strength, muscle imbalance and tightness, ligamentous laxity and central motor control. Psychological and psychosocial factors as well as general mental ability are also factors in predisposition to injury. Some of these factors are modifiable, such as strength and movement technique, which means we can make intrinsic modifications that can alter the risk associated with that factor. For example, we can modify our risk for muscle strength by undertaking a strengthening programme targeted towards the at risk areas. However, many intrinsic factors are considered non-modifiable. Age, sex and injury history are examples of these types of factors. With non-modifiable factors, there are no adjustments we can make to reduce the risk associated with that factor. However, by understanding the risk associated with these factors we can adjust related factors such as workloads, equipment and movement technique that in turn may reduce the risk of injury to that individual. In the following sub-sections, we will look at age, sex, previous injury history, anatomy, and movement technique as examples of intrinsic risk factors in athletes. We will look at the types of injuries most associated with these risks and relevant mechanical factors involved.

Age (non-modifiable risk factor)

Age is a non-modifiable risk factor for sports injury. In this section, we will focus on two particular at-risk populations, the paediatric athlete and the mature or masters athlete. Both these groups have unique risk factors related to their age and maturing musculoskeletal system.

The paediatric athlete

A child's vulnerability to sports injury is heightened by immature reflexes, an inability to recognise and evaluate risks, underdeveloped coordination, susceptible growth plates, the non-linear nature of growth, their limited thermoregulatory systems, and the vast variability in biological maturity status among children of similar age. In this sub-section, we will focus on commonly reported childhood sports injuries and the mechanical factors related to them.

Forearm fractures are the most common fractures in children, representing 40–50% of all childhood fractures and 75–84% of forearm fractures occur in the distal third of

Figure 3.1 Types of forearm fractures found in children: (a) greenstick fracture of distal radius; (b) torus fracture of the distal radius.

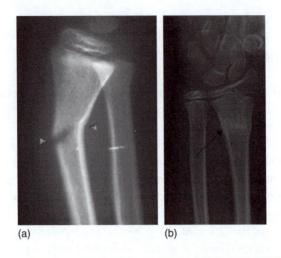

(a)   (b)

the radius or ulna. Torus (Figure 3.1(b)) and greenstick (Figure 3.1(a)) fractures occur most frequently in children under the age of 10 years and complete fractures occur more frequently in children between 10 and 15 years. It is likely that adolescents tend to experience complete fractures because of the increased body mass in relation to a relatively low bone mineral content during periods of rapid growth and development, which allows for higher rates of loading, that is, higher energy impacts.

In the growing athlete, the open epiphysis and soft articular cartilage are vulnerable. The epiphyseal plate is less resistant to torsional or shear stress than the surrounding bone, and epiphyseal plate damage can lead to growth disturbances (Meyers, 1993). The bones of children can undergo plastic deformation or bending instead of fracturing, and this can lead to long-term deformity. The greater strength of the joint capsule and ligaments, in comparison with the epiphyseal plate in children, can mean that loads that would dislocate an adult joint will fracture a child's epiphyseal plate. The distal portions of the humerus, radius and femur are particularly vulnerable to epiphyseal plate fracture, as the collateral ligaments attach to the epiphysis not the metaphysis (Meyers, 1993). More osteochondrotic diseases occur during periods of rapid growth in adolescence because muscle strength lags behind skeletal growth and the muscle-tendon unit is relatively shortened, reducing flexibility (MacIntyre and Lloyd-Smith, 1993). The occurrence of epiphyseal injury in young athletes also peaks at the rapid growth spurts, supporting the view that collision sports and intense training should be avoided at those times (e.g. Meyers, 1993).

The long bones of a child are divided into three parts, the diaphysis or shaft of the bone in the middle, and two epiphyses on either end of the bone (Figure 3.2). In a growing human, the epiphysis is separated from the diaphysis by a layer of hyaline cartilage called the growth plate (Figure 3.2). In an immature skeleton, there is primary ossification, which occurs prenatally; these are the bones as they are at birth (Figure 3.3).

Figure 3.2 The anatomy of the long bone (femur) of a child.

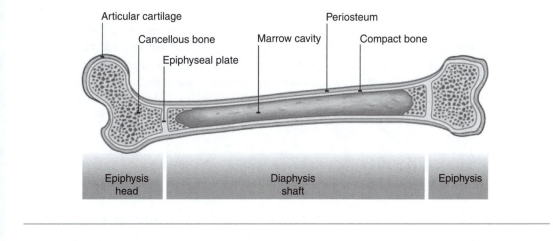

Figure 3.3 Primary and secondary ossification centres as they appear in embryos, youth and adults.

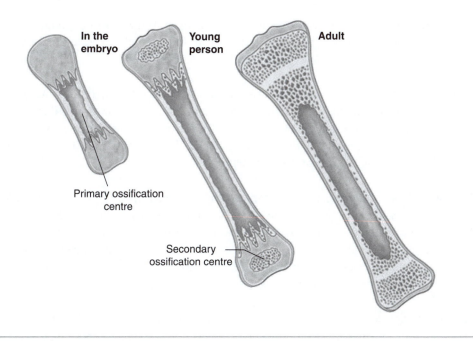

During the growing years from birth to approximately 18 years of age, secondary ossification occurs. Secondary ossification is the area of ossification that appears after the primary ossification centre (the diaphysis) has already appeared – most of which will appear during the postnatal and adolescent years – and occurs in the epiphysis and apophysis (Figure 3.3).

Longitudinal growth occurs as new trabecular bone is created at the primary and secondary ossification centres; the cartilaginous centre of the growth plate is replaced by bone on the diaphysis side thus pushing the epiphyseal plate further away from the shaft (Figure 3.3). This process of new bone formation is unique to children, while in adults bone growth occurs through the process of modelling. When the cells at the growth plate stop dividing, the epiphysis fuses with the shaft of the long bone and the skeleton achieves its adult form. The existence of growth plates poses particular threats to young athletes because they represent weak points along the length of bone and are particularly vulnerable to shear and tensile stress.

BOX 3.2 THE SALTER–HARRIS CLASSIFICATION OF GROWTH PLATE INJURIES

Type I Fracture through the growth plate: The epiphysis is completely separated from the end of the bone or the metaphysis, through the deep layer of the growth plate. The growth plate remains attached to the epiphysis. Unless there is damage to the blood supply to the growth plate, the likelihood that the bone will grow normally is excellent.

Type II Fracture through the growth plate and metaphysis: This is the most common type of growth plate fracture. It runs through the growth plate and the metaphysis, but the epiphysis is not involved in the injury.

Type III Fracture through the growth plate and epiphysis: This fracture occurs only rarely, usually at the distal tibia. It happens when a fracture runs completely through the epiphysis and separates part of the epiphysis and growth plate from the metaphysis. Surgery is sometimes necessary to restore the joint surface to normal. The prognosis for growth is good if the blood supply to the separated portion of the epiphysis is still intact.

Type IV Fracture through the growth plate, metaphysis and epiphysis: This fracture runs through the epiphysis, across the growth plate, and into the metaphysis. This injury occurs most commonly at the end of the humerus (the upper arm bone) near the elbow. Surgery is frequently needed to restore the joint surface to normal and to align perfectly the growth plate. Unless perfect alignment is achieved and maintained during healing, prognosis for growth is poor, and angulations of the bone may occur.

Type V Compression fracture through the growth plate: This uncommon injury occurs when the end of the bone is crushed and the growth plate is compressed. It is most likely to occur at the knee or ankle. Prognosis is poor, since premature stunting of growth is almost inevitable.

A newer classification, called the Peterson classification, adds a Type VI fracture, in which a portion of the epiphysis, growth plate and metaphysis is missing. This usually occurs with open wounds or compound fractures, and often involves lawnmowers, farm machinery, snowmobiles, or gunshot wounds. All Type VI fractures require surgery. Bone growth is usually stunted. Ogden has also added to the Salter–Harris classification with Types VI and VII (Figure 3.4(a)). Type VI is an injury to the peripheral zone of Ranvier at the edge of the physis and may eventually form an osseous bridge causing an angular deformity in that area. Type VII involves only the epiphysis; the fracture runs through the cartilage of the epiphysis or the epiphyseal ossification centre.

Figure 3.4 Examples of growth plate injuries: (a) the Salter–Harris classifications of growth plate injuries Types I–V and Ogden Types VI and VII; (b) example of resulting growth disturbance caused by disruption to the growth plate in the tibia. The injured tibia has become significantly shorter as the child grows.

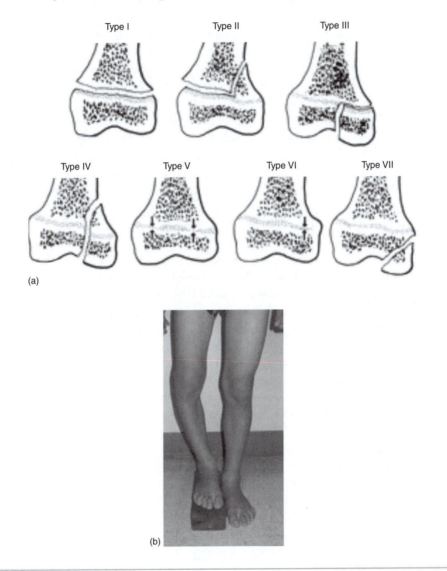

Biomechanical literature on the stress tolerance of the human growth plate is lacking. Nevertheless, we assume that, as the growth plates represent an area of weakness in the developing bone and as tissue-failure usually occurs at the weakest point, the growth plate poses a threat to the growing athlete (Figure 3.4(a)). Most common mechanisms of injury are site dependent and may be either acute or overuse in onset. Approximately 15–30% of all childhood fractures are growth plate fractures and most often occur in children over 10 years of age. Growth plate fractures occur twice as often in boys as in girls, because girls' bodies mature earlier than boys' do. One-third of all growth plate injuries occur in competitive sports such as American football, rugby, basketball, or gymnastics, while about 20% of growth plate fractures occur as a result of recreational activities such as biking, sledging, skiing, or skateboarding. The upper extremities particularly the phalanges (30%) and radius are the most commonly affected followed by the tibia and fibula of the lower leg.

Damage to the growth plate can result in premature closing or asymmetrical closing of the growth plate resulting in significant anatomical deformities once the skeleton reaches full maturation (Figure 3.4(b)). Growth deformity occurs in 1–10% of all growth plate injuries and studies have shown the growth plate to be susceptible to excessive repetitive stresses. For example, studies conducted on gymnasts have shown significant bone length discrepancies suggesting the occurrence of growth delay and cessation of physeal growth secondary to excessive repetitive loading.

A periosteal membrane that supplies nutrients to the underlying tissues covers bone. In children, this membrane is tightly adhered to the metaphyseal and epiphyseal region through fibrous and ligamentous insertions. Studies have shown that the perichondrial complex (periosteal membrane plus fibrous and ligamentous components) increases both the shear and tensile strength of the growth plate, although the amount varies according to the age of the child and the site of the growth plate. In fact, it has been estimated that by excising the perichondrial complex the growth plate would lose 50% of its shear strength.

Bone density and bone porosity in children are lower than in adults. Compared to adult bone, the bone in a growing skeleton has a lower modulus of elasticity and bending strength. Thus, a given stress applied to an area of paediatric bone will result in more strain than the same stress applied to adult bone. For this reason, the paediatric bone absorbs more energy before breaking and the bone may still absorb energy even after fracture. Thus, bone fractures in children tend to be incomplete fractures in which partial continuity of the bone remains. Thus, fractures such as greenstick (Figure 3.1(a)) and torus (Figure 3.1(b)) fractures are seen almost exclusively in children. Both greenstick and torus fractures occur as either the result of bending or compression stress on the bone, seen in such incidents as falling on an outstretched arm (FOOSH). The difference between greenstick and torus fractures is the mechanical mechanism. In a greenstick fracture, commonly the bone splinters on the side under tensile stress while in a torus fracture the side of the bone under compression buckles and breaks first (Figure 3.1).

Children often experience periods of rapid growth, referred to as a growth spurt. Growth spurts pose a particular problem to young athletes by affecting their coordination and strength. Mechanical causes for impairment to coordination are the crucial time lags between increased bone length, increased muscle length, increased muscle strength and increased bone mineral content. Typically, a growth spurt is marked by a rapid increase in stature caused by increased length in the long bones. The growth spurt occurs around 13.45 years in boys and around 11.80 years in girls (Rauch *et al.*, 2004). The rapid increase in bone length applies a mechanical tension to the muscles and the increased tension signals the muscle to adapt its length. Once the muscle has adapted in length it must also adapt to the new strength requirements of the longer, heavier limb. Once again, there is a time delay while the muscle responds to the increased mechanical load by increasing the cross-sectional area of the muscle. With greater muscle force applying increased mechanical load to the bones, there is an adaptive response that increases bone mineral content. The process of bone and muscle adaptation may take from a few months to a year to occur.

There are two mechanical reasons for overuse injuries in children that stem from the adolescent growth spurt. The first has to do with the increased tension in the musculotendinous unit and the resulting loss in flexibility. Linked to this increase in tensile stress are three types of chronic connective tissue problems in adolescents.

- Perception of increased pain in a joint on the opposing side to an excessively tight muscle. Such generalised joint pains are often referred to as growing pains in children.
- Excessive tensile stress in a muscle that crosses over a bony prominence can cause increased pressure in the muscle directly over the prominence. Due to the increased pressure on the muscle, there is an increase in the friction component between the muscle and the bony prominence. The combination of pressure and friction can cause irritation, inflammation, and thickening of the muscle or tendon as seen in overuse syndromes such as iliotibial band syndrome or 'snapping hip' syndrome.
- Finally, the increased tensile stress can also cause increased strain at the tendon–bone junctions. Because some tendon–bone junctions are not fully fused, that is they have growth plates or apophyses, the excessive strain may cause pain, inflammation or disruption of the growth plate called traction apophysitis, for example Sever's disease (Table 3.1).

Table 3.1 Common sites of apophysitises

LOCATION	MEDICAL NAME	ANATOMICAL REGION
Elbow	Little League elbow	Medial epicondylar apophysis
Knee	Osgood Schlatter's disease	Tibial tuberosity
Heel	Sever's disease	Calcaneal apophysis
Foot	Iselin's disease	Base of the 5th metatarsal attachment of peroneus brevis

The second mechanical reason for overuse injuries in children related to growth spurt has to do with the change in body segment parameters and the lag in muscle cross-sectional area that occur during a growth spurt. The significant increase in limb length that can occur with a growth spurt will also have a significant effect on the limb mass and moment of inertia, which will affect the force output requirements of the muscle. Hawkins and Metheny (2001) estimated that after a 4 cm increase in lower limb length, a child would need to develop about 30% more force to produce the same lower leg angular acceleration during a kicking movement as before the growth spurt.

The masters athlete

Placing an age bracket on the masters athlete is somewhat difficult as there is a big difference between chronological age and physiological age. As we age, our tissues begin to lose strength, compliance, density and energy-carrying capacity; however, the ageing process has different effects on different individuals. A 65-year-old athlete may have tissues with better mechanical properties than those of a 47-year-old athlete. Nevertheless, while athletes in their 20s tend to suffer more from acute injuries, athletes in their 40s and older tend to suffer more from overuse injuries. Most probably, this is because masters age athletes are more likely to participate in non-contact sports, train at slower paces and enter more long distance competitions than do their younger counterparts. Care must be taken to discriminate between the effects of ageing and those of physical inactivity. However, ageing athletes have to work closer to their physiological maximum to maintain a particular standard of performance, heightening the risk of injury. In ageing athletes, sports injuries are usually overuse rather than acute, for example, tendinopathy, fasciitis, bursitis and capsulitis as well as arthritis. Such injuries can occur not only through current training and competing but also as a recurrence of injuries sustained when younger.

Adult bone strength is dependent upon two factors, first the peak bone mass reached during early adulthood and second the rate of bone loss. Throughout childhood bone mass, that is bone mineral content, increases with skeletal growth with a rapid increase in density during puberty. An adult usually reaches peak bone mass sometime during the third decade of life. Beyond that age, the loss of mass is about 1–2% annually for postmenopausal women and 0.5–1% for men. The average reductions per decade with age in the 20–102 year range are 5% and 9% for ultimate tensile stress and strain respectively, and 12% for energy absorption to failure (Nigg and Grimston, 1999). As bones age they experience a decrease in compressive strength and fracture more easily; this is more marked in females than in males. The loss of strength is a combination of the bones becoming thinner and an increasing number of calcified osteons leading to brittleness (Edington and Edgerton, 1976). Although fractures are not considered a common injury in masters athletes when they do occur, the older athlete tends to suffer from complete fractures of bone rather than stress fractures.

The decrease in stiffness and the lower failure load with ageing for ligaments, for example, may be linked to a decrease in physical activity. Frank and Shrive (1999) cited a decrease of 60% in the ultimate tensile stress of the anterior cruciate ligament from young adulthood to the age of 65 years, but regular exercise may retard the decline with ageing by as much as 50% (Hawkins, 1993). Degeneration begins early, with the central artery disappearing from tendons as early as the age of 30. Changes in the mechanical properties of connective tissue with ageing mean that the masters athlete is prone to overuse injuries, particularly tendinopathies.

Tendinopathies and incidence of tendon rupture have a tendency to increase with age. As discussed in Chapter 2, from middle age the attachments of tendons begin to weaken. There are physiological changes within the tendon that stem from a reduced rate of metabolism. The tendon begins to lose viscosity and gain more collagen cross-bridges, making the collagen fibres less compliant. However, while collagen becomes less compliant, the elastin component increases, which makes the tendon itself more compliant when compared to younger tendons. The increased tendon compliance in older adults may slow the rate of force development in the muscle, affecting the time necessary to decelerate a moving limb. Overall, this means that older tendons are less capable than younger tendons of transmitting large forces from muscles to bones. Furthermore, the increased tendon compliance would result in larger strains at any given force, which could increase the risk of tendon strain injury in older athletes.

The most common tendinopathies in masters athletes are located in the tendons of the rotator cuff and the gastrocnemius. Achilles tendinopathy is commonly reported by athletes involved in activities that include running and jumping. Kujala et al. (2005) found that the lifetime cumulative incidence of Achilles tendinopathy among former endurance runners was 52%. Other studies have shown that Achilles tendon injury accounted for about 20% of all injuries seen in the 30–60-year-old group and up to 4% of those resulted in complete ruptures of the Achilles tendon; the peak age for rupture is between 30 and 40 years for both men and women.

Sex (non-modifiable risk factor)

Sex differences in anatomy, physiology, endocrinology, sociology, and activity patterns often see one sex at greater or lesser risk of certain injuries. Because of anatomical differences, women are often thought to be more susceptible to injury than are men. The reasons given for this include the altered hip- and knee-loading resulting from the wider female pelvis and greater genu valgum, greater stresses in the smaller bones and articular surfaces, and less muscle mass and greater body fat content. Males are at greater risk of tendinopathy (e.g. rotator cuff and Achilles tendon) than females but little research appears to focus on these disparities. Only one study could be found that even compared the mechanical properties of the Achilles tendon between the sexes. Kubo et al. (2003) found that male Achilles tendons were generally stiffer and had higher hysteresis than female tendons. Perhaps there is a mechanism in this greater hysteresis but no one has followed up on this factor. Thus, because of the lack of data available on male injury mechanisms, the following section is heavily biased toward female injury, specifically stress fracture and anterior cruciate ligament (ACL) injury.

Stress fractures

Stress fractures are common in both sexes; a gender disparity is not conclusive outside military recruits and long distance runners. However, stress fractures in female athletes appear to be more often associated with low bone mineral density. Studies have shown significant effects of intense training on the concentrations of hormones such as testosterone in men and oestrogen in women. Observations of the current research suggest a direct relationship between a low oestrogen concentration and bone loss in female athletes. We have long known that intense training may cause menstrual irregularities in female athletes which have a detrimental effect on the concentrations of oestrogen in the blood, which in turn affects the regulation of bone remodelling. Several studies have shown that the lower an athlete's oestrogen concentration and the longer her menstrual irregularity persists, the greater the deficits in her bone density. Amenorrheic or oligomenorrheic athletes may have 8-31% lower bone density than normally-menstruating athletes, and 3-24% lower bone density than non-exercising, normally-menstruating women. Particularly at risk are endurance athletes and athletes participating in aesthetic sports such as dancing, gymnastics and figure skating. The research on male athletes is not as conclusive, meaning direct links between reduced testosterone and decreased bone mineral density have not been established. However, some findings have been clear, particularly for male endurance athletes. Negative correlations have been found for running distance and bone mineral density in the lumbar spine, for example, distance runners averaging 92 km per week were found to have around 9.7% lower bone density in the lumbar spine than a group of non-runners (MacDougall *et al.* 1992). Therefore, it appears that there are different mechanisms at work for reduced bone mineral density in males and females. It seems that female athletes tend to have hormonally-driven reduced bone mineral density while decreased bone mineral density in male athletes may be directed by homeostatic imbalance in the remodelling process, potentially linked to overtraining. Clearly, there is a need for further research into how bone mineral density affects the incidence of stress fractures.

Anterior cruciate ligament (ACL) injuries

As discussed in the previous chapter, ACL injuries are a common problem in both male and female athletes. Mechanically, ACL injury occurs when an excessive tensile load is applied to the ACL. Research by Boden *et al.* (2000) has shown several common characteristics underlying the non-contact ACL mechanism. According to their research at the time of injury, 35% of patients were decelerating, 31% were landing, 13% were accelerating, and 4% were falling backward. Female athletes between the ages of 15 and 20 have a disproportionately larger risk (four to eight times) than males of the same age for non-contact ACL injury. Many studies have found that women, with a history of ACL injury, have smaller knee flexion angles (<30°), more knee valgus, greater quadriceps activation and reduced hamstring activation when compared to males during landing and the stance phase of athletic cutting manoeuvres. However, the mechanism of ACL injury is still quite controversial and researchers are still divided, probably because the true mechanism is multifactorial and has a strong component of individual and situational variability. Whatever the true answer, at present there are several hypotheses for potential anatomical, hormonal and neuromuscular factors that may be to blame. Because this text is focused on biomechanics, we will focus on the biomechanical factors related to ACL injury. Biomechanical hypotheses for ACL injury fall into one of two broad categories: those related to muscle force and excessive tibial translation and those related to movement analysis focusing on sagittal plane or multiplane movement errors.

The muscle force hypotheses for ACL injury are entrenched in the theory that the predominant forces that affect strain in the ACL are anteriorly directed shear forces applied to the tibia and that the shear force generated by the quadriceps is inversely proportional to the knee flexion angle. Studies based on the quadriceps force hypotheses tend to use *in vitro* or computational modelling approaches. Within this group of studies, there are two main overarching arguments: the first is that ACL injury is the result of excessive forces purely within the sagittal plane; the second argument centres on multiplane force requirements. The first group of authors (e.g. Yu *et al.*, 2006) postulates that ACL disruption is the result of aggressive quadriceps loading (either eccentric or concentric) applying large shear forces to the anterior tibia causing excessive translation of the tibia and subsequent rupture of the ACL. When the ACL fails, there will be greater displacement of the lateral tibial plateau resulting in internal rotation of the tibia and, with further axial load, the knee will collapse into excessive valgus. Thus, according to this group of authors the appearance of internal tibial rotation and knee valgus is due to mechanical failure of the ACL not a cause of ACL injury. Studies have shown that valgus torque can only increase strain on the ACL after failure of the medial collateral ligament has occurred. In contrast, the second group of authors (e.g. Shimokochi and Shultz, 2008) argue that excessive forces from the quadriceps create an anterior shear force at the proximal end of the tibia; when combined with either a knee internal rotation or valgus moment, the result is a significantly greater strain in the anterior medial bundle of the ACL than for an anterior shear force at the proximal end of the tibia alone. Thus, according to this group of authors the appearance of internal tibial rotation and knee valgus is a mechanical cause of failure of the ACL due to excessive tensile load.

The second group of hypotheses around the gender disparity in ACL injury is entrenched in movement analysis. Studies based on the movement error hypotheses tend to use video analysis of human participants and kinematic data to draw their conclusions. Historically, within this group of researchers there have been two main arguments: the multiplanar argument and the sagittal plane argument. However, recent sex-specific evidence may lead to a middle ground between these two arguments, presenting a mainly sagittal plane mechanism for males and a multiplanar mechanism for females (Quatman and Hewett, 2009). Specifically, males adopt a more upright body posture with neutral hips, flexion of the knee and minimal tibial rotation, while females experience 'valgus collapse' (Figure 3.5). The body posture of valgus collapse is marked by increased forward flexion and rotation of the trunk, adduction with internal rotation of the hip, less than 30° knee flexion with pronounced knee valgus and internal or external tibial rotation (Olsen *et al.*, 2004). Most evidence for body position at moment of injury comes from

Figure 3.5 Example of altered frontal plane kinematics, termed valgus collapse, that has been considered a sex-related issue in anterior cruciate ligament injury.

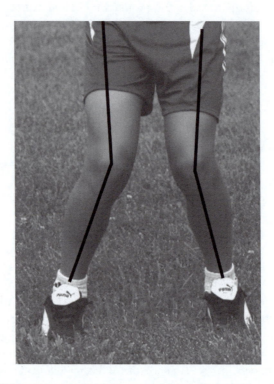

video analysis of athletes taken at the moment of injury and often relies on video footage taken for broadcasting purposes rather than laboratory studies. Therefore, many predictions and assumptions are made about the exact instant injury occurs without supporting biomechanical evidence. Biomechanical support does come from studies that have used inverse dynamics to calculate the stress on the ACL. These studies have shown that sagittal plane forces alone are not great enough to cause injury to the ACL and, furthermore, that dangerous valgus loads occur more frequently in women than in men, during side-cutting manoeuvres (McLean, 2008; McLean *et al.*, 2005).

Anatomy

Some anatomical abnormalities such as leg length asymmetries or limb misalignments are considered non-modifiable risk factors for injury because the fault cannot be corrected with exercise or equipment modifications. Leg length discrepancy is an anatomical risk factor for overuse injury to the lower extremity. It is mediated through compensatory excessive pronation or supination of the foot, and it is strongly associated with low-back pain (MacIntyre and Lloyd-Smith, 1993). An angle between the neck and shaft of the femur of less than the normal 125° (coxa vara) causes impaired functioning of the hip abductors because of the closeness of the ilium and greater trochanter. Anteversion – the angulation of the neck of the femur anterior to the long axis of the shaft and femoral condyle – greater than the normal value of 15° can also lead to injury. Because of the need to align the femoral head with the acetabulum, anteversion can cause, for example, excessive internal rotation at the hip, genu varum, pes planus, and excessive foot pronation (MacIntyre and Lloyd-Smith, 1993). At the knee, genu varum or genu valgum can lead to excessive pronation or supination depending on foot type. Tibial varum of more than 7° has the same effect as genu varum (MacIntyre and Lloyd-Smith, 1993).

During running, the neutral foot requires little muscular activity for balance. The pes planus foot is flat and flexible, and susceptible to excessive pronation through midstance, with a more medial centre of pressure at toe-off. These factors can lead to an excessively loaded rear foot valgus, internal tibial torsion, genu valgum and increased internal femoral rotation. Pes planus is implicated in many overuse injuries, including sacroiliac joint dysfunction, patellofemoral pain syndrome, iliotibial band syndrome, and tarsal stress fractures. Shin splints are more common in athletes with pes planus (Best and Garrett, 1993). Pes cavus (high arched and rigid foot) leads to greater supination with a more lateral loading and centre of pressure at toe-off. The effects are the opposite to those of pes planus. It is implicated in overuse injuries such as irritation of the lateral collateral knee ligament, metatarsal stress fractures, peroneal muscle tendinitis and plantar fasciitis (MacIntyre and Lloyd-Smith, 1993); it has been reported that 20% of injured runners presented with pes cavus. Other anatomical abnormalities can also predispose to sports injury, for example the positions of the muscle origins and insertions, and compartment syndromes.

Other anatomical factors, such as those related to fitness, flexibility and body composition may be improved with training and nutrition and are, therefore, considered to be modifiable factors. A lack of fitness, along with increased body weight and body fat, may lead to an increased risk of injury. Inflexibility, muscle weakness and strenuous exercise all contribute to overuse injury (Kibler and Chandler, 1993). No direct and unambiguous proof of the effects of flexibility on injury exists (MacIntyre and Lloyd-Smith, 1993) despite the popularity of stretching and the benefits often claimed for it. However, examples do exist of links between lack of flexibility and injury. For example, tightness of the iliotibial band has been associated with patellofemoral pain syndrome, and tightness of the triceps surae with plantar fasciitis (MacIntyre and Lloyd-Smith, 1993). The tendency of athletes to have tightness in muscle groups to which tensile loads are applied during their sports may predispose to injury. For example, tennis players often show a reduced range of internal shoulder rotation but greater external rotation than non-players. This relates to a development of increased internal rotator strength without a balancing strengthening of external rotators (Kibler and Chandler, 1993). Despite conflicting evidence, stretching is often considered to be beneficial if performed properly. The finding that runners who stretched were at higher risk than those that did not (Jacobs and Berson, 1986) should be viewed cautiously as it does not imply cause and effect. It may well be that the runners who stretched did so because they had been injured (Taunton, 1993). Hamstring strains have been reported to be more common in soccer teams that do not use special flexibility exercises for that muscle (Best and Garrett, 1993). Many investigations of stretching have found an increase in the range of motion of the joint involved, and have shown stretching and exercise programmes to prevent much of the reduction in joint range of motion with ageing (e.g. Stanish and McVicar, 1993). Attempts to assess the relative efficacy of the various types of stretching (ballistic, static, proprioceptive) have proved inconclusive. Ballistic stretching can be dangerous and may have reduced efficacy because of the inhibitory effects of the stretch reflex (Best and Garrett, 1993). Also, as rapid application of force to collagenous tissue increases its stiffness, the easiest way to elongate the tissues is to apply force slowly and to maintain it, as in static and proprioceptive stretching (Stanish and McVicar, 1993). Although some investigators have suggested that stretching (and warm-up) can reduce the risk of sustaining a severe injury, laboratory and clinical data to show that these procedures do prevent injury are lacking (Best and Garrett, 1993).

Some evidence supports an association between lack of muscle strength and injury; for example, weakness of the hip abductors is a factor in iliotibial band syndrome (MacIntyre and Lloyd-Smith, 1993). Hamstring strains have been thought to be associated with an imbalance between the strength of the hamstring and quadriceps femoris muscles, when the hamstrings have less than 60% of the strength of the quadriceps. Although some research supports this, the evidence is inconsistent (e.g. Kibler et al., 1992). A contralateral hamstring or quadriceps imbalance of more than 10% has also been reported to be linked to an increased injury risk (Kibler et al., 1992). Neuromuscular coordination is also an important factor in hamstring strains in fast running where the muscles decelerate knee extension and cause knee flexion. A breakdown of the fine balance between, and motor control of, the hamstrings and quadriceps femoris, possibly caused by fatigue, may result in injury (MacIntyre and Lloyd-Smith, 1993).

Muscle strength imbalances may arise through overtraining. Swimmers have been reported to develop an imbalance between the lateral and medial rotators of the shoulder such that those reporting pain had a mean muscle endurance ratio of less than 0.4, while those without pain had a ratio above 0.7 (Kibler and Chandler, 1993). Resistance strength training has been claimed to help prevent injury by increasing both strength and, when using a full range of movement and associated stretching exercises, flexibility. Resistance training also strengthens other tissues around a joint, such as ligaments and tendons, possibly helping to prevent injury (Kibler and Chandler, 1993). However, few specific studies show a reduced rate of injury with resistance training (Chandler and Kibler, 1993).

Previous injury history (non-modifiable risk factor)

There is strong evidence that previous injury, especially when followed by inadequate rehabilitation, places an athlete at increased risk for re-injury. Research demonstrates that after any serious injury there may be certain structural deficits as well as psychological problems that persist. These problems may make it difficult for athletes to regain their full strength and ability before returning to play. Some structural deficits will always remain even after an athlete has undergone a full rehabilitation programme. Sometimes structural deficits remain because the rehabilitation programme was inadequate or incorrect. An inadequate rehabilitation programme may miss important aspects of reconditioning, such as eccentric strengthening. At other times structural deficits remain because of the severity of the injury. For example, if ligament is completely ruptured the ends may not rejoin and the integrity of the ligament is lost, in turn reducing the stability of the associated joint. Severely injured tissue will require a lengthy healing period and a specialist may not be aware of techniques to train them. In the following paragraphs, we will familiarise ourselves with the phases of tissue healing and the mechanical properties of healing tissue. Then we will examine specific injuries linked with high rates of recurrent and frequent injury in athletes.

Once an athlete has suffered a significant injury, tissue requires time to return to its pre-injury state. This may take more than a year, depending upon the grade of injury. The issue for athletes is that healing tissue does not have the same mechanical properties as healthy, non-injured tissue and is, therefore, more vulnerable to re-injury during the remodelling phase of the healing process. There are three phases of tissue healing as outlined in Figure 3.6; these phases are fluid, meaning they may overlap and may have a great deal of individual variation in their timing. However, there are certain physiological events that mark each phase and must occur before the next phase can begin.

The first phase is the inflammatory response, which begins immediately after injury and is critical to the entire healing process. Inflammation is a cellular reaction to tissue damage; this protective mechanism uses chemical mediators to localise and dispose of injury by-products through phagocytosis, and to protect the injured area through clot formation. The five cardinal signs of inflammation are redness, swelling, tenderness,

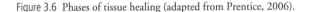

Figure 3.6 Phases of tissue healing (adapted from Prentice, 2006).

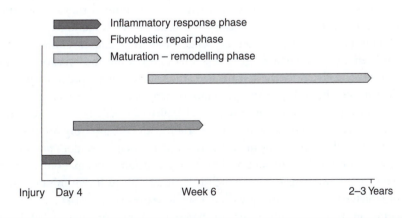

Inflammatory response phase
Fibroblastic repair phase
Maturation – remodelling phase

Injury Day 4 Week 6 2–3 Years

increased temperature and loss of function. Problems arise when the acute inflamma-tory response does not respond sufficiently to eliminate the damaged cells and restore tissue to its normal physiological state. When this happens, low-grade inflammation persists, causing damage to connective tissue through tissue necrosis and fibrosis that prolong the healing process. Persistent low-grade inflammation transitions into chronic inflammation where granulation tissue and fibrous connective tissue develop within the injured tissue site. Causes for chronic inflammation are not entirely understood but it does appear that cumulative microtrauma from overuse or chronic overloading may be a significant factor (King *et al.*, 2009).

The second phase of tissue healing is called the fibroblastic repair phase and is marked by scar tissue formation. Scar tissue is made from collagen fibres that are deposited randomly throughout the injured tissue. There are many different types of collagen tissue in the human body (around 16) but the most common are Types I, II and III. Type I is found in skin, bone, tendon, ligament and cartilage while Type II is found in hyaline cartilage and vertebral disks. Type III collagen is most commonly found in smooth muscle, nerves and blood vessels and in scar tissue during the fibroblastic repair phase of tissue healing (Seeley *et al.*, 2006). The tensile strength of Type III fibres is lower than that of the most common tendon and ligament collagen fibres (Type I), which makes the newly-formed scar tissue highly susceptible to re-injury from tensile loading. As the collagen continues to proliferate during phase two of healing, the tensile strength of the scar increases. With increasing tensile strength the number of fibroblasts reduces, signalling the start of the maturation phase.

The third phase of tissue healing is the maturation or remodelling phase. This phase is the longest of all the phases and is when the scar tissue becomes realigned, reorganised and remodelled into normal Type I fibres. Remodelling and realignment of fibres is dependent upon the tensile stresses applied to the injured area during the healing process. Scar tissue is laid down randomly with haphazardly arranged cross-linkages; it looks and functions differently than the highly organised healthy tissue surrounding it. Because of this, the presence of scar tissue tends to reduce flexibility and suppleness in the healing tissue, which ultimately reduces the range of motion at the associated joints. While the collagen fibres are transforming, the cross-linkages and bonds between them are weak. As the collagen fibres mature they begin to transform to Type I fibres and the cross-linkages between them become stronger. Therefore, to improve flexibility, range of motion and tissue suppleness, range of motion and flexibility exercises should commence within the first three weeks after injury, while the linkages are weak and may be broken easily. Once the scar tissue matures, it becomes more resistant to change and the effects on flexibility and range of motion may become permanent (Houglum, 2005).

Some of the most common recurrent injuries in athletes are muscle strains, lateral ankle sprains and concussion. Muscle strains can be frustrating for athletes and clini-cians alike. They are problematic because the recurrence risk does not appear to reduce significantly until many weeks after return to sport participation. In particular, the hamstring muscles appear to be high-risk muscles for recurrent injury, with up to 30% of athletes injuries recurring within a single season (Orchard *et al.*, 1997). The most common problem with recurrent hamstring injury is poor rehabilitation before reengagement in competitive sporting activity. Croisier (2004) found that certain factors related to rehabilitation had a high degree of involvement with recurrent hamstring injury. Specifically, reduced flexibility or tightness in the affected hamstring muscle, eccentric agonist–antagonist muscle imbalance, and incomplete or overly aggressive rehabilitation practices were found to be highly related to recurrent injury. Croisier *et al.* (2002) identified 18 individuals who had a significant deficiency in at least one of the following parameters: concentric bilateral asymmetries, eccentric bilateral asymmetries, concentric flexors-to-quadriceps ratio, and eccentric flexors-to-concentric quadriceps ratio (Figure 3.7). They implemented an individually tailored rehabilitation programme based on each individual's isokinetic profile, which included eccentric and concentric isokinetic training. Once athletes attained bilateral symmetry in their isokinetic profile, they were allowed to return to play. On a 12-month follow-up, none of the athletes had suffered from further hamstring strains.

Previous injury history is considered a strong predictor for recurrent joint injury particularly in the knee, ankle and shoulder. Ligaments may take up to one year to return to their normal mechanical function and further disruption of ligamentous material has been shown to create partial deafferentation that can reduce neuromuscular control of the joint. Therefore, reduced mechanical and functional stability will make certain joints, such as the ankle and knee, susceptible to recurrent injury. It has been suggested that 20–75% of athletes who experience lateral ankle sprain will suffer recurrent ankle sprains and a further 25% report 'frequent sprains' (i.e. more than two per season). The re-injury rates to the ACL-reconstructed knee within five years varied by

Figure 3.7 The strength ratio of hamstring to quadriceps in healthy (shaded areas) and injured (white and black dots) hamstrings. Comparisons are shown between slow concentric (C_{60}/C_{60}), fast concentric (C_{240}/C_{240}) and eccentric to concentric (E_{30}/C_{240}). The diagram shows that the injured group differ from the healthy group in eccentric to concentric ratio in the injured hamstring (adapted from Croisier, 2004).

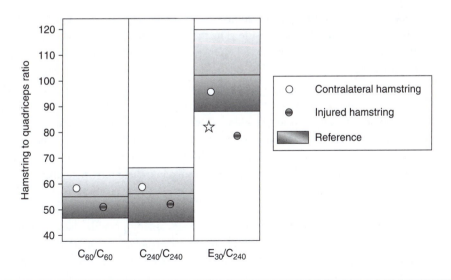

age: for the under 18 group, the rate was 8.7%; for ages 18–25, it was 2.6%; for those older than 25, the rate was 1.1% (Shelbourn *et al.*, 2009). A sex disparity is also present in ACL re-injury with females experiencing twice the rate of re-injury of men. For the shoulder, approximately 59% of those athletes who experience shoulder dislocation will experience subsequent shoulder injury and dislocation.

Recurrent mild traumatic brain injury or concussion in athletes is problematic because it may result in long-term cognitive decline. Mild traumatic brain injury can alter the brain's physiology for hours to weeks, setting into motion various pathological events that may interfere with brain function. The metabolic processes that follow concussion are reversed in most of the affected brain cells but some cell death is expected after the injury (Iverson, 2005). High recurrent concussion risk has been reported in professional wrestling, soccer, rugby, skydiving, horse-racing and boxing. The major risk or conse-quence of repetitive concussive and sub-concussive blows to the brain is chronic trau-matic brain injury, also known as dementia pugilistica, chronic traumatic encephalopathy, or the 'punch drunk' syndrome (Rabadi and Jordan, 2001: McCrory, 2011). Little is known about the mechanism for recurrent concussion or why an athlete's concussion risk increases after initial injury (Guskiewicz *et al.*, 2003). The period associated with greatest risk of recurrent concussion within the same season was 7–10 days after initial injury. It is thought that injury risk is heightened during this time because altered brain physiology has not returned to baseline and as a result, the athlete may suffer deficits that make them less coordinated or affect their decision-making abilities, which may put them at greater risk for re-injury. Research in younger athletes has shown that recurrent concussion risk can be reduced by instituting a 10–14 day no-play period after the initial injury.

Movement technique (modifiable risk factor)

Sport and exercise participants subject their bodies to loads that are well beyond the stresses and strains of sedentary life. The movement techniques used even when consid-ered 'correct' may cause injury. Therefore, the use of many repetitions of these tech-niques in training should not be undertaken lightly; the risk of injury may well override beneficial motor learning considerations. The use of an incorrect movement technique is usually considered to exacerbate the injury potential of sports. This has rarely been verified scientifically, although indirect evidence can often be deduced (Mallon and Hawkins, 1994). The sport and exercise scientist should seek to identify incorrect move-ment techniques to prevent injury. Training to improve movement technique and acquire appropriate strength and flexibility is likely to help to reduce injury as well as to improve performance. Some exercise activities, such as aerobics, have changed from high- to low-impact to reduce the incidence of injury. However, movement techniques in many sports are determined by the activity, reducing possible changes to movement technique, particularly at high standards of performance (Nigg, 1993). Some injuries (such as gouging in rugby) are caused by illegal techniques and will not, generally, be discussed in this chapter; nor will most aspects of strength and flexibility training. The following provides an overview of the relationship between movement technique and injury using selected examples.

Throwing

Most throwing injuries are caused by overuse. As discussed in Chapter 2, during the cocking phase, the shoulder externally rotates and the humeral head translates anteriorly; as the thrower's body moves forward, the inertial force on the arm creates further external rotation. In a forceful or high speed throw (or throw-like action) the inertial force is greater, therefore there is greater external rotation force placed on the shoulder. During this over-rotation stretch placed on the anterior soft tissues of the shoulder, the posterior rotator cuff may become impinged between the glenoid labrum and the humeral head; long term this can cause degeneration of the superior labrum and the rotator cuff tendons. A more rare but possible injury is spiral fracture of the humerus caused by high inertia and large accelerations. Elbow injury is possible, particularly towards the end of the preparation phase, where the maximum valgus stress on the elbow occurs (Figure 3.8). In overarm throwing, it appears that to achieve the goal of the movement (maximum ball or implement speed) the desire to avoid injury is relegated to second place.

Atwater (1979) proposed that sidearm as opposed to overarm throws incur an increased injury risk. This is well established for the javelin throw (Kuland, 1982), where a roundarm throw, rather than throwing with the classic elbow lead position, can lead to sprains of the medial collateral elbow ligament, paralysis of the ulnar nerve or fractures of the olecranon. This can result from a poor movement technique starting with an incorrect position of the wrist after withdrawal, and a wrong line of pull followed by pronation during the final elbow extension in an attempt to reduce javelin flutter.

Figure 3.8 Examples of overarm throwing that places excessive stress on the elbow at the end of the preparatory phase: (a) baseball pitch; (b) overhead smash in tennis.

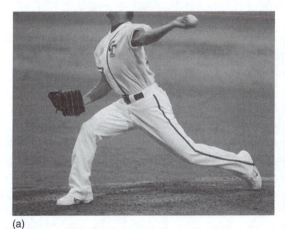

(a)

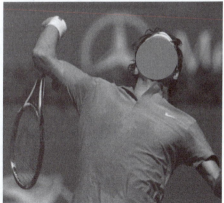

(b)

Hyperextension of the elbow can damage the olecranon process; incorrect alignment of the javelin before the start of the throw can rupture the pronator teres. A faulty grip on the binding can injure the extensor pollicis longus (Reilly, 1992).

Incorrect timing of the shot-put can lead to injury to any of the rotator cuff muscles. Various tears of the tendon of the long head of the biceps brachii, and the wrist and finger flexors and extensors originating from the humeral epicondyles, are associated with several shot-put technique faults. These include poor coordination of arm and trunk muscles, the putting elbow too low or ahead of the shot, and 'dropping' the shoulder on the non-throwing side. Incorrect positioning of the thumb can injure the extensor pollicis longus (Reilly, 1992). Timing errors in the discus and hammer throws can also result in similar injuries to those in the shot-put.

Low-back pain, its causative factors, and lumbar spine injuries in fast bowlers in cricket were touched on in Chapter 2. The incidence of spondylolysis (stress fracture of one or both neural arches) and other lumbar abnormalities in fast bowlers is a good example of the association between movement technique and injury. The major factor appears to be the use of the 'mixed technique'. In this, the bowler counter-rotates the shoulders away from the hips, from a more front-on position at back-foot strike in the delivery stride, to a more side-on position at front foot strike (see Figure 8.7(a) in Chapter 8). A relatively low incidence of spondylolysis has been reported amongst genuine side-on or front-on bowlers. A study of the 20 members of the Western Australian fast bowling development squad (mean age 17.9 years) grouped the bowlers into those showing: no abnormal radio-logical features; disc degeneration or bulging on an MRI scan; and bony abnormalities.

Bony abnormalities included spondylolysis, spondylolisthesis (forward subluxation of one vertebral body on another, usually after bilateral spondylolysis) or pedicle sclerosis (an increase in bone density of the pedicle or neural arch). The only significant difference was that between group 1 and the other two groups for the change in shoulder alignment from back foot impact to the minimum angle, a clear indication of a mixed bowling technique (Elliott *et al.*, 1992). This supported earlier research at the University of Western Australia (for example, Foster *et al.*, 1989). It might be hypothesised that overcoaching in early years has been inappropriate. British coaches and teachers have long been taught that the side-on technique is the correct one. However, as the less coached West Indians might be held to demonstrate, the front-on technique may be more natural. Several intervention studies that have sought to reduce the incidence of the mixed technique are discussed in Chapter 8.

Racket sports

Injuries in tennis commonly occur to inexperienced players owing to flawed movement techniques arising from too little emphasis being placed on the lower body (Nirschl and Sobel, 1994). The insertion tendons of pectoralis major and the anterior deltoid can be strained by forced stretch in the preparation for the badminton clear and tennis serve. Impact and follow through may traumatise the fully stretched scapular origins of the posterior deltoid, rhomboideus major and the long head of triceps brachii. Sprain owing to incorrect foot placement (40%) and strain from excessive movement (38%) have been most clearly associated with traumatic badminton injuries. Injury can result from not training the correct stroke movements, for example the medial and lateral rotation of the upper arm and pronation and supination of the forearm (Jørgensen and Hølmich, 1994). Constant repetitions of shoulder movements can cause bicipital tenosynovitis, particularly in real and lawn tennis (Tucker, 1990).

Reported injury rates for elbow injury in tennis are high ranging from 39 to 57%. The incidence of tennis elbow is 2 to 3.5 times higher in the over-40 age group than for those under 40, and higher among athletes who played more than two hours a day than among those who play less than two hours a day. Many factors are associated with tennis elbow for players of club standard and below; poor movement technique is a significant contributor. A faulty backhand stroke has been implicated, for example, using an Eastern forehand grip or a 'thumb behind the handle' grip and a high, hurried backswing. Also involved is poor use of weight transfer, with too much of the power for the stroke coming from elbow extension, ulnar deviation of the wrist and pronation of the forearm. These actions cause friction between the extensor carpi radialis brevis and the lateral epicondyle of the humerus and head of the radius. In addition, repeated stress on the origin of the wrist extensors produces microtears. The results are adhesions between the annular ligament and the joint capsule. Chan and Hsu (1994) considered good approach footwork, use of the whole body in the stroke, and use of the two-handed backhand to be elements of technique that guard against tennis elbow. Tucker (1990) supported the feelings of many coaches and players that tennis elbow is most common in those players who put a great deal of top spin on the backhand. This is worse for inexperienced players who have more mis-timing errors and off-centre hits, and who tend to keep a tight grip for too long, instead of just for impact.

Swimming

The movements of complete arm circumduction in front crawl and backstroke can lead to 'swimmer's shoulder', also known as impingement syndrome, and including tendinitis of the rotator cuff muscles, particularly the supraspinatus. Shoulder injuries are the most common complaint in swimming with incidence ranging from 6.5 to 21 injuries per 100 participant years. During the front crawl and backstroke, the rotator cuff muscles contract strongly to contain and stabilise the glenohumeral joint (Fowler, 1994), which can lead to this overuse injury. Impingement injuries of supraspinatus and biceps brachii tendons can be caused by the movement technique or lack of strength and flexibility (Tucker, 1990; Fowler, 1994). An important factor is often not enough body roll to achieve a high elbow position during the recovery phase of the front crawl, with use of shoulder muscle activity to compensate for this defect in movement technique (Fowler, 1994).

'Breaststroker's knee' involves a grade 1 medial (tibial) collateral ligament sprain caused by the knee extending from a flexed position while subject to valgus stress with the tibia laterally rotated in the whip-kick. Breaststroker's knee is most problematic in breaststroke specialists, with up to 47% of participants in one study reporting the problem (Rovere and Nichols, 1985). While significant links between training distances and injury severity have been identified, problems may also be caused by a faulty movement technique. One technique fault occurs when a swimmer fails to adduct the hips during recovery and then rapidly extends the knees with the legs apart, instead of keeping the heels together in the recovery and only moving the knees slightly apart in the thrust. However, because of the severity of the loading and the number of repetitions, the whip-kick can predispose to injury even with a good movement technique (Fowler, 1994). Strain of adductor longus can arise from powerful adduction of the legs from a position of considerable abduction with knees and ankles fully extended. Chronic overuse of the feet in the fully plantar-flexed position can cause tendinitis of the extensor tendons on the dorsum of the foot in all the strokes (Tucker, 1990; Fowler, 1994).

Team sports

Injuries caused by the trunk twisting or turning while excessive friction fixes the foot were considered in 'The Ankle', page 59. A movement technique factor is also involved. Where possible, twists and turns should be executed while the body is accelerating downward; this technique, known as unweighting, reduces the normal component of ground contact force, for example in hammer- and discus-throwing. The movement techniques involved in abrupt changes in speed or direction can dislocate the ankle joint or cause stress fractures of the tibia and fibula.

In hockey, the ergonomically unsound running posture with spinal flexion is a contributory factor. The sidestep swerve stresses the ligaments on the medial aspect of the planted knee such that the twist of the planted leg and contraction of the quadriceps femoris at push-off may laterally dislocate the patella. The crossover swerve stresses the lateral ligaments of the knee, while the tibia rotates inwards stressing the anterior cruciate ligament. If tackled at this time, complete rupture of this ligament can occur, leading to haemarthrosis of the knee. This movement technique, along with straight-leg landing and single-step stops, accounts for most non-contact injuries to the anterior cruciate ligament (Henning et al., 1994).

In tackling techniques in, for example, soccer and rugby, soft tissues can be injured owing to the high impact loads. The ligaments and cartilage of the knee and ankle are particularly vulnerable accounting for up to 53.8% of tackling injuries (Andersen et al., 2004). In soccer, overstretching for the ball or poor kicking technique can strain the hamstrings or the quadriceps femoris. Tackling with a fully extended knee can tear collateral ligaments. Before impact in kicking, the leg contains about 900 J of energy, of which about 85% is absorbed after impact by the hamstrings; strain is a common injury, particularly with many repetitions. The poor movement technique often used by learners, trying to kick with the medial aspect of the foot, can strain the medial hamstrings (Kuland, 1982).

As outlined in Chapter 2, the rugby scrum has been indicated in significant spinal injuries because of the large magnitude of impact force during engagement. Recall that the magnitude of force applied by one pack upon the other is proportional to the mass of the pack and the pack acceleration at the moment of impact. The impact forces during engagement have been measured at 8 kN in professional players (Milburn, 1990). The importance of vertebral column alignment in the transfer of force from one player to another is well recognised. Axial loading of the vertebral combined with bending or shear is a common mechanism of injury to the spine and poor engagement technique may place excessive loads on certain parts of the spine (Figure 3.9).

Figure 3.9 Examples of scrum technique and its effect on reaction forces in the spine of individual players: (a) This player does not have a straight back, the flexion in the thoracic spine will create a moment on the motion segments in that section of spine, increasing the risk of thoracic spine injury; (b) This player has his shoulders too low and will be experiencing a large moment on the lower lumbar spine; (c) An example of good scrum posture, this athlete is trying to maintain a straight back and shoulders, thus reducing rotation moments about individual spinal motion segments.

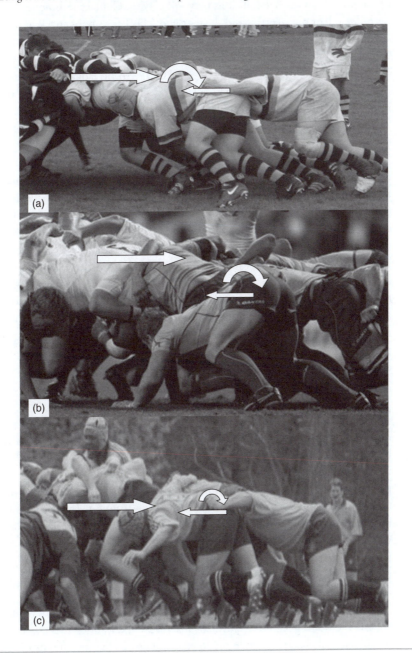

Maintaining the alignment of the spine and shoulders during engagement reduces the reaction moment about the spine, which reduces the potential for shearing loads between vertebral segments.

Contact sports, such as rugby, American football and ice hockey carry an extra risk of intended high impact collisions between players. Contact technique is important for both the ball or puck carrier and the tackler or checker. A poor check or tackle can cause serious injury particularly to the head, neck or spine (McIntosh and McCrory, 2005). Rugby union has a particularly high incidence of tackle-related injuries (91 injuries per 1000 player match hours) (Brooks et al., 2005). An investigation of contact events in rugby union has shown that high tackles and shoulder tackles are most likely to cause injury to the head and spine (Fuller et al., 2010).

Jumping

Poor landing technique can cause chronic bruising of the soft tissue of the heel, repetitive jumping can cause patellar tendinitis, and repeated forced dorsiflexion can lead to bony outgrowths in the calf or shin. Landing on a leg twisted under the player, as after an airborne knock, can lead to tears of the medial cartilage and anterior cruciate ligament. Poor landing technique in the long and triple jumps can lead to groin, as well as lower back, injuries. Uncontrolled landings between the phases of the triple jump can cause damage to the meniscus of the knee of the landing leg if the leg is torsionally loaded while the knee is flexed (McDermott and Reilly, 1992). Overconcern for the airborne technique in the Fosbury flop can lead to a tendency to plant the take-off foot in an abducted and everted position, damaging the deltoid ligament. Large forces in the plantar flexors at take-off in the pole vault can cause a total rupture of the Achilles tendon (McDermott and Reilly, 1992).

Running

Running technique may be important in preventing injury. For example, an across-the-body arm swing accentuates pelvic rotation, which can lead to inflammation of the muscle attachments on the iliac crest. In sprinting, fast and powerful but poorly coordinated contractions when fatigued can lead to muscle tears, for example of the hamstrings or hip flexors. Overstretching to maintain stride length at top speed is implicated in injuries, particularly of two-joint muscles; this can also occur in the long and triple jump when reaching for the board. Because of the acute femoral shaft inclination, some young female runners tend to recover the leg to the lateral side of an anteroposterior plane through the hip. This should be avoided as it causes additional stresses on the medial aspect of the knee at ground contact.

In hurdling, a good hurdle clearance technique without hitting the hurdles is preferable. If the trailing leg hits a hurdle it may cause the lead leg to land early with forced dorsiflexion of the ankle while the knee is fully extended, possibly tearing the gastrocnemius. An imbalanced clearance technique, with the thigh in forced abduction on landing, can lead to adductor magnus or gracilis tears. An imbalanced landing on an inverted and inwardly rotated foot can damage the lateral collateral ligament and possibly cause a fracture of the lateral malleolus (McDermott and Reilly, 1992).

Weight-lifting

The strain on the knee as the lifter sits into and then rises from the deep squat or split position in the 'Olympic lifts' is enormous (Tucker, 1990). Any such full squat technique, in which the posterior aspects of the calf and thigh make contact, causes overstretching of the knee ligaments, which may result in long-term damage. The lateral meniscus might also be trapped between the femoral condyle and tibial plateau. Full squats with weights are therefore to be discouraged as a regular exercise, with half squats being preferred (e.g. Tucker, 1990). Weight-lifting activities can impose unacceptable loads on the spine, particularly if performed incorrectly. The movement technique usually recommended is the 'knee lift' technique where the athlete looks straight ahead with a straight back and knees initially flexed. The weight is kept close to the body as the lift is made with knee then hip extension. This movement technique should be used for lifting any weight from the ground. The 'Olympic lifts' both involve two phases in which the large muscles of the legs are used to lift the weights with an intermediate, positioning phase to enable the second lifting phase to occur.

Weight training techniques can also cause spinal injury. Several activities should be avoided because of high loads on the lumber intervertebral discs already forced into an abnormal curvature. These include: bent rowing with knees fully extended; biceps curls involving spinal hyperextension; sit-ups with feet fixed (which recruits the hip flexors), or fully extended knees (passive tension in the posterior thigh muscles).

EXTRINSIC RISK FACTORS RELATED TO INJURY

Extrinsic risk factors are those factors that influence the load characteristics applied to the tissues within the athlete, such as environment, equipment, climate, training errors and rules of the game. As with intrinsic risks, some of these factors are modifiable, such as equipment and training errors. Some modifiable risks, such as equipment, have limitations due to sporting rules and regulations, but usually there is a choice available within the equipment range that will allow for an improved player–environment–position fit. For example, the shape, orientation, length, and number of studs on rugby boots may be modified to suit different surface conditions and different player positions. Some extrinsic factors are considered non-modifiable, such as surfaces, climate and rules of the game. Nonetheless, adjustments can be made to equipment or player movement technique that may minimise these risks. For example, playing tennis on concrete surfaces brings an increased risk due to higher repetitive ground impacts and higher energy return shots. We cannot change the tennis playing surface but modifications can be made to cushioning within the player's shoes and tightness in the racquet strings that can reduce these risks to the athlete. In the following section, we will look at sports surfaces, equipment and training errors as examples of extrinsic risk factors in athletes. Where possible we will look at the types of injuries most associated with these risks and relevant mechanical factors involved.

Environment (non-modifiable risk factor)

Sports surfaces

Sports surfaces are often complex structures with several layers, all of which contribute to the overall behaviour of the surface. The following characteristics are important for the behaviour of surfaces for sport and exercise and have the greatest association with injury.

Friction and traction

The friction or traction force between a shoe or other object and a surface is the force component tangential to the surface. In friction, for 'smooth' materials, the force is generated by 'force locking', and the maximum friction force depends on the coefficient of sliding friction (µ) between the two materials in contact. Traction is the term used when the force is generated by interlocking of the contacting objects, such as spikes penetrating a Tartan track, known as 'form locking'. This friction or traction force is particularly important in, for example, running, for which the coefficient of friction or traction should exceed 1.1, and for changes of direction as in swerves and turns. For sports surfaces, the coefficient of friction or traction should be independent of temperature, weather and ageing. Friction or traction can be too high as well as too low and has an association with injury. Friction is about 10–40% greater on artificial turf than on grass. It is debatable whether spikes are necessary on a clean, dry, synthetic surface. If used, they should not excessively penetrate the surface, otherwise energy is required to withdraw the spike and damage is caused to the surface. Friction also affects the rebound and rolling characteristics of balls, such as in tennis and golf.

Compliance

Compliance, the inverse of stiffness, relates to the deformation of the sports surface under load and may have an optimum value for the performer. Although it is widely believed that stiffer surfaces can enhance performance in, for example, sprinting, training on such surfaces can increase the risk of injury owing to larger impact accelerations. A too-compliant surface, however, is tiring to run on. Compliance has no specific connection with resilience. For example, a crash mat has a high compliance and low resilience, and concrete has a low compliance but high resilience.

(Rebound) resilience

Resilience is a measure of the energy absorbed by the surface that is returned to the striking object. The resilience, or rebound resilience (R), is the square of the coefficient of restitution (*e*) between the object and surface ($R = e^2$). For an inanimate sports object, the rebound resilience is the kinetic energy of the object after impact divided by that before impact. It relates to the viscoelastic behaviour of most surfaces for sport and exercise, where the viscous stresses are dissipated as heat, not returned to the striking object. Again, this has a relation to injury; a lack of resilience causes fatigue. Resilience is important in ball sports (ball bounce resilience) and relates to the description of a surface as fast or slow (for cricket $R < 7.8\%$ is classified as slow, $R > 15.6\%$ as very fast). Specified ranges of rebound resilience for some sports include (Bell *et al.*, 1985; Sports Council, 1978 and 1984): hockey 20–40%; soccer 20–45%; cricket 20–34%; tennis (grass) 42%; tennis (synthetic court) 60%.

Hardness
Strictly, the hardness of a material is the resistance of its surface layer to penetration. This property is closely related to compliance: hard sports surfaces tend to be stiff and soft ones tend to be compliant, to such an extent that the terms are often interchangeable in common use. Because of their close association with stiffness, hard surfaces are closely associated with injury (Denoth, 1986).

Force reduction
This is a surface characteristic specified by the German Standards Institute (DIN). It expresses the percentage reduction of the maximum force experienced on a surface compared with that experienced on concrete; this is also called impact attenuation. Concrete is an extremely stiff surface that causes large impact forces; a surface with good force reduction will reduce this impact force, one important factor in injury. The International Amateur Athletics Federation (IAAF) specifies a force reduction of between 35% and 50% for athletic tracks. Interestingly, the track for the Olympic Games in Atlanta in 1996 only just attained these limits with a force reduction of 36%. This was a fast track not intended for training, as the use of the stadium changed from athletics to baseball soon after the games. Nevertheless, similar tracks were used for the 2004 and 2008 Olympic Games in Athens and Beijing.

Force reduction is closely related to shock absorbency, a term that, although frequently used, is not unambiguously defined and may be associated with the peak impact force, the force impulse or the rate of change of force.

Natural surfaces
These are surfaces formed by the preparation of an area of land and include turf (grass), loose mineral layers (such as cinders), ice and snow. In many respects, grass is the ideal sports surface. A greater attenuation of the impact force can be obtained by switching from running on asphalt to running on grass than could be achieved by any running shoe on asphalt (Nigg, 1986b). If allowed enough recovery after each use, and if properly maintained, grass has a life-span that far exceeds that of any alternative as it is a living material. Frequency of use is limited, otherwise wear damage can be considerable, and grass does not weather particularly well.

Artificial surfaces

Artificial surfaces are becoming the norm in today's sporting environments, particularly where new stadiums make it impossible to maintain natural surfaces. Playing surfaces that have a major polymeric component (such as artificial turf and various elastomeric surfaces) are called synthetic surfaces. Synthetic surfaces are composite structures of several layers, often divided into the 'surface system' and the 'foundation' (Figure 3.10). The foundation generally comprises an engineered sequence of porous bound macadam (up to 65 mm thick), overlying crushed rock (up to 300 mm thick typically) and the natural soil. Each of the components of the system has been designed to interact in a way that provides the optimal aspects of performance required, typically ball rebound, adequate compression resistance or deformation, and safety characteristics related to foot-surface and possibly head-and skin-surface interactions dependent upon the sport for which the pitch is intended.

For field sports, the surface system starts with synthetic grass, called pile. Today synthetic grass is typically made from polypropylene or polyethylene, whereas it used to be mostly nylon. Synthetic grass pile may range from 16 mm to 65 mm in length depending on the sports requirement, and is woven into a primary cloth or backing. Polypropylene grass tends to be stronger and is used for sports where skin to ground contact is minimal, as in tennis. Polyethylene grass is a softer material and is, therefore, less likely to cause skin burn. Thus, this type of synthetic grass is recommended for sports where skin-to-ground contacts are more likely, such as American football, soccer or baseball. Synthetic grass systems require some sort of in-fill, usually a combination of sand and rubber pellets that help the grass maintain its vertical position (Figure 3.10(a and b)). The sand adds weight to the system and the rubber aids traction. Underneath the synthetic grass and its backing, there is usually a shock pad, which is constructed of high density foam (Figure 3.10(b)). The purpose of the shock pad is force reduction to make the surface safe for player impacts and to reduce overuse injuries.

Rubberised or polyurethane surface systems have been utilised for athletic tracks since the mid 1960s. Polyurethane surfaces allow for a range of spring stiffness to provide faster running speeds by decreasing foot contact time and increasing step length. Typically, a polyurethane surface is made up of rubber granules mixed with an artificial binder that is poured in place. However, Mondo, an Italian company that built Beijing's Olympic track, believes it can get better quality control by making the track in a factory and unrolling it on site, in strips. However, there is still some argument about the optimal surface stiffness for running tracks. Because the track at the Atlanta Games was considered very stiff and produced many fast track times this has lead some athletic coaches to believe that stiffer tracks are better. However, it has been reported that as surface stiffness increased, there was a proportional increase in a runner's leg displacement, which also increased the metabolic cost of running. In their research, with runners performing at a constant intermediate speed, the surface with the lowest stiffness produced the most economical running pattern. Clearly, more research is needed to determine optimal stiffness characteristics for running tracks.

Figure 3.10 Synthetic grass systems: (a) example of synthetic grass showing infill; (b) a transverse section showing the different types of fibres included into the weave of synthetic grass, the infill and foundation of the system; (c) shows how the system is constructed, the shock pad would be underneath the backing of the system.

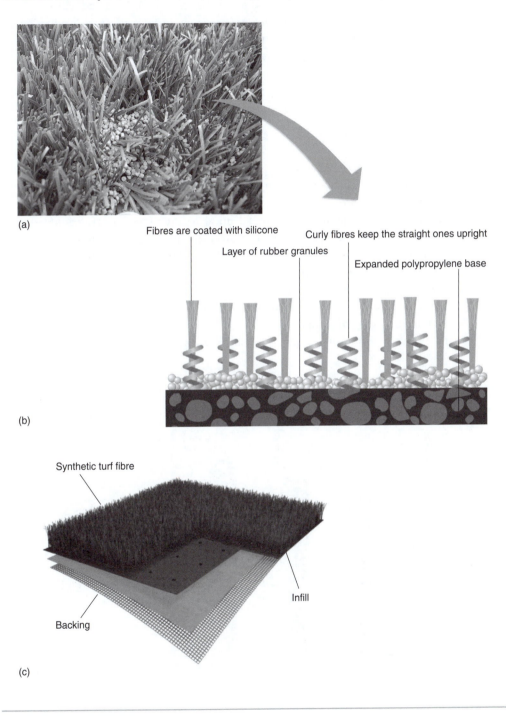

(a)

Fibres are coated with silicone

Layer of rubber granules

Curly fibres keep the straight ones upright

Expanded polypropylene base

(b)

Synthetic turf fibre

Infill

Backing

(c)

Biomechanical assessment of surfaces

Various functional standards for playing surfaces have been developed (for example see Tipp and Watson, 1982; Kolitzus, 1984; Bell *et al.*, 1985). Nigg and Yeadon (1987) provided a review of the methods of assessing how surfaces affect the loading on the body of an athlete. They noted that load assessment methods differ for horizontal and vertical loads and depending on whether the surface exhibits point or area elasticity. In the former, the deformation is only at the impact point, and in the latter, the area of deformation is larger than the impact area, distributing the forces. Furthermore, some tests are standard materials tests; others involve humans.

Vertical load assessment

For assessment of vertical loads on point elastic surfaces, the materials tests, which offer the advantage of reliability, include the use of 'artificial athletes' and simpler drop tests, where a weight is dropped on to the surface mounted either on a rigid base or on a force platform. The methods should give identical results for point elastic surfaces. The 'Artificial Athlete Stuttgart' is an instrumented drop test mass-spring system that produces a contact time of around 100–200 ms. This is similar to the ground contact time that occurs for the performer in many sports. Other similar devices are also used, such as the 'Artificial Athlete Berlin'. All drop test results also depend on the striking speed, mass, shape and dimensions of the test object. Changing the values of these may even alter which surface appears to be best (Figure 3.11). Tests with humans usually take place with the surface mounted on a force platform. Nigg and Yeadon (1987)

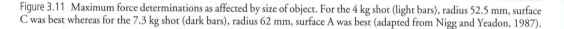

Figure 3.11 Maximum force determinations as affected by size of object. For the 4 kg shot (light bars), radius 52.5 mm, surface C was best whereas for the 7.3 kg shot (dark bars), radius 62 mm, surface A was best (adapted from Nigg and Yeadon, 1987).

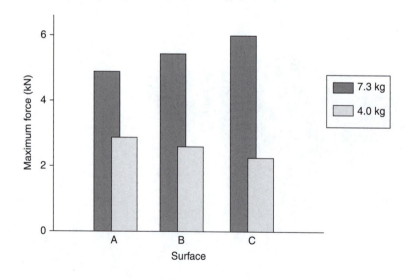

provided results from a range of studies comparing human and materials tests, and reported correlations as low as 0.34 between the vertical force peaks from the two.

For area elastic surfaces, such as sprung wooden floors, drop tests similar to those above are also used. Other methods use accelerometers or filming of markers mounted on the surface (Nigg and Yeadon, 1987). These authors noted the size limitations for force platform testing of area elastic surfaces. Errors in drop tests because of the inertia of the surface and further errors in the use of the 'artificial athletes' because of the test system inertia render these methods inappropriate for such surfaces. These deflection-time methods provide information about the deformation of the surface, but the relationship between that deformation and force has not been established (Nigg and Yeadon, 1987). For both types of surface, there has been little, if any, validation of the use of results from materials tests as indicators of the potential of surfaces to reduce load on the human body. This led Nigg and Yeadon (1987) to conclude that materials tests cannot be used to predict aspects of loading on humans.

Horizontal load assessment

For assessment of horizontal (frictional) loads on both point and area elastic surfaces, a survey of the methods used to measure translational and rotational friction and some results of such tests was provided by Nigg and Yeadon (1987). They questioned the use of rotational tests and challenged the assumption that frictional test measurements are valid in sporting activities. Although these tests provide information on the material properties of the shoe–surface interface, they do not directly indicate the effects of these properties on the sports performer.

Assessment of energy loss

Again, drop tests such as 'artificial athletes' are used and the energy loss is calculated from a force–deformation curve (Figure 3.12). Confusion can be caused by viscoelastic

Figure 3.12 Representation of energy loss as the area enclosed by the hysteresis loop for a force–deformation curve.

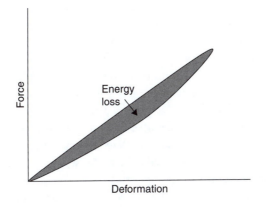

surfaces tending to give different results for single and repeated impacts, and by the effect that the properties of the impact object have on the surface ranking (see above). Difficulties arise when using humans in energy loss tests because of the two distinct systems involved – human and surface – each of which can be represented as a mass-spring-damper.

INJURY ASPECTS OF SPORTS SURFACES

Many types of surface are implicated in different injuries but the footwear–surface interface is the crucial factor in lower extremity injuries. There appears to be an optimal compliance for a surface, both for performance and for reduction of injury, which is about two to three times that of the runner (Greene and McMahon, 1984). Nigg (1986a) reported that impact forces are implicated in damage to cartilage and bone, and are involved in shin splints. Although non-compliant surfaces, which increase the impact loading, are mostly implicated in injury, excessively compliant surfaces can lead to fatigue, which may also predispose to injury. Kuland (1982) suggested that, for running, the best surfaces are grass, dirt paths and wood chips as they provide the desirable surface properties of resilience, smoothness, flatness and reasonable compliance. Hard, non-compliant surfaces are by far the worst for lower extremity injury and lower back pain and Kuland (1982) identified asphalt roads, pavements and wood as the worst surfaces.

Synthetic surfaces are also implicated in joint and tendon injuries owing to the stiffness of the surface. Macera *et al.* (1989) found the only statistically significant predictor of injury for females to be running at least two-thirds of the time on concrete. The important impact variables would appear to be peak vertical impact force, the time to its occurrence, peak vertical loading rate and the time to its occurrence (Figure 3.13(a)). It is, however, not clear which of these ground reaction force measures are most important. The peak vertical impact force and peak loading rate are likely to relate to the shock wave travelling through the body (Williams, 1993). All of these variables are made worse by non-compliant surfaces. For example, on a non-compliant surface such as asphalt, the tendency is for a high impact peak, about two and a half times greater than that on a compliant surface such as grass. However, on compliant surfaces, the active force peak tends to be about 20% larger than on non-compliant surfaces, and it may exceed the impact force (Figure 3.13(b)). It is possible that these larger duration, and sometimes higher magnitude, active forces are important for injury (Williams, 1993) as they have a greater force impulse (average force multiplied by its duration) than the impact. Kuland (1982) reported that the repeated impact forces experienced when running on non-compliant surfaces might cause microfractures of subchondral bone trabeculae, leading to pain and a reduction in their shock-absorbing capacity on healing. This leads to an increased demand for shock absorbency from cartilage, leading eventually to cartilage damage and arthritis.

Hard grounds also account for an increased incidence of tendon injuries and inflammation of the calf muscles because of increased loading as the surface is less compliant.

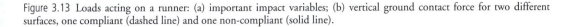

Figure 3.13 Loads acting on a runner: (a) important impact variables; (b) vertical ground contact force for two different surfaces, one compliant (dashed line) and one non-compliant (solid line).

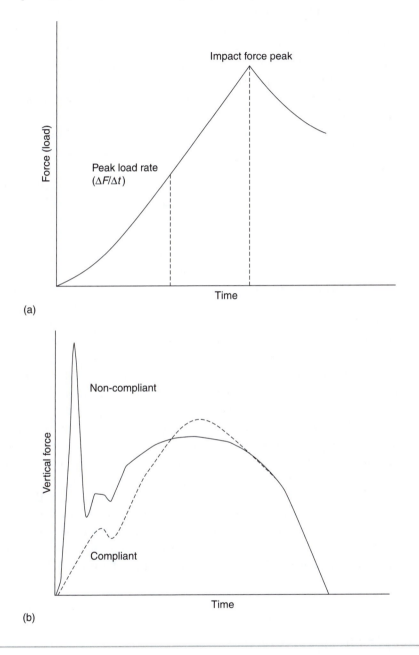

Hard mud-based grounds increase the likelihood of inversion injuries of the ankle joint owing to surface ruts and ridges (O'Neill, 1992).

Surface stiffness is important for sports in which vertical movements dominate; the frictional behaviour of the surface is of great importance when large horizontal movements occur (Nigg, 1993). Artificial surfaces may reduce or eliminate sliding and impose a higher resistance to rotation. For example, the incidence of injury has been reported to be at least 200% more frequent for tennis surfaces that do not allow sliding, such as asphalt and synthetics, than for those that do, such as clay and synthetic sand (Nigg, 1993). The frictional behaviour of the surface is also important and has in the past been indicated in the increased frequency of injury on artificial compared with natural turf. Technology for artificial turf has come a long way in the last ten years, third generation turf is made from relatively softer materials and incorporates some pile coating that reduces the friction coefficient. Indeed, recent studies have shown that there are no major differences in the incidence, severity, nature or cause of match injuries sustained on new generation artificial turf and grass by either male or female soccer players (Fuller *et al.*, 2007). In fact, one injury survey found that injury frequency, as assessed in terms of primary injury type, revealed a higher injury incidence in ligament tears on natural grass compared to third generation artificial turf (Meyers and Barnhill, 2004). In the past, high friction coefficients were cited as a problem with artificial surfaces: reducing the friction coefficient increases sliding, which allows for a reduction in loading because of the increased deceleration distance as well as a reduction in the rotational stress placed on the knee and ankle.

The inclination of the surface also affects the risk of injury. Uphill running imposes greater stress on the patellar ligament and quadriceps femoris tendon and on the ankle plantar flexors at push-off, as the foot has to be lifted to clear the ground. The anterior pelvic tilt and limited hip flexion increase the stress on the muscles of the lumbar spine, which can lead to lower back pain (Kuland, 1982). Downhill running requires a longer stride length, which causes a greater heel strike impact force and imposes greater strain on the anterior muscles of the thigh. In addition, the quadriceps femoris, contracting eccentrically to decelerate the thigh, presses the patella against the articular cartilage of the femur (Kuland, 1982) and the increased pressure can lead to chondromalacia patellae. Downhill running can also lead to low back pain owing to posterior pelvic tilt and spinal hyperextension. Running on flat turns causes adduction of the inside hip and increased foot pronation. The stride length of the outside leg increases, leading to a more forceful heel strike and greater stress on the lateral aspect of the foot; these are exacerbated by banked tracks. A severe camber on tracks and roads increases the pronation of the outside foot and increases the load on the inside leg, leading to Achilles tendon, ankle and knee joint injury (McDermott and Reilly, 1992); this can also occur when running on beaches, as the firm sand near the sea is also 'cambered'.

Equipment (modifiable risk factor)

Protective equipment

In most sporting environments, protective equipment is required to protect the athlete from impacts. There are two types of sporting impacts that require protective equipment, the high speed, low mass impact, caused by direct contact from a ball or puck, and the low speed, high mass impact, caused by collisions with other players or with the ground. For protective equipment to be mechanically effective, it should play the role of shock absorber (creating a time delay of an impact) and be a source of temporary energy storage and absorption to reduce impulsive force directed to the anatomy. Protective equipment is worn to reduce the effect of potential injurious forces by: transferring or dispersing impact force; reducing the friction coefficient between contact surfaces; absorbing energy of an impact; and limiting excessive movement at a joint.

The optimal material for impact protection varies depending on the sport, body part and size of the athlete. Generally, protective padding is selected based on the optimal energy absorption offered by the material and required by the type of impact most likely experienced during the sporting endeavour. Two mechanical properties most important in designing protective equipment are material resilience and energy absorption. Recall that resilience is a measure of the energy absorbed by a material that is returned when the load is removed; it is related to the elastic and plastic behaviour of the material and to its hysteresis characteristics. A highly resilient material quickly retains its original shape after an impact whereas a less resilient material may take some time to return to its initial configuration. Thus, highly resilient materials tend to be used to protect areas of the body that may be subject to repeated impacts during an activity. Both energy absorption and resilience of a given material can be affected by the thickness, density and temperature of the material at the time of impact. Typically, protective padding is made up of either low density or high density material. Low density material tends to be light and more comfortable to wear but only effective in low intensity impacts; rugby Shock Top® (Protective Sports Apparel Ltd., New Zealand) shoulder pads are a good example of this kind of equipment. High density material tends to be less flexible and heavier and, therefore, less comfortable for the athlete to wear, but it will also offer greater protection in high intensity impacts as it will absorb more energy through deformation. Equipment made out of high density, highly resilient materials, such as high density foam and thermomoldable plastics, are often used to protect areas most likely to be affected by high intensity repeated impacts such as the shins in soccer, hockey or rugby, or to protect more vulnerable areas such as the genitalia and head.

In field sports, such as rugby, soccer and hockey, high energy impacts to the shins are commonplace causing contusions, hematomas and even fractures. The midshaft of the tibia is particularly vulnerable because of the lack of soft tissue covering that usually helps to dissipate impact loads. Forces required to fracture the tibia are in the range of 3 to 7 kN and can occur during missed kicks and tackles when the opposing player's foot contacts the midshaft of the tibia. Shin guards are typically constructed of a plastic or fibreglass shell and a foam lining and have a much lower bending stiffness and second moment of area than the human tibia. Thus, the shin guard is easily deformed, making it impossible for this construction to disperse the loads that cause significant injury to the tibia. But shin guards are quite good at reducing lower impact forces of around 2 kN, which would cause significant contusions without the protection of a guard (Mills, 2006).

Helmets

Among people aged 15 to 24 years, participation in sport is the leading cause of traumatic brain injury after motor vehicle accidents (Sosin *et al.*, 1991). In many sports, particularly those where high energy impacts are common, the brain, head and face are particularly susceptible to injury. For example, in skiing and snowboarding, head injury is the most frequent reason for hospital admission and the most common cause of death (Furrer *et al.*, 1995; Hackam *et al.*, 1999). Wearing of helmets to protect the head and brain has been shown to reduce the risk of injury in cycling, in-line skating and skiing by as much as 60%.

Helmets, scrum caps, face guards and glasses have been designed to suit the specific needs of individual sports, such as cycling, ice hockey, lacrosse, softball, rugby, skiing, snowboarding and American football. Thus, a piece of headgear designed for one sport cannot offer protection from the kind of impacts experienced in another. Scrum caps, for example, were designed to reduce the coefficient of friction between two players in a scrum and therefore, reduce injuries to the ears and scalp: they were not designed to reduce impact forces. There are several different testing standard authorities responsible for setting the safety standards and testing protocols for protective equipment including helmets, for example, the Canadian Standards Association (CSA), the British and European Standard (BSEN), the American Society for Testing of Materials (ASTM) and the National Operating Committee on Standards for Athletic Equipment (NOCASE). Studies conducted at the CSA laboratory on rugby scrum caps found that peak headform accelerations were reduced by 11–20% at drop heights of one metre, whereas helmets designed for ice hockey and American football reduced these accelerations by 56–62%. Their conclusion was that rugby scrum caps only provide a slight impact resistance and should not be relied upon for concussion protection. This finding is not surprising considering rugby scrum caps are made of relatively thin, low to medium density foam, and ice hockey helmets are constructed out of polyethylene and high density foam.

Probably the most commonly used helmet worldwide is the one designed for cycling. Traumatic brain injury and concussion account for 6% of cycling related injuries (Caine *et al.*, 1996). The wearing of a cycling helmet has been shown to decrease the incidence of head injuries in Australian cyclists by 60–70% (Caine *et al.*, 1996). There are three protective components to a cycling helmet, the thermoplastic shell, the foam liner and the chin strap (Figure 3.14 (a and b)). The shell is 0.3 mm thick and constructed of thermoplastic, it is designed to prevent breakage of the foam liner and to decrease the coefficient of friction between the rider's head and road surface. By allowing the head to slide on the road surface, the helmet reduces the risk of injury to the cervical spine from excessive rotational loading. It should be noted that the thermoplastic shell is not designed to absorb excessive energy during an impact. The foam liner on the other hand, constructed of polystyrene bead moulding, ranging in density from 50–100 kg/m^3, is designed to compress by 90% during impact (Mills and Gilchrist, 2006). Mills and Gilchrist (2006) also found that the impact force was predicted to vary with liner crush in the same linear manner, meaning that the peak impact force is linearly proportional to the normal component of the impact velocity and the foam crushing distance (until of course the foam reaches its compression limit). This construction has a very low resilience and will never return to its original shape; for this reason, once impacted the helmet should be discarded. The chin strap is designed to ensure that the liner maintains good congruence with the wearer's head and, therefore, should be adjusted as tightly as is bearable by the wearer. If the chin-strap is not tight, the helmet may come off or move during a collision and, therefore, may not fulfil its protection potential.

Other common helmets are those used by ball sports to protect the wearer's head from low mass, high speed impacts during batting, for example, in softball, baseball and cricket (Figure 3.14 (c and d)). Unfortunately, there has not been enough research conducted on the relationship between helmet usage and head trauma reduction in these sports, so one has to assume they must help. Unlike a cycling helmet, a batting helmet has a thick fibreglass or polyethylene shell that is designed to disperse localised

Figure 3.14 Examples of different types of protective helmets: (a) typical cycling helmet; (b) cycling helmet usually used for BMX riding; (c) typical softball or baseball helmet; (d) helmet used for cricket, including face shield.

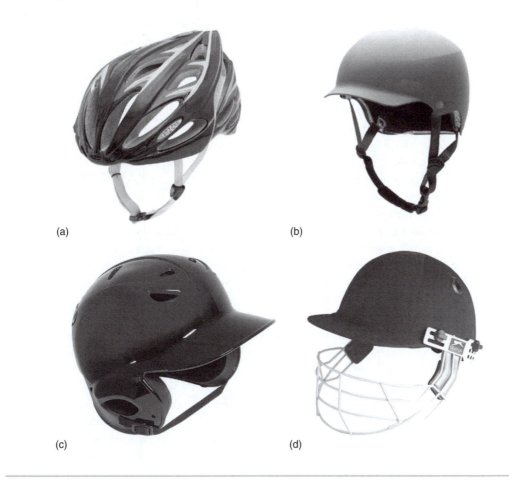

(a)

(b)

(c)

(d)

forces from ball impacts. A cricket helmet consists of a relatively stiff shell 3–4 mm thick and a thin 8–10 mm foam liner, whereas baseball helmets have a 2 mm high density polyethylene shell and a thicker 38 mm lower density foam liner. Tests conducted by McIntosh and Janda (2003) showed that the baseball helmet was better at absorbing energy at higher speed impacts (27 m/s) than the stiffer, thinner cricket helmet. This may not be an issue for amateur or younger athletes but in elite cricket, ball speeds may reach 30–45 m/s, so this helmet construction may not offer the best protection at this standard of the sport. According to Stretch *et al.* (2000) the likelihood of ball-to-head impacts may be greater at the higher speeds because of the reduced response time.

Wrist guards

As discussed in Chapter 2 wrist injury is a common sports problem. The most common acute injuries to the wrist are the scaphoid fracture, the Colles fracture (distal radius fracture), the scapholunate ligament sprain and injuries to the distal radioulnar joint and triangular fibrocartilage complex. The most common mechanism for wrist injury is falling on an outstretched hand (FOOSH). Thus, in sports where fall incidence is high, such as in-line skating, snowboarding and skateboarding, protective equipment for the wrist is highly recommended. Snowboarding in particular has a large problem with wrist injury. According to O'Neill (2003), almost a quarter of snowboarding injuries occur during a person's first snowboarding experience and half in their first season; furthermore, wrist fractures account for 20% of all snowboard injuries. There are many wrist guards on the market at the moment. Most are designed to supplement wrist strength by using a rigid volar plate, which reduces the impact force transmission by local load sharing and energy shunting and also increases the bending stiffness so as to reduce the likelihood of bending failure (Verdejo and Mills, 2004). However, if the wrist guards cover only the distal forearm region with a short rigid volar plate (Figure 3.15(a)), the impact force may be transmitted to the proximal forearm and, thereby, energy shunting may be localised to the proximal forearm region. This design feature may save the scaphoid from fracture but has a higher risk of causing Colles fracture. One way around this problem is to wear a longer wrist guard that covers the forearm to the midshaft of the radius and ulna (Figure 3.15(b)). However, Verdejo and Mills (2004) argued that the problem with wrist guard design could be overcome if the guards were constructed to allow more effective impact energy absorption which can only occur with a material that offers more deformation upon impact, for example an air bladder or other such compliant material on the palm. Their study showed that an air bladder on the palm of the hand reduced the impact force transmitted to the hand to less than 45% of the bare hand value (e.g. from 4253 N to 1752 N for a drop height of 51 cm). To date few wrist guard manufacturers are incorporating this feature into their design. The wrist guard in Figure 3.15(c) has incorporated palmer padding between the volar plate and palm of the hand but this padding is constructed of cotton duck, which would offer little energy absorption as compared to high density foam or an air bladder as shown by Verdejo and Mills (2004).

Figure 3.15 Examples of different types of wrist guards commonly used for snowboarding, skateboarding and rollerblading: (a) has a short volar plate that covers only the distal forearm; (b) is a longer wrist guard that covers to the midshaft of the radius and ulna; (c) is a short guard that has incorporated palmer padding between the volar plate and palm of the hand.

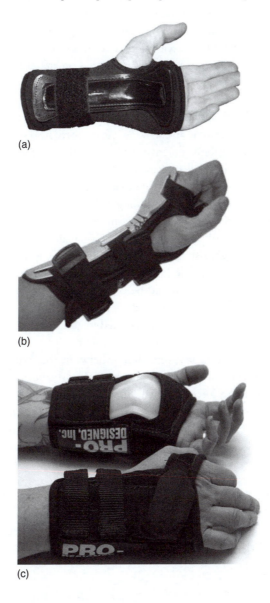

(a)

(b)

(c)

Footwear

In general, athletic footwear has several common characteristics that are important for improving performance and reducing the risk of injury. The first is to provide protection to the surfaces of the foot from the terrain and the elements. The second is to provide traction between the sporting surface and shoe, which allows optimal propulsion, braking and change of direction. The third characteristic is motion control during movement, either control of the rear and midfoot as in running or the forefoot in field and court sports. Finally, athletic shoes should provide some cushioning to attenuate impact forces. The shoe–surface interface is an important modifiable factor in lower extremity injuries. Abrupt changes in velocity – acceleration, deceleration, changes in direction, twisting – are common in sport and exercise and put great stress on ankles and knees in particular. The shoe–surface interface can be modified to reduce some of the injury risk to the performer by first selecting the correct shoe for the desired activity and individual performer. Shoes are manufactured with specific activities in mind; in general, there are several categories of athletic shoe, such as running and walking, court sports, field sports, athletics, and specialty (e.g. golf and dance shoes). For many activities, there are even more specific footwear adjustments that can be made for weather and surface conditions and some of these adjustments will be discussed further in the following relevant sub-sections. In the next subsection, we will focus on shoes for running, field sports and court sports because these are the most popular shoe types, and the ones most commonly associated with injury risk.

We briefly discussed the concepts of friction and traction in the sub-section on environmental extrinsic risk factors earlier in this chapter. Particularly when discussing court and field shoes, the friction component becomes immensely important. There are two types of friction we should be concerned with in understanding shoe–surface interaction – translational friction and rotational friction. Translational friction determines how much horizontal force is required to allow the shoe to slide over the surface. In translational friction, the coefficient of friction (μ) is measured as the ratio of the horizontal force required to cause sliding between the two surfaces and the normal force. On a horizontal surface in a static condition, the normal force (N) is equal to the vertical component of force and the horizontal component (F_f) is identified as the frictional force, $F_f = \mu_s N$ (static friction). To solve for μ_s, we rearrange the equation so that $\mu_s = F_f/N$. Therefore, if a person with a mass of 80 kg is standing on a surface with a μ of 0.8, it will take 80% of their weight, or 628 N, in a horizontal direction to initiate sliding. Once two surfaces start sliding it is easier to increase or maintain the velocity of sliding. The coefficient of sliding friction, also called dynamic friction (μ_d), is expressed using a similar formula to that for static friction. However, the coefficient of sliding or dynamic friction is usually lower than the coefficient of static friction (μ_s) but how much lower will depend upon the characteristics of the two surfaces in question. The coefficients of friction for some common sporting surfaces are presented in Table 3.2.

Table 3.2 Translational friction coefficients for athletic shoes on different surfaces

EQUIPMENT	SURFACE	FRICTION COEFFICIENT
Tennis shoes	Synthetic grass	1.3–1.8
Basketball shoes	Wooden floor	1.0–1.2
Cleated shoes	AstroPlay, Fieldturf	0.54–1.45
Skates	Ice	0.003–0.007

Rotational friction determines the moment of force required to cause a shoe to rotate on a surface. Often referred to as the free moment of rotation between shoe and surface, it appears that rotational friction is a necessary consequence of sliding friction. In other words a higher translational friction coefficient usually means a higher rotational coefficient and vice versa. Measurement of rotational friction relies on relative values of free moments of rotation between the shoe and surface. The rotational friction component of various shoe and surface combinations is described as the peak free moment of ground reaction force. Greater peak moments of ground reaction force are associated with surface–shoe combinations that have higher rotational friction when performing a pivot manoeuvre. For example, performing a pivot on a wooden court surface in an athletic sock would produce a peak moment of about 3 N·m and the same performer wearing a basketball shoe and performing the same pivot manoeuvre on the same wooden surface would produce a peak moment of about 13 N·m. Therefore, the shoe–surface combination can greatly affect the rotational friction component.

Running

The running shoe industry is probably one of the most prolific sporting goods industries in modern society with over 200 new models released each season. Running shoes have become highly technologically advanced with many shoe companies vying to offer the running enthusiast novel designs that purport to reduce injury risk and improve running economy. Manufacturers produce models for specific foot types, gait patterns, and training styles. The categories of running shoes are extensive and growing, with shoes designed for motion control, racing, trail running, light weight, cushioning and even 'free' or 'five-finger' running shoes based on barefoot technology (Figure 3.16).

Figure 3.16 Example of a five-finger running shoe.

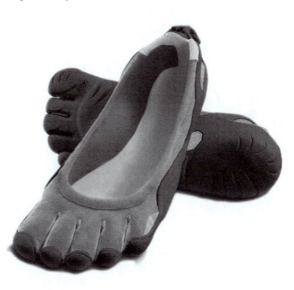

The most common complaint by runners is knee pain accounting for as much as 48% of reported injuries (Caine *et al.*, 1996; Taunton *et al.*, 2002). The most common problems causing knee pain are patella femoral pain syndrome, iliotibial band syndrome, and meniscal injuries. After knee injuries, the most common complaints of runners are tibial stress syndrome, Achilles tendinopathy and tibial stress fractures. These most common injuries in runners are associated with overuse mechanisms and often clinically linked to accumulated impact loads. A runner experiences between 500 and 1200 impacts per kilometre, with peak impact forces of several times body weight. Although the relationship between running impact and injury has not been conclusively established, running shoes have been designed to attenuate the impact force during the initial contact and stance phases of running.

The vertical force component for heel-toe running has two peaks. The first occurs between 5 to 30 ms after initial ground contact and is referred to as the 'vertical impact force peak' (Figure 3.17) (Nigg and Herzog, 2007). This force peak is the result of the collision between the runner's foot and the ground. The time of occurrence and magnitude of the impact force peak are dependent on several factors, including running speed, material properties of the shoe heel, shape of the shoe heel, and running style. For instance, the vertical force peaks are greater in heel-toe runners than for midfoot and forefoot strikers. It is believed that forefoot strikers are able to use the eccentrically contracting plantar flexors to prevent a heel-first contact and absorb shock. The control

Figure 3.17 Typical ground reaction force curve during heel-toe running showing the vertical impact force peak, active vertical force peak and toe-off.

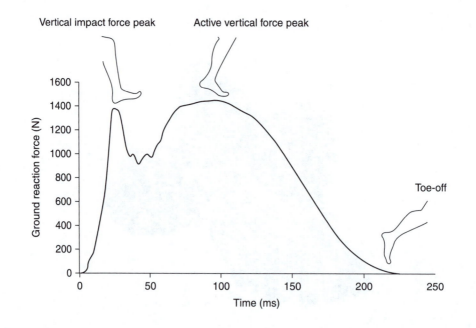

of the lowering of the rest of the foot, because of more joints in the kinetic chain, allows a prolonged period of force dissipation. The time occurrence of peak force is earlier in habitually shod runners when barefoot running than when they run in shoes (Lieberman *et al.*, 2010), and also earlier in hard soled shoes than in soft sole shoes. A second peak in the vertical force curve is called the 'active vertical force peak' (Figure 3.17) and is controlled by muscular activity. This peak generally occurs between 100 and 300 ms after the initial ground contact (Nigg and Herzog, 2007).

The vertical impact force peak is a high frequency force (> 30 Hz) that is not consciously affected by the runner owing to the 30 ms muscle latency period. The remainder of the force–time trace, including the active vertical force peak, is an active propulsion force of low frequency (< 30 Hz). The body's passive mechanisms are important in attenuating higher frequency components and the active ones are more important at low frequencies. Some evidence shows that the use of shock absorbing materials in shoes can reduce injury, yet many runners prefer uncushioned shoes for racing and there has been a recent resurgence in barefoot running. This is perhaps because too much shock absorbency slows the runner down, reduces rear foot control, and distorts feedback mechanisms (Pratt, 1989). The hardness, for example, of running shoes can influence aspects of movement technique, with runners responding to the physical characteristics of the shoe. The probability of heel-first contact, for example, has been reported to decrease as the force of impact increases through reduced surface compliance or increased running speed. Such adaptations can lead to smaller measured differences in ground contact forces than would be expected from the shoe's material properties.

Manufacturers have tended to pay more attention to shock absorbency, or cushioning, than to other shoe characteristics. This has resulted in many innovations including air-filled chambers, gels, hydroflow and other devices. However, several pieces of research have shown only a slight relationship between peak vertical impact forces and midsole hardness. Nigg and Cole (1991) reported results from tests with seven runners and three different running shoes differing only in midsole hardness. Using a pressure insole and a six-segment foot model, they calculated internal bone-on-bone contact forces and tendon forces. All their results showed little effect of midsole hardness, and greater internal forces during the propulsive phase than during the impact phase. The authors proposed that the cushioning properties of the running shoe are not important for loading within the foot, and, therefore, injury reduction, but may be important for comfort or for fine tuning of muscle-tendon units. Segesser and Nigg (1993) noted that, despite evidence and speculation linking impact loading to cartilage degeneration, stress fractures and shin splints, no prospective study existed that analysed the link between the aetiology of sports injury and external or internal impact forces. In fact Milner *et al.* (2006) found that the magnitude of the free moment was a better predictor of tibial stress fractures in female distance runners than vertical impact force peak. The free moment has been defined as the torque about the vertical axis due to the friction between the foot and ground during stance (Holden and Cavanagh, 1991).

If pronation is excessive, or prolonged into the propulsive phase, it produces an increased medial rotation of the tibia; this is transferred along the kinetic chain causing greater loading on many tissues of both the leg and lumbar spine (e.g. Craton and McKenzie, 1993). Because of the increased loads involved, overpronation has been heavily implicated in a wide range of injuries, including lateral compartment syndrome of the knee, iliotibial band syndrome, Achilles tendinitis and posterior tibial tendinitis (e.g. Nigg, 1986a); it may, indeed, be the cause of lower extremity pain in many runners. However, further understanding of the mechanism of injury involving excessive or rapid pronation is needed, along with the establishment of the relationship between lower extremity structure and pronation. Evidence is lacking to indicate how much reduction in overpronation is needed to relieve symptoms and it has not been demonstrated that appropriate footwear will remove symptoms (Williams, 1993). Arguments that footwear creates overpronation have been used by barefoot running enthusiasts; however, research using bone implanted markers has shown little difference in rear foot motion between shod and unshod runners (Reinschmidt *et al.*, 1997). Nevertheless, shoes with inappropriate heel flare can increase pronation or supination twofold or threefold, because of greater mediolateral forces and bending moments (Nigg, 1993). As overpronation is thought to damages ligaments, tendons and muscles, sports shoes should seek to reduce this risk.

Shoe design changes can influence moment arms (as in Figure 3.18) between the forces acting on the shoe and the joints of the body, and can change the way in which external forces affect internal forces. Shoe designs that increase the moment arms between the joints and the ground will generally reduce impact forces but increase pronation or supination (Nigg, 1993). For example, a reduction of the flare of the midsole on the lateral aspect of the heel can obviously decrease the moment about the subtalar joint (Stacoff and Luethi, 1986). Thick-soled shoes with broad-flared heels and wedged midsoles can protect the Achilles tendon from injuries caused by large impact

Figure 3.18 Schematic representation of how the moment arm (r) and moment of force (M) as they appear in (a) might increase as a result of: (b) a change in heel flare; (c) a change in midsole thickness. If force (F) remains the same in all conditions, we see an increase in r as well as M in (b) and (c)

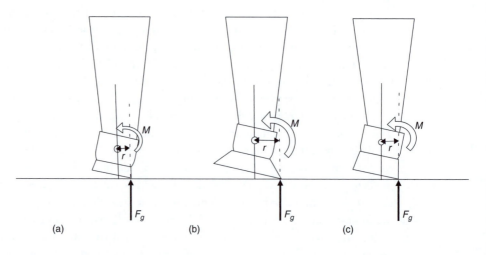

forces in many runners. Indeed, thick and soft shoe soles would appear to give best impact attenuation. However, such soles would hinder rear foot control, by generating excessive moments in the leg and ankle, owing to the increased moment arm for the impact force occurring on first contact with the outer border of the shoes (see Figure 3.18). Pratt (1989) reported that the heel base should not be wider than 75 mm to prevent too rapid pronation and that bevelling the lateral border would also be beneficial. Rear foot control in sports footwear owes much to thermoplastic heel counters that stabilise the subtalar joint and limit excessive pronation. Enhanced torsional stability around the longitudinal axis of the shoe can also be achieved by the use of firm materials placed between the upper and midsole, a technique known as board-lasting (Craton and McKenzie, 1993). To obtain a compromise between impact attenuation and rear foot control, the material of the lateral side of the midsole, which absorbs shock, is often softer than that used on the medial side, which is reinforced with a higher density material. This reduces any tendency for the shoe to collapse on the medial side, thereby controlling excessive pronation. The use of a straight last, rather than the earlier curved last (see Box 3.3), also helps to reduce pronation (Craton and McKenzie, 1993).

BOX 3.3 ANATOMY OF A RUNNING SHOE

Figure 3.19 Parts of a running shoe.

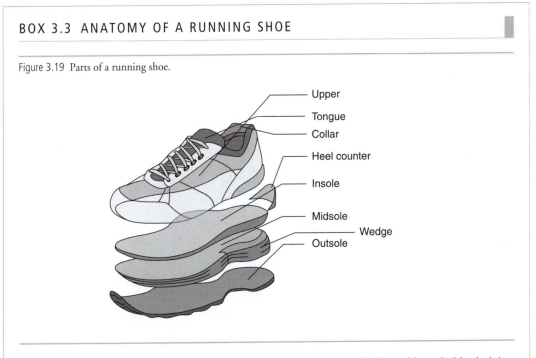

Upper It may be made of a compound synthetic material that is light and breathable, helping to release heat from the foot inside. The upper usually consists of a layer of foam that provides perspiration absorption and padding for comfort and protection. The tongue of the upper should be padded to cushion the top of the foot against the pressure from the laces. The collar is stitched around the side and back of the upper to prevent rubbing and irritation against the Achilles tendon and malleolus. Hard or high collars can cause inflammation of the tendon or peritendon. Covering the foam padding is a woven nylon taffeta that supplies the strength while a cotton weave backing helps to prevent the nylon from tearing or snagging.

Midsole and heel wedge These are the critical parts of the shoe for shock absorption. The most commonly used materials are closed-cell polymeric foam (EVA – ethylene vinyl acetate) although manufacturers may also use polyurethane or dual density EVA as well. Closed-cell foams absorb energy by compression of the pockets of air trapped in the cells and secondarily from deformation of the cell walls. These foams are 80% gaseous with thin (<10 mm) walls. Closed-cell foams regain their original dimensions more quickly than open cell foams. Long term durability of these foams is unknown, but all foams form a compression-set, which is a permanent deformation due to repetitive stress. Compression-set occurs through fracturing and buckling of the cell walls of the foam material, which reduces the ability of the material to absorb shock. This is why runners are recommended to replace their running shoes after 3–6 months, depending upon their mileage.

Insole board and last Some shoe designs, known as 'board-lasted' shoes, incorporate an insole board that provides the rigid base for the rest of the shoe and gives excellent stability but limited flexibility. In modern running shoes, fibreboard is usual; this is composed of cellulose fibres embedded in an elastomeric matrix with additives to prevent fungal and bacterial growths. Other shoes, known as 'slip-lasted' shoes, do not have an insole board and the upper is fitted directly to the last giving flexibility but with limited stability. Combination-lasted shoes have the rear part of the shoe board-lasted and the forefoot part slip-lasted: this represents a good compromise between rear foot stability and shoe flexibility. The last is a three-dimensional copy of a foot; therefore, the shape and fit of the shoe is dependent upon the shape of the last. Different lasting shapes and combinations create shoes that may be straight, curved or semi-curved. A straight last provides more support to the medial aspect of the foot and is recommended to athletes with a low arch or no arch and who tend to overpronate. The curved last tends to be fitted to athletes with high arches and a neutral foot because it provides less support to the medial foot but allows for greater flexibility in a more rigid foot. In between is the semi-curved last, which provides more support to the medial arch than the curved last and is, therefore, recommended to athletes with low arches who may tend towards pronation.

Insole Usually made from moulded polyethylene foam with a laminated fabric cover, this should help to reduce impact shock, absorb perspiration and provide comfort. It should provide good friction with the foot or sock to prevent sliding and consequent blistering.

Inserts A wide variety of 'inserts' are available. Some may be built into the shoe, others can be either added loosely or glued in position. Various materials are used, including foam rubbers with few air cells to reduce compression set. Sorbothane, a viscoelastic material, is popular and, supposedly, reduces the skeletal accelerations associated with repeated impacts. Other investigators have suggested that inserts do no more than provide a tight fit. Certainly, they should not raise the heel of the foot so much that rear foot control is hindered because of an increased moment arm of the ground contact force.

Heel counter This is an important part of the shoe as it contributes to shoe and rear foot stability, cradling the calcaneus and limiting excessive pronation. Rigid, durable materials are needed for this purpose and a sheet of thermoplastic is normally incorporated in the heel counter. External counter stabilisers are also used to reduce excessive rear foot movement. The design of the heel counter has a profound effect on the stiffness of the fatty heel pad and, therefore, on impact attenuation.

Outsole This has a tread for traction, flex grooves for flexibility, and protects from dirt and rocks. The outsole is made of two materials; carbon rubber for durability and blown rubber which is lighter, more flexible and aids in shock absorption.

Figure 3.20 Examples of three different types of last: (a) curved; (b) semi-curved; (c) straight.

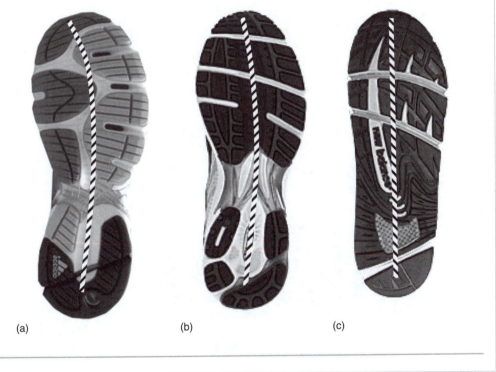

(a)　　　　　　　　　　(b)　　　　　　　　　　(c)

Court sports
Court sports include indoor racquet sports (badminton, squash, and racquetball), tennis, basketball, volleyball and European handball. Court sports tend to involve plenty of starting, stopping and side-to-side motion whereas running requires only forward motion. Therefore, court shoes differ from running shoes in the necessity for

mediolateral movement. One of the most important characteristics of court shoes is the construction of the outer sole. Patterns on the outer sole are designed to enhance stability and provide the optimal traction for given sport and surface requirements. Traction provided by the outsole is an important consideration in the design of a court shoe and is directly related to the ability of the shoe to develop frictional forces with the playing surface. The amount of traction required depends upon the specific sports being played and specific surface conditions (Figure 3.21). In this sub-section we will discuss

Figure 3.21 Different tennis shoe sole patterns for different playing surfaces: (a) hard surface shoe; (b), (c) and (d) clay court shoes; (e) and (f) grass court shoes.

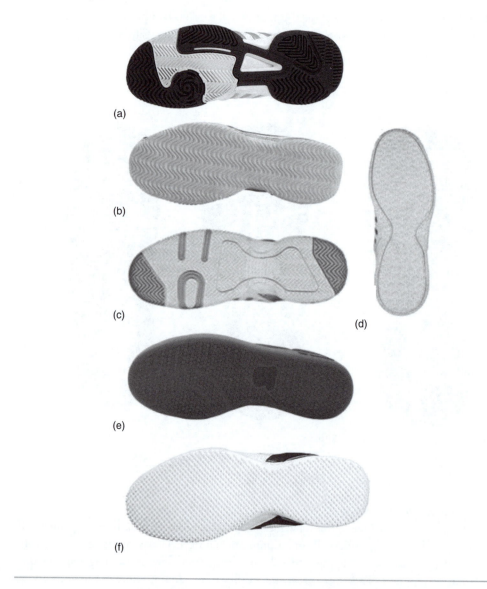

(a)

(b)

(c)

(d)

(e)

(f)

basketball and tennis as particular examples of court shoe design and the effect of the shoe design on the shoe–surface interface and the incidence of lower limb injury.

Basketball is a popular sport worldwide. Most injuries in basketball occur to the lower limb, particularly the ankle, knee and foot. Ankle injuries are the most common injuries in basketball and the single greatest cause for missed time due to injury (53.7%) (McKay *et al.*, 2001). High-top basketball shoes have been designed specifically for the sport to augment ankle support and provide increased resistance to ankle rotation in the frontal plane. Research has shown that high-top basketball shoes are more protective than low-top shoes, and that athletes may be able to generate up to 29.4% greater resistance to ankle inversion with a firmly-laced three quarter-top shoe than with a low-top shoe (Ottaviani *et al.*, 1995). High-top shoes are recommended to reduce the incidence of ankle injuries. However, if a player already suffers from ankle sprain, studies have shown that low-top shoes combined with rigid (e.g. air cast) or semi-rigid (e.g. laced) ankle supports are best at protecting the ankle from further injury.

Basketball is a multidirectional sport, thus a player is required to perform forward, backward and mediolateral accelerations. The sport may be played on a wooden floor or on a synthetic rubberised surface. To support the foot and provide the best traction in all directions, a basketball shoe should provide mediolateral support, have a flat sole with a slight heel wedge and a large firm heel counter. Soles with multiple-edge patterns offer better traction than herringbone designs. Studies on tread pattern have indicated that the surface compliance and traction characteristics will have a greater effect on the performer than the compliance and traction characteristics of the shoe. For instance, wood floors tend to allow more sliding than synthetic floors regardless of tread type. It is for this reason that synthetic floors have been indicated as a potential risk for increased incidence of ACL injuries. Often in sports like basketball or handball, athletes wear the same shoes regardless of the type of surface they are playing on; this is poor practice and may increase injury risk. It is recommended that athletes choose different shoes for each surface, particularly a shoe with less traction on a synthetic surface and more traction on a wooden one will allow for the best shoe–surface traction combination.

Tennis is another court sport that is played on a wide range of court types, such as clay, synthetic grass, natural grass and various other forms of hard court. Players tend to prefer a court that suits their particular style of play, for example, a serve-and-volley player will play best on a fast court whereas a consistent baseline player will play better on a slow court. The type of court should determine a player's choice of tennis shoes. Excessive friction between the shoe and court can cause excessive rotational loading to the ankle as seen in Figure 2.12. Epidemiological studies on elite tennis players have found that 35–50 of all injuries were to the lower extremities. Overuse injuries, such as Achilles tendinosis, patellar tendinosis (jumper's knee) and iliotibial band syndrome, are common. However, there are also frequent acute injuries such as tennis leg (rupture of the medial head of gastrocnemius) and lateral ankle sprain. For tennis players, selecting the correct shoe for the surface as well as the surface condition is crucial in reducing injury risk.

Similarly to basketball shoes, tennis shoes should be chosen based on the type of court being played. Because of the quick side-to-side movements as well as sprinting and jumping, a tennis shoe should provide good lateral support and have a flat outer sole with a good heel wedge. Sole design as well as the construction material will affect traction with the surface of the court. Soft court tennis shoes are specifically made for clay tennis courts. Their soles have a characteristic herringbone pattern that gives the utmost traction without scuffing the clay surfaces (Figure 3.21(b–d)). Grass tennis shoes have characteristic dimpled soles for maximum traction on slippery grass (Figure 3.21(e and f)). Grass tennis shoes also tend to be low cut to enhance mobility. Hard-court tennis shoes are designed for concrete playing surfaces. Their soles feature the combination of the herringbone and dimpled patterns for traction and mobility (Figure 3.21(a)). Fewer injuries appear to occur during play on courts that allow greater sliding, such as clay, than during games played on courts with less sliding, such as grass. This may seem contradictory, because a clay surface has the highest frictional coefficient with the ball. However, the loose surface particles on a clay court reduce the frictional coefficient with the player as the particles tend to roll under the foot, allowing for easier sliding. As discussed previously, sliding allows the player more time to decelerate and thus come to a more gradual stop, which results in a lower stress peak.

Field sports

Field sports such as soccer, rugby, American football and hockey combine multidirectional movement with a variable amount of body contact and may be played on natural grass or synthetic surfaces. Sports played on natural turf (e.g. rugby) require the use of boots with longer blunt studs while sports played on artificial turf (e.g. hockey) require a turf shoe with many short plastic or rubber cleats. In field sports, boots tend to have relatively flat soles with little arch support. Cleated or studded boots may have flat, short, blade or mixed cleat designs. The cleats or studs have been incorporated to increase the traction between the boot and the surface; however, traditionally very little thought was put into the locations of the cleats and the effect this might have on the performer. Frequently, studs coincide with the metatarsal heads and may cause unnecessary localised high loads. An athlete should never be able to feel the cleats or studs through the sole of the boot and the cleats, ideally, should be positioned under the major weight bearing joints of the body.

The interaction between the grass and cleat may lead to the production of high frictional and rotational forces, which may lead to excessive shearing or rotational load on the knee and ankle (Orchard and Powell, 2003; Livesay et al., 2006). High frictional forces lead to insufficient rotational freedom between the surface and footwear. In violent twisting or turning movements, as in some tackles and swerves, the foot remains fixed to the ground while the trunk rotates. This has been termed the cleat catch mechanism. Cleat design and layout has also been associated with increased instances of cleat catch and rotational loading on the knee and implicated as a potential risk for ACL injuries (Lambson et al., 1996). Boots with longer irregular cleats at the peripheral margin of the sole, with smaller pointed cleats in the middle of the sole, produced higher torsional resistance on grass surfaces (Lambson et al., 1996).

For sports such as rugby several choices of stud design are available. Soft ground rugby boots typically consist of a six or eight stud design with screw in studs that come in various lengths. Longer studs are recommended for soft wet grounds and shorter studs are recommended for harder dry grounds. The choice of six or eight studs is mostly dependent upon the position being played. The six stud configuration has less surface area penetrating the ground so will offer reduced traction and increased mobility compared to the eight stud design. Therefore, six studs may be best suited to backs or loose forwards. The eight stud design has more studs penetrating the ground in the forefoot region, which allows greater pressure distribution and traction. Thus, eight stud designs may be best suited to forwards, particularly the tight five forwards. Firm ground boots or 'mouldeds' have more short rubber or plastic studs; this works very well on hard grounds because of the greater surface area, which increases force dispersion compared to soft ground studs.

Training errors (a modifiable risk factor)

Training errors are often cited as the most frequent cause of injury and can be described as overtraining, training on inappropriate surfaces or excessive workload. A training programme should avoid training errors by close attention to the principles of progression, overload and adaptation, with appropriate periods of rest to allow for the adaptation. It should also be individual and sport-specific. Some examples of training errors are persistent high-intensity training, sudden increases in training mileage or intensity, a single severe training or competitive session, and inadequate warm-up. These account for at least 60% of running injuries. For the ten most common running injuries, the effect of training errors is exacerbated by malalignment or strength–flexibility imbalances. The underlying mechanism has been proposed to be local muscle fatigue decreasing the muscular function of shock absorption and causing more structural stress to the bone, leading to an increase of osteoclastic bone remodelling. Without balancing osteoblastic activity during rest and recovery, a stress fracture could occur. Training errors were also cited as the main aetiological cause of over 75% of overuse tendon injuries by Leadbetter (1993), mostly through a sudden increase in mileage or too rapid a return to activity. In throwing and bowling sports, excessive workloads have been associated with both acute and overuse injuries. In the following sub-section, we will look more closely at the issue of workload in throwing sports, such as cricket and baseball.

Workload in cricket and baseball

Cricket
Epidemiological studies conducted on both the South African and Australian cricketers have shown that bowlers are most likely to sustain an injury that causes them to miss a match, followed by batsmen and then fielders. Lower back injuries account for most of the loss of playing time in professional cricket. Fast bowlers show a relatively high prevalence of degeneration of the lumbar spine discs and stress patterns in the lumbar spine compared to active controls as determined by magnetic resonance imaging (MRI) (Ranson *et al.*, 2005). The most common cause of low back pain in fast bowlers is a lumbar stress

fracture. These injuries often occur in the posterior bony elements, the pedicles and pars interarticularis of the lower lumbar vertebrae (L3–L5) on the opposite side to the bowling arm. Bowling workload has been significantly correlated to injuries in fast bowlers (Dennis *et al.*, 2003). Early indications from that study indicate that number of bowling sessions per week, whether they are training or match, is the factor which most strongly correlates with injury risk. They found that bowlers with an average of less than two days between bowling sessions and bowlers with an average of five or more days between sessions had a significantly increased risk of injury compared to bowlers with an average of 3–3.99 days between sessions. Analysing by the number of deliveries, less than 123 or more than 188 per week showed that the bowlers may be at an increased risk of injury. Injuries were described as being caused by 'gradual bowling', which was defined as an overuse mechanism due to bowling, but body position or bowling technique was not reported.

Other factors that may contribute to lower back injury in fast bowlers include: overbowling, particularly of young bowlers whose epiphyses are not yet closed; poor footwear and hard surfaces, particularly in indoor nets; lack of physical conditioning; relatively high ball release positions; poor hamstring and lower back flexibility; and a straight front knee from front foot impact to ball release (see also Bartlett *et al.*, 2006; Elliott *et al.*, 1995; and Chapter 8 of this book).

The incidence of shoulder injuries in Australian cricketers is around one injury per 10,000 playing hours, which seems fairly low. However, a study of English cricketers showed that 23% reported shoulder injury in a single season. Saw *et al.* (2011) found that players suffering from shoulder injuries threw 40 extra throws per week and 12.5 extra throws per day than their uninjured team-mates and that throwing greater than 75 throws per week put them at 1.73 times the risk of injury.

Often the same players will play several grades and types of cricket matches, which will increase their individual workloads and potential for injury. For instance, including Twenty20 matches in the cricket calendar has increased the seasonal injury incidence rates, resulting in higher annual injury prevalence rates, with an average of 10%, and fast bowlers exceeding 18% (Orchard *et al.*, 2010).

Baseball

Little league elbow is caused by excessive valgus stress at the elbow (Banks *et al.*, 2005). In a study of youth baseball pitchers by USA Baseball in 1999, pitching biomechanics did not correlate to elbow pain, but pitches per game and per season did correlate. Pitch type (sliders and curve ball) were correlated with shoulder and elbow pain. Recommendations were introduced, limiting 9–14-year-old pitchers to 75 pitches per game and a maximum of 600 per season. The USA Baseball Medical and Safety Advisory Committee has recommended that 8 to 10-year-olds be limited to 50 pitches per game, 11 to 12-year-olds to 75 pitches per game, 13 to 14-year-olds to 75 pitches per game, 15 to 16-year-olds to 90 pitches per game, and 17 to 18-year-olds to 105 pitches per game (Benjamin and Briner, 2005).

The risk factors for shoulder injury in youth baseball pitchers include arm fatigue during the game, throwing more than 75 pitches per game, and fewer than 300 pitches per season (Lyman *et al.*, 2001). Elbow injury risk factors include arm fatigue during the game, playing baseball outside the league games, and throwing fewer than 300 or more than 600 pitches per season (Lyman *et al.*, 2001). This shows a relationship similar to the one found for cricket by Dennis *et al.* (2003). Pitch type (curve balls and sliders) as well as the number of pitches thrown during the game and during the season are significantly related to shoulder injury in young (9–14-year-old) baseball pitchers (Lyman *et al.*, 2002).

Olsen *et al.* (2006) compared 95 adolescent baseball pitchers who underwent surgery for shoulder or elbow injuries against 45 adolescent pitchers who had not had a significant injury related to pitching. They found the injured pitchers had a higher workload in several measures: months per year, games per year, innings per game, pitches per game, pitches per year, and warm-up pitches per year. Other associated factors were pitch speed and pitching in showcase games.

SUMMARY

In this chapter, we looked at some common intrinsic and extrinsic risk factors associated with athletic injuries. Assessing injury risk is a complex problem as many factors do not act in isolation and some may be quite individual specific. Intrinsic factors are those related to the athlete such as age, sex, anatomy, previous injury history and movement technique. Highest risk athletes are the very young (paediatric) and the more mature (masters), while female athletes are at greater risk of ACL sprains and tibial stress fractures. We learned that inadequate rehabilitation and neuromuscular imbalances were most commonly responsible for risk associated with previous injury history, specifically with respect to ankle sprains and hamstring strains. We also covered various movement technique faults related to injury in a variety of sports. We then looked at extrinsic factors related to injury, such as playing surfaces, equipment and training errors. We learned that some factors, such as the shoe–surface interface, might be modified in such a way as to prevent or reduce the risk of injury. Other factors, such as the surface, cannot be modified as easily: players must play on the surface provided and attempt to adjust other equipment to suit the present surface make-up and conditions. Nevertheless, designers of artificial playing surfaces have been working hard over the past ten years to develop surfaces that significantly reduce athlete risk. Protective equipment can be crucial in reducing athlete injuries as long as it is in good working order and is fitted properly. Finally, we found that training errors such as overtraining and excessive workload might increase the incidence in overuse injury in runners, cricketers and baseball players.

STUDY TASKS

1 Identify the intrinsic risk factors related to shoulder overuse injury in swimming and pitching. What are the similarities and differences?

2   Identify the intrinsic and extrinsic risk factors related to ACL injuries in basketball players. How do the risks differ between males and females?

3   You purchase a second-hand cycling helmet, you notice it has a dent on the side. Will the dent affect the efficacy of the helmet? If so, how?

4   List four of the most important factors related to shoe selection for each of the following activities: running, court sports and field sports.

5   What are the three phases of tissue healing and how are they pertinent to injury risk? What tissue characteristics are most important to restore during the rehabilitation process to reduce injury recurrence?

6   The coefficient of friction between a tennis shoe and synthetic grass is 1.3 and a player weighs 74 kg. Approximately, how much horizontal force is required to initiate sliding between his or her shoe and the synthetic surface?

7   What are the most common injury problems related to athlete–surface interactions? What are the mechanical factors that are important for injury risk related to surfaces? Explain clearly your answer to each question.

8   Age and the environment are considered to be non-modifiable injury risks, yet there are things we can do, in certain circumstances, to reduce risks associated with these factors. Using the examples of baseball and soccer, outline some of the measures that may be taken to reduce the risks associated with age and the environment.

GLOSSARY OF IMPORTANT TERMS

Accelerometer A device for measuring acceleration of an object. An accelerometer measures the acceleration of the free-fall reference frame (inertial reference frame) relative to itself.

Apophysis The type of growth plate that occurs between a tubercle (e.g. tibial tuberosity) and parent bone (e.g. tibia).

Bone mineral content The measure of the total mineral content in bone, measured in grams.

Bone mineral density (BMD) The measure of mineral content in a volume of bone, measured as area bone mineral density (g/cm^2) or volumetric bone mineral density (g/cm^3).

Bursitis Inflammation of the fluid-filled sac that lies between a tendon and skin, or between a tendon and bone.

Chondromalacia patellae The softening and breakdown of the cartilage that lines the underside of the patella.

Coefficient of restitution The measure of elasticity of an object is a fractional value representing the ratio of velocities after and before an impact.

Headform An instrumented system for testing head impacts.

Hemarthosis Bleeding or extravasation of blood into the joint spaces.

Hematoma An extravasation of blood outside the blood vessels, usually in liquid form within the tissue and generally the result of a haemorrhage.

Injury incidence The number of new cases of an injury within a specified time period divided by the size of the population initially at risk.

Injury prevalence Defined as the total number of cases of the injury in the population at a given time, or the total number of cases in the population, divided by the number of individuals in the population.

Inverse dynamics Inverse rigid-body dynamics is a method for computing forces and moments of force (torques) based on the kinematics of a body and the body's inertial properties (mass and moment of inertia).

Muscle latency period Refers to the lack of visible change that occurs in the muscle fibre during (and immediately after) the action potential.

Musculotendinous unit A muscle tendon unit functions as a single system, whose two components contribute to force production at different times. The force is produced by a combination of muscle actions and a release of elastic energy from the tendon component.

Osteochondrotic diseases Characterised by interruption of the blood supply of a bone, in particular to the epiphysis, followed by localised bony necrosis and, later, regrowth of the bone.

Pes cavus Also known as a 'high arch' is a human foot type in which the sole of the foot is distinctly hollow when bearing weight.

Pes planus Also known as 'flat footed' is a condition in which the arch or instep of the foot collapses and comes in contact with the ground.

Phagocytosis A specific form of endocytosis involving the vesicular internalisation of solid particles, such as bacteria, and is the body's mechanism used to remove pathogens and cell debris after injury.

Plantar fasciitis An irritation and swelling of the thick tissue (fascia) on the bottom of the foot.

Polyethylene A type of polymer that is classified as a thermoplastic, meaning that it can be melted to a liquid and remoulded as it returns to a solid state. Polyethylene is chemically synthesised from molecules that contain long chains of ethylene, a monomer that provides the ability to double bond with other carbon-based monomers to form polymers.

Polypropylene A thermoplastic polymer used in a wide variety of applications. It is an addition polymer made from the monomer propylene and it can serve as both a plastic and a fibre.

Polyurethane Any polymer consisting of a chain of organic units joined by urethane links. It is an incredibly resilient, flexible, and durable manufactured material. It is made by combining a diisocyanate and a diol, two monomers, through a chemical reaction. This makes a basic material whose variations can be stretched, smashed, or scratched, and remain fairly indestructible.

Porous bound macadam The foundation layer of most artificial sports surfaces, the term macadam refers to the method of laying the stone and sand aggregates that are sprayed with the porous binding material.

Proprioceptive stretching Proprioceptive neuromuscular facilitation (PNF) is a more advanced form of flexibility training that involves both the stretching and contraction of the muscle group being targeted. Exercises are based on the stretch reflex which is caused by stimulation of the Golgi tendon and muscle spindles. This stimulation results in impulses being sent to the brain, which leads to the contraction and relaxation of muscles. After an injury, there is a delay in the stimulation of the muscle spindles and Golgi tendons resulting in weakness of the muscle. PNF exercises are used in rehabilitation programmes to re-educate the motor units that are lost due to the injury.

Rotator cuff The group of muscles (supraspinatus, infraspinatus, teres minor and subscapularis) that act to stabilise the shoulder. The four muscles of the rotator cuff, along with the teres major and the deltoid, make up the six scapulohumeral muscles.

Shin splints The more common term for 'medial tibial stress syndrome', which is a slow healing and painful condition in the anterior medial tibia.

Superior labrum The labrum is a lip-like piece of cartilage that deepens the glenoid of the shoulder joint that aids in stabilising the shoulder joint. The labrum is divided into superior, inferior, anterior and posterior parts.

Thermomoldable plastics A type of plastic that can be moulded using a heat source such as a heat gun or special oven.

Tibia varum A frontal plane deformity where the distal third of the tibia is angled closer to the mid-sagittal plane than the proximal end.

Ultimate tensile stress The maximum stress that a material can withstand while being stretched or pulled before necking, which is when the injury occurs.

REFERENCES

Andersen, T.E., Tenga, A., Engebretsen, L. and Bahr, R. (2004) Video analysis of injuries and incidents in Norwegian professional football. *British Journal of Sports Medicine*, 38, 626.

Atwater, A. (1979) 'Biomechanics of overarm throwing movements and of throwing injuries', in R.S. Hutton and D.I. Miller (eds) *Exercise and Sport Sciences Reviews*, Vol. 7, New York: Franklin Institute Press, pp. 43–85.

Banks, K.P., Ly, J.Q., Beall, D.P., Grayson, D.E., Bancroft, L.W. and Tall, M.A. (2005) Overuse injuries of the upper extremity in the competitive athlete: magnetic resonance imaging findings associated with repetitive trauma. *Current Problems in Diagnostic Radiology, 34,* 127–142.

Bartlett, R., Gratton, C. and Rolf, C. (eds) (2006) *Encyclopedia of International Sports Studies.* London: Routledge.

Bell, M.J., Baker, S.W. and Canaway, P.W. (1985) Playing quality of sports surfaces: a review. *Journal of the Sports Turf Research Institute, 61,* 26–45.

Benjamin, H.J. and Briner, W.W. Jr. (2005) Little league elbow. *Clinical Journal of Sports Medicine, 15,* 37–40.

Best, T.M. and Garrett, W.E. (1993) 'Muscle–tendon unit injuries', in P.A.F.H. Renström (ed) *Sports Injuries: Basic Principles of Prevention and Care,* London: Blackwell Scientific, pp. 71–86.

Boden, B.P., Dean, G.S. and Feagin, J.A. (2000) Mechanism of anterior cruciate ligament injury. *Orthopedics 23,* 573–578.

Brooks, J.H.M., Fuller, C.W., Kemp, S.P.T. and Reddin, D.B. (2005) Epidemiology of injuries in English professional rugby union: Part 1 match injuries. *British Journal of Sports Medicine*, *39*, 757–766.

Caine, D.J., Caine, C.G. and Lindner, K.J. (1996) *Epidemiology of Sports Injuries*. Champaign, IL: Human Kinetics.

Chan, K.M. and Hsu, S.Y.C. (1994) 'Elbow injuries', in P.A.F.H. Renström (ed) *Sports Injuries: Basic Principles of Prevention and Care*, London: Blackwell Scientific, pp. 46–62.

Chandler, T.J. and Kibler, W.B. (1993) 'Muscle training in injury prevention', in P.A.F.H. Renström (ed) *Sports Injuries: Basic Principles of Prevention and Care*, London: Blackwell Scientific, pp. 252–261.

Craton, N. and McKenzie, D.C. (1993) 'Orthotics in injury prevention', in P.A.F.H. Renström (ed) *Sports Injuries: Basic Principles of Prevention and Care*, London: Blackwell Scientific, pp. 417–428.

Croisier, J.L. (2004) Factors associated with recurrent hamstring injuries. *Sports Medicine, 34,* 681–695.

Croisier, J.L., Forthomme, B.N, Namurois, M.H., Vanderthommen, M. and Crielaard, J.M. (2002) Hamstring muscle strain recurrence and strength performance disorders. *The American Journal of Sports Medicine, 30*, 199–203.

Dennis, R.J., Farhart, R., Goumas, C. and Orchard, J. (2003) Bowling workload and the risk of injury in elite cricket fast bowlers. *Journal of Science and Medicine in Sport, 6*, 359–367.

Denoth, J. (1986) 'Load on the locomotor system and modelling', in B.M. Nigg (ed.) *Biomechanics of Running Shoes*, Champaign, IL: Human Kinetics, pp. 63–116.

Edington, D.W. and Edgerton, V.R. (1976) *The Biology of Physical Activity*. Boston, MA: Houghton Mifflin Company.

Elliott, B.C., Burnett, A.F., Stockill, N.P. and Bartlett, R.M. (1995) The fast bowler in cricket: a sports medicine perspective. *Sports Exercise and Injury, 1*, 201–206.

Elliott, B.C., Hardcastle, P.H., Burnett, A.F. and Foster, D.H. (1992) The influence of fast bowling and physical factors on radiologic features in high performance young fast bowlers. *Sports Medicine, Training and Rehabilitation, 3*, 113–130.

Foster, D.H., Elliott, B.C., Ackland, T. and Fitch, K. (1989) Back injuries to fast bowlers in cricket: a prospective study. *British Journal of Sports Medicine, 23*, 150–154.

Fowler, P.J. (1994) 'Injuries in swimming', in P.A.F.H. Renström (ed) *Clinical Practice of Sports Injury: Prevention and Care*, London: Blackwell Scientific, pp. 507–513.

Frank, C.B. and Shrive, N.G (1999) 'Ligament', in B.M. Nigg and W. Herzog (eds) *Biomechanics of the Musculo-skeletal System* (3rd edn), Hoboken, NJ: John Wiley & Sons, pp. 107–126.

Fuller, C.W., Ashton, T., Brooks, J.H.M., Cancea, R.J., Hall, J. and Kemp, S.P.T. (2010) Injury risks associated with tackling in rugby union. *British Journal of Sports Medicine, 44*, 159–167.

Fuller, C.W., Dick, R.W., Corlette, J. and Schmalz, R. (2007) Comparison of the incidence, nature and cause of injuries sustained on grass and new generation artificial turf by male and female football players. Part 1: Match injuries. *British Journal of Sports Medicine, 41(Suppl 1)*, i20–i26.

Furrer, M., Erhart, S., Frutiger, A., Bereiter, H., Leutenegger, A. and Ruedi, T. (1995) Severe skiing injuries: a retrospective analysis of 361 patients including mechanism of trauma, severity of injury, and mortality. *Journal of Trauma, 39*, 737–741.

Greene, P.R. and McMahon, T.A. (1984) 'Reflex stiffness of man's anti-gravity muscles during kneebends while carrying extra weights', in E.C. Frederick (ed.) *Sports Shoes and Playing Surfaces*, Champaign, IL: Human Kinetics, pp. 119–137.

Guskiewicz, K.M., McCrea, M., Marshall, S.W., Cantu, R.C., Randolph, C., Barr, W., Onate, J.A. and Kelly, J.P. (2003) Cumulative effects associated with recurrent concussion in collegiate football players. *JAMA: The Journal of the American Medical Association*, *290*, 2549–2555.

Hackam, D.J., Kreller, M. and Pearl, R.H. (1999) Snow-related recreational injuries in children: assessment of morbidity and management strategies. *Journal of Pediatric Surgery*, *34*, 65–68.

Hawkins, D. (1993) 'Ligament biomechanics', in M.D. Grabiner (ed.) *Current Issues in Biomechanics*, Champaign, IL: Human Kinetics, pp. 123–150.

Hawkins, D. and Metheny, J. (2001) Overuse injuries in youth sports: biomechanical considerations. *Medicine & Science in Sports & Exercise*, *33*, 1701–1707.

Henning, C.E., Griffis, N.D., Vequist, S.W., Yearout, K.M. and Decker, K.A. (1994) 'Sport-specific knee injuries', in P.A.F.H. Renström (ed.) *Clinical Practice of Sports Injury: Prevention and Care*, London: Blackwell Scientific, pp. 164–178.

Holden, J.P. and Cavanagh, P.R. (1991) The free moment of ground reaction in distance running and its changes with pronation. *Journal of Biomechanics*, *24*, 887–889, 891–897.

Houglum, P.A. (2005) *Therapeutic Exercise for Musculoskeletal Injuries* (2nd edn.). Champaign, IL: Human Kinetics.

Iverson, G.L. (2005) Outcome from mild traumatic brain injury. *Current Opinion in Psychiatry*, *18*, 301–317.

Jacobs, S.J. and Berson, B. (1986) Injuries to runners: a study of entrants to a 10 000 meter race. *American Journal of Sports Medicine*, *14*, 151–155.

Jørgensen, U. and Hølmich, P. (1994) 'Injuries in badminton', in P.A.F.H. Renström (ed.) *Clinical Practice of Sports Injury: Prevention and Care*, London: Blackwell Scientific, pp. 475–485.

Kibler, W.B. and Chandler, T.J. (1993) 'Sport specific screening and testing', in P.A.F.H. Renström (ed.) *Sports Injuries: Basic Principles of Prevention and Care*, London: Blackwell Scientific, pp. 223–241.

Kibler, W.B., Chandler, T.J. and Stracener, E.S. (1992) Musculoskeletal adaptations and injuries due to overtraining. *Exercise and Sport Science Reviews*, *20*, 99–126.

King, K., Davidson, B., Zhou, B.H., Lu, Y. and Solomonow, M. (2009) High magnitude cyclic load triggers inflammatory response in lumbar ligaments. *Clinical Biomechanics*, *24*, 792–798.

Kolitzus, H.J. (1984) 'Functional standards for playing surfaces', in E.C. Frederick (ed.) *Sports Shoes and Playing Surfaces*, Champaign, IL: Human Kinetics, pp. 98–118.

Kubo, K., Kanehisa, H. and Fukunaga, T. (2003) Gender differences in the viscoelastic properties of tendon structures. *European Journal of Applied Physiology*, *88*, 520–526.

Kujala, U.M., Sarna, S. and Kaprio, J. (2005) Cumulative incidence of Achilles tendon rupture and tendinopathy in male former elite athletes. *Clinical Journal of Sport Medicine*, *15*, 133–135.

Kuland, D.N. (1982) *The Injured Athlete*, Philadelphia, PA: Lippincott.

Lambson, R.B., Barnhill, B.S. and Higgins, R.W. (1996) Football cleat design and its effect on anterior cruciate ligament injuries. *The American Journal of Sports Medicine*, *24*, 155–159.

Leadbetter, W.B. (1993) 'Tendon overuse injuries: diagnosis and treatment', in P.A.F.H. Renström (ed.) *Sports Injuries: Basic Principles of Prevention and Care*, London: Blackwell Scientific, pp. 449–476.

Lieberman, D.E., Venkadesan, M., Werbel, W.A., Daoud, A.I., D'Andrea, S., Davis, I.S., Mang'Eni, R.O. and Pitsiladis, Y. (2010) Foot strike patterns and collision forces in habitually barefoot versus shod runners. *Nature*, *463*, 531–535.

Livesay, G.A., Reda, D.R. and Nauman, E.A. (2006) Peak torque and rotational stiffness developed at the shoe–surface interface. *The American Journal of Sports Medicine*, *34*, 415–422.

Lyman, S., Fleisig, G.S., Andrews, J.R. and Osinski, E.D. (2002) Effect of pitch type, pitch count, and pitching mechanics on risk of elbow and shoulder pain in youth baseball pitchers. *The American Journal of Sports Medicine*, *30*, 463–468.

Lyman, S., Fleisig, G.S., Waterbor, J.W., Funkhouser, E.M., Pulley, L., Andrews, J.R., Osinski, E.D. and Roseman, J.M. (2001) Longitudinal study of elbow and shoulder pain in youth baseball pitchers. *Medicine & Science in Sports & Exercise*, *33*, 1803–1810.

MacDougall, J.D., Webber, C.E., Martin, J., Ormerod, S., Chesley, A., Younglai, E.V., Gordon, C.L. and Blimkie, C.J. (1992) Relationship among running mileage, bone density, and serum testosterone in male runners. *Journal of Applied Physiology*, *73*, 1165–1170.

Macera, C.A., Pate, R.R., Powell, K.E., Jackson, K.L, Kendrick, J.S. and Kraven, T.E. (1989) Predicting lower extremity injuries among habitual runners. *Archives of International Medicine*, *49*, 2565–2568.

MacIntyre, J. and Lloyd-Smith, R. (1993) 'Overuse running injuries', in P.A.F.H. Renström (ed.) *Sports Injuries: Basic Principles of Prevention and Care*, London: Blackwell Scientific, pp. 139–160.

Mallon, W.J. and Hawkins, R.J. (1994) 'Shoulder injuries', in P.A.F.H. Renström (ed.) *Clinical Practice of Sports Injury: Prevention and Care*, London: Blackwell Scientific, pp. 27–45.

McCrory, P. (2011) Sports concussion and the risk of chronic neurological impairment. *Clinical Journal of Sport Medicine*, *21*, 6–12.

McDermott, M. and Reilly, T. (1992) 'Common injuries in track and field athletics – 1. Racing and jumping', in T. Reilly (ed.) *Sports Fitness and Sports Injuries*, London: Wolfe, pp. 135–144.

McIntosh, A.S. and Janda, D. (2003) Evaluation of cricket helmet performance and comparison with baseball and ice hockey helmets. *British Journal of Sports Medicine*, *37*, 325–330.

McIntosh, A.S. and McCrory, P. (2005) Preventing head and neck injury. *British Journal of Sports Medicine*, *39*, 314–318.

McKay, G.D., Goldie, P.A., Payne, W.R. and Oakes, B.W. (2001) Ankle injuries in basketball: injury rate and risk factors. *British Journal of Sports Medicine*, *35*, 103–108.

McLean, S.G. (2008) The ACL injury enigma: we can't prevent what we don't understand. *Journal of Athletic Training*, *43*, 538.

McLean, S.G., Andrish, J.T. and van den Bogert, A.J. (2005) Comment on: Aggressive quadriceps loading can induce noncontact anterior cruciate ligament injury. *American Journal of Sports Medicine*, *33*, 1106.

Meeuwisse, W.H., Tyreman, H., Hagel, B. and Emery, C. (2007) A dynamic model of etiology in sport injury: the recursive nature of risk and causation. *Clinical Journal of Sport Medicine*, *17*, 215–219.

Meyers, J.F. (1993) The growing athlete, in P.A.F.H. Renström (ed) *Sports Injuries: Basic Principles of Prevention and Care*, London: Blackwell Scientific, pp. 178–193.

Meyers, M.C. and Barnhill, B.S. (2004) Incidence, causes, and severity of high school football injuries on field turf versus natural grass. *The American Journal of Sports Medicine*, *32*, 1626–1638.

Milburn, P.D. (1990) The kinetics of rugby union scrummaging. *Journal of Sports Sciences*, *8*, 47–60.

Mills, N. (2006) 'Protective equipment: shin guards and gloves', in R.M. Bartlett, C. Gratton and C.G. Rolf (eds) *Encyclopedia of International Sports Studies*, London: Routledge, pp. 1081–1183.

Mills, N. and Gilchrist, A. (2006) Bicycle helmet design. *Proceedings of the Institution of Mechanical Engineers, Part L: Journal of Materials: Design and Applications*, *220*, 167–180.

Milner, C.E., Davis, I.S. and Hamill, J. (2006) Free moment as a predictor of tibial stress fracture in distance runners. *Journal of Biomechanics*, *39*, 2819–2825.

Nigg, B.M. (1986a) 'Biomechanical aspects of running', in B.M. Nigg (ed.) *Biomechanics of Running Shoes*, Champaign, IL: Human Kinetics, pp. 1–26.

Nigg, B.M. (1986b) 'Some comments for runners', in B.M. Nigg (ed.) *Biomechanics of Running Shoes*, Champaign, IL: Human Kinetics, pp. 161–165.

Nigg, B.M. (1993) 'Excessive loads and sports-injury mechanisms', in P.A.F.H. Renström (ed) *Sports Injuries: Basic Principles of Prevention and Care*, London: Blackwell Scientific, pp. 107–119.

Nigg, B.M. and Cole, G. (1991) The effect of midsole hardness on internal forces in the human foot during running, *Second IOC World Congress on Sport Sciences*, Barcelona: COOB, pp. 118–119.

Nigg, B.M. and Grimston, S.K. (1999) 'Bone', in B.M. Nigg and W. Herzog (eds) *Biomechanics of the Musculo-skeletal System* (2nd edn), Hoboken, NJ: John Wiley & Sons, pp. 64–85.

Nigg, B.M. and Herzog, W. (2007) *Biomechanics of the Musculo-skeletal System* (3rd edn), Hoboken, NJ: John Wiley & Sons.

Nigg, B.M. and Yeadon, M.R. (1987) Biomechanical aspects of playing surfaces. *Journal of Sports Sciences*, *5*, 117–145.

Nirschl, R.P. and Sobel, J. (1994) 'Injuries in tennis', in P.A.F.H. Renström (ed.) *Clinical Practice of Sports Injury: Prevention and Care*, London: Blackwell Scientific, pp. 460–474.

Olsen, O.E., Myklebust, G., Engebretsen, L. and Bahr, R. (2004) Injury mechanisms for anterior cruciate ligament injuries in team handball. *The American Journal of Sports Medicine*, *32*, 1002–1012.

Olsen, S.J., Fleisig, G.S., Dun, S., Loftice, J. and Andrews, J.R. (2006) Risk factors for shoulder and elbow injuries in adolescent baseball pitchers. *The American Journal of Sports Medicine*, *34*, 905–912.

O'Neill, D.F. (2003) Wrist injuries in guarded versus unguarded first time snowboarders. *Clinical Orthopedics*, *409*, 91–95.

O'Neill, T. (1992) 'Soccer injuries', in T. Reilly (ed.) *Sports Fitness and Sports Injury*, London: Wolfe, pp. 127–132.

Orchard, J., James, T., Kountouris, A. and Portus, M.R. (2010) Changes to injury profile (and recommended cricket injury definitions) based on the increased frequency of Twenty20 cricket matches. *Open Access Journal of Sports Medicine*, *1*, 63–76.

Orchard, J., Marsden, J. and Lord, S. (1997) Preseason hamstring weakness associated with hamstring muscle injury in Australian footballers. *American Journal of Sports Medicine*, *25*, 81–85.

Orchard, J. and Powell, J.W. (2003) Risk of knee and ankle sprains under various weather conditions in American football. *Medicine & Science in Sports & Exercise*, *35*, 1118–1123.

Ottaviani, R.A., Ashton-Miller, J.A., Kothari, S.U. and Wojtys, E.M. (1995) Basketball shoe height and the maximal muscular resistance to applied ankle inversion and eversion moments. *The American Journal of Sports Medicine*, *23*, 418–423.

Pratt, D.J. (1989) Mechanisms of shock attenuation via the lower extremity during running. *Clinical Biomechanics*, *4*, 51–57.

Prentice, W.E. (2006) *Arnheim's Principles of Athletic Training: A Competency-based Approach*. New York: McGraw-Hill.

Quatman, C.E. and Hewett, T.E. (2009) The anterior cruciate ligament injury controversy: Is valgus collapse a sex-specific mechanism? *British Journal of Sports Medicine*, *43*, 328–335.

Rabadi, M.H. and Jordan, B.D. (2001) The cumulative effect of repetitive concussion in sports. *Clinical Journal of Sport Medicine*, *11*, 194–198.

Ranson, C.A., Kerslake, R.W., Burnett, A.F., Batt, M.E. and Abdi, S. (2005) Magnetic resonance imaging of the lumbar spine in asymptomatic professional fast bowlers in cricket.
Journal of Bone and Joint Surgery, 87-B, 1111–1116.

Rauch, F., Bailey, D.A., Baxter-Jones, A., Mirwald, R. and Faulkner, R. (2004) The muscle-bone
unit during the pubertal growth spurt. *Bone, 34,* 771–775.

Reilly, T. (1992) 'Track and field – 2. The throws', in T. Reilly, (ed.) *Sports Fitness and Sports
Injuries,* London: Wolfe, pp. 145–151.

Reinschmidt, C., van den Bogert, A.J., Murphy, N., Lundberg, A. and Nigg, B.M. (1997)
Tibiocalcaneal motion during running, measured with external and bone markers. *Clinical
Biomechanics, 12,* 8–16.

Rovere, G.D. and Nichols, A.W. (1985) Frequency, associated factors, and treatment of breaststroker's knee in competitive swimmers. *The American Journal of Sports Medicine, 13,*
99–104.

Saw, R., Dennis, R.J., Bentley, D. and Farhart, P. (2011) Throwing workload and injury risk in
elite cricketers. *British Journal of Sports Medicine, 45,* 805–808.

Seeley, R.R., Stephens, T.D. and Tate, P. (2006) *Anatomy & Physiology* (7th edn), Boston, MA:
McGraw-Hill.

Segesser, B. and Nigg, B.M. (1993) Sport shoe construction: orthopaedic and biomechanical
concepts, in P.A.F.H. Renström (ed.) *Sports Injuries: Basic Principles of Prevention and Care,*
London: Blackwell Scientific, pp. 398–416.

Shelbourne, K.D., Gray, T. and Haro, M. (2009) Incidence of subsequent injury to either knee
within 5 years after ACL reconstruction with patellar tendon autograft. *American Journal of
Sports Medicine, 37,* 246–251.

Shimokochi, Y. and Shultz, S.J. (2008) Mechanisms of noncontact anterior cruciate ligament
injury. *Journal of Athletic Training, 43,* 396–408.

Sosin, D.M., Sniezek, J.E. and Thurman, D.J. (1991) Incidence of mild and moderate brain
injury in the United States. *Brain Injury, 10,* 47–54.

Sports Council (1978 and 1984) *Specification for Artificial Sports Surfaces – parts 1–3,* London:
The Sports Council.

Stacoff, A. and Luethi, S.M. (1986) 'Special aspects of shoe construction and foot anatomy', in
B.M. Nigg (ed.) *Biomechanics of Running Shoes,* Champaign, IL: Human Kinetics, pp.
117–137.

Stanish, W.D. and McVicar, S.F. (1993) 'Flexibility in injury prevention', in P.A.F.H. Renström
(ed.) *Sports Injuries: Basic Principles of Prevention and Care,* London: Blackwell Scientific,
pp. 262–276.

Stretch, R.A., Bartlett, R. and Davids, K. (2000) A review of batting in men's cricket. *Journal of
Sports Science, 18,* 931–949.

Taunton, J.E. (1993) 'Training errors', in P.A.F.H. Renström (ed.) *Sports Injuries: Basic Principles
of Prevention and Care,* London: Blackwell Scientific, pp. 205–212.

Taunton, J.E., Ryan, M.B., Clement, D.B., McKenzie, D.C., Lloyd-Smith, D.R. and Zumbo,
B.D. (2002) A retrospective case-control analysis of 2002 running injuries. *British Journal of
Sports Medicine, 36,* 95–101.

Tipp, G. and Watson, V.J. (1982) *Polymeric Surfaces for Sport and Recreation,* London: Applied
Science.

Tucker, C. (1990) *The Mechanics of Sports Injuries: an Osteopathic Approach,* Oxford: Blackwell.

van Mechelen, W., Hlobil, H. and Kemper, H.C.G. (1992) Incidence, severity, aetiology and
prevention of sports injuries: A review of concepts. *Sports Medicine,, 14,* 82–99.

Verdejo, R. and Mills, N.J. (2004) Heel–shoe interactions and the durability of EVA foam
running-shoe midsoles. *Journal of Biomechanics, 37,* 1379–1386.

Williams, K.R. (1993) 'Biomechanics of distance running', in M.D. Grabiner (ed.) *Current Issues in Biomechanics*, Champaign, IL: Human Kinetics, pp. 3–31.

Yu, B., Lin, C.F. and Garrett, W.E. (2006) Lower extremity biomechanics during the landing of a stop-jump task. *Clinical Biomechanics*, *21*, 297–305.

FURTHER READING

Hong, Y. and Bartlett, R. (2008) *Routledge Handbook of Biomechanics and Human Movement Science*, London: Routledge. Section IV, 'Engineering technology and equipment design', contains interesting studies of the biomechanical aspects of footwear, the study of sports surfaces and the relationship between energy and performance in sports equipment. Section VI 'Injury, orthopaedics and rehabilitation', contains studies on specific injuries to the upper and lower extremity as well as an interesting paper on biomechanical methods for *in vivo* study for injury prevention.

Ujihashi, S. and Haake, S. (2002) *The Engineering of Sport 4*, Malden, MA: Blackwell Science. Section 2, 'Materials', has many sophisticated mechanical studies of sporting materials including vibration in cricket bats, the footwear–surface interface for different sole constructions, as well as many other interesting studies. Section 3, 'Impact,' also has further interesting information about shock attenuation of sports surfaces, as well as the effect of tennis court surfaces on playing performance.

4 Calculating the loads on the body

Roger Bartlett and Melanie Bussey

Knowledge assumed
Basic understanding of
algebra
Basic understanding of
geometry
Familiarity with Newton's laws
of motion

INTRODUCTION – ESTIMATING FORCES IN THE MUSCULOSKELETAL SYSTEM

BOX 4.1 LEARNING OUTCOMES

After reading this chapter you should be able to:

- understand and evaluate simplifications made in 'inverse dynamics modelling'
- explain the terms in the equations for calculating joint reaction forces and moments for single segments, and for a segment chain, in planar motions
- understand how multiple-segment systems can be analysed to calculate joint reaction forces and moments
- appreciate the difficulties of calculating the forces in muscles and ligaments arising from the indeterminacy (or redundancy) problem (too few equations to solve for the number of unknowns)
- describe and compare the various approaches to solving the indeterminacy problem
- understand the method of inverse optimisation, and evaluate the various cost functions used
- appreciate the uses and limitations of electromyography (EMG) in estimating muscle force.

This chapter is intended to provide an understanding of how the forces in the musculoskeletal system can be estimated. To understand injury or to correct movement technique faults it is important to know what muscles are doing. In particular, we want to know about the timing of muscle contractions, the amount of force generated, and the power of the contraction. Our problem is that these structures are internal to the body and, at present, technology limits our direct measures to externally applied forces. Because we, as yet, have no way to measure forces internally in the human body we must determine these forces indirectly from the kinematics of the movement and the anthropometrical and inertial properties of the moving body. This process of determining the joint and muscle forces that act to create a given movement from the measured kinematics of the movement is called inverse dynamics (Figure 4.1). The method of inverse dynamics is a crucial first step towards estimating the forces in muscles and ligaments and establishing injury mechanisms. For the sports biomechanist, an insight into the musculoskeletal dynamics that generate the observed characteristics of sports movements is also vital for a full understanding of those movements. Inverse dynamics variables are derived using the equations of motion (Newton–Euler equations) from Newton's second law of motion where the resultant force is partitioned into known and unknown forces (Figure 4.1). These equations describe the behaviour of a mathematical model of the limb called a link-segment model. Because of the complexity of calculating forces and moments of force (also known as a torque) in three dimensions, the examples considered in this chapter will be two-dimensional, or planar (for a consideration of the more general three-dimensional, or spatial, case, see Robertson *et al.*, 2004 or Winter, 2005).

Figure 4.1 A schematic representation of the inverse dynamics approach (Buchanan *et al.*, 2004). We begin with motion tracking specifically tracking markers on adjacent limb segments. The data are used to calculate relative position and orientation of the segments, and from these the joint angles are calculated. We then differentiate these data to obtain velocities and accelerations. The accelerations and force plate recordings are then input to the equations of motion to compute the corresponding joint reaction forces and moments. We may estimate muscle forces by including musculoskeletal geometry but partitioning these forces can be complex.

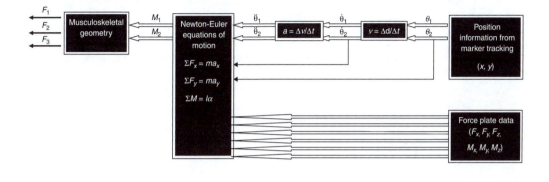

THE BASICS OF INVERSE DYNAMICS

When conducting an inverse dynamics analysis a picture is worth a thousand words. A free body diagram can make it easier to understand the forces, and torques or moments, acting on a system and how they may work in relation to one another. We also use free body diagrams to suggest the proper theory to apply in order to find the solution to a problem. When constructing free body diagrams there are some simple guidelines to follow that will help ensure all relevant information is included, irrelevant information is excluded and the appropriate assumptions are made.

First it helps to divide the body into kinetic chains, and then divide those chains into segments. Convention dictates that we start our analysis with the terminal segment of the chain. This is because the terminal end is closest to the direct force measures (i.e. ground reaction force for foot or hand reaction force for hand). Before we begin, we must acknowledge that this model is based on several assumptions. Our first assumption is that each segment is a rigid body with its mass concentrated at the centre of mass. A rigid body cannot be deformed and has no moving parts; this is a convenient assumption because it means that we can also assume the mass moment of inertia, length and centre of mass of each segment remains constant throughout a movement. Second, we assume that each joint is a rotationally frictionless pin or hinge joint. Because the analysis is two dimensional, rotation can only take place about a single axis orthogonal to the plane of motion. Third, we assume air friction is minimal. And finally, we assume that joint forces and moments are equal and opposite about a joint. Of course we know that none of these assumptions is completely accurate in the case of the human body, but the assumptions make the mathematics easier and the estimates made from these types of models are just as informative, although not completely correct.

We begin with a sketch of the free body of interest and include only as much detail as necessary. Free body diagrams are so named because the diagram isolates the body of interest from all other interacting sources to focus on one specific segment at a time. All external contacts, constraints, and body forces are indicated by vector arrows labelled with appropriate descriptions (Figure 4.2). The arrows show the direction and scale magnitude of the various forces. Where possible, the arrows should indicate the point of

Figure 4.2 Creating and interpreting a free body diagram: (a) diving board example from Chapter 1; (b) resulting free body diagram; (c) right-hand rule.

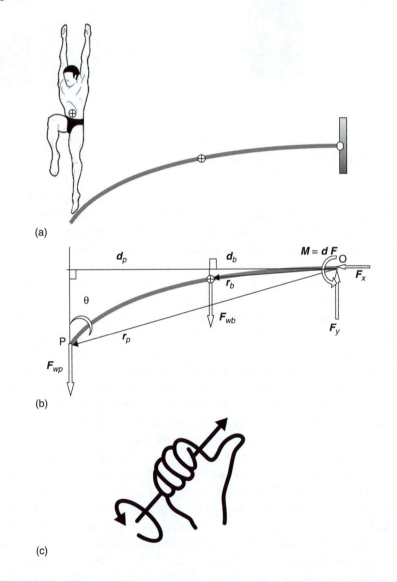

application of the force. If the chain is a closed-chain, meaning that it is in contact with the ground, then the ground reaction forces must be known (i.e. measured with an external measurement device). If we do not know the external forces we must begin with the segment at the proximal end of the chain.

A model will generally include several types of forces. Gravitational forces will act downward through the centre of mass of each segment and are equal to the product of the mass of the segment and acceleration due to gravity (9.81 m/s^2) (Figure 4.2). Ground reaction forces are external forces that may be measured directly and usually act on a point called the centre of pressure. Muscle forces in a model are typically expressed in terms of a net muscle force (agonist and antagonist), their actions expressed by a single force arrow. By combining muscle actions into a net muscle force we reduce the number of force variables in our equations and also reduce the number of arrows in the free body diagram, which tends to keep the diagrams and mathematics much clearer. Forces from ligaments are calculated for extreme ranges of motion and they will subtract or add to the net muscle force. Finally, joint reaction forces are calculated when individual segments within a kinetic chain are examined in isolation from one another. Because each segment is separated from the next by a joint, a part of the puzzle is missing: how one joint affects the other. According to Newton's third law of motion, for every action there is an equal and opposite reaction, so we apply the appropriate reaction force to each joint based on the action of the distal segment. For a general segment, there will be a reaction force at each end, one from the next most distal segment and one from the next most proximal segment.

In a two-dimensional or planar analysis a segment or object has three degrees of freedom, two translational degrees (horizontal and vertical) and one rotational degree (orthogonal to the translational plane). Thus, three equations of motion can be written for each segment in the kinetic chain $\Sigma F_x = m\,a_x$, $\Sigma F_y = m\,a_y$, $\Sigma M = I\,\alpha$. The equations of motion are derived from Newton's second law. The first two are the translational form, which states that the sum (Σ) of all forces (F) acting on the segment is equal to its mass (m) times its acceleration (a). The third equation is derived from the angular analogue of Newton's second law stating that the sum (Σ) of all moments of force (M) acting on a segment is equal to the mass moment of inertia (I) of the segment times its angular acceleration (α). This third equation may also be written from the Euler expression, where $M = dL/dt$ ($M\,\Delta t = I\,\Delta\omega$) using the time ($t$) derivative ($d/dt$) of angular momentum ($L$), which is equivalent to the mass moment of inertia (I) times the change in angular velocity ($\Delta\omega$). The information required to solve these equations includes:

- the linear velocity (V) and acceleration (a) of the centre of mass of each segment relative to a global inertial reference frame;
- the angular position (θ), velocity (ω) and acceleration (α) of each segment relative to a global inertial reference;
- the location of the centre of mass, the mass (m) and mass moment of inertia (I) of each segment relative to the segment's centre of mass (Siegler and Wen, 1997).

Once we have all the necessary data we can solve the equations for the unknown forces. Note the sum symbol (Σ) on the left side of the equation. This means that each equation may combine many forces and moments but each should have only one unknown net force or moment to solve for. Unfortunately, because we have many muscles acting on a joint or segment we often end up with more than three unknowns. When you have more unknowns than equations to solve them you face the problem called indeterminacy. We deal with this problem later in the chapter, but essentially we must reduce the number of unknowns or increase the number of equations. There are several methods available to reduce the number of unknowns, such as: calculating joint reaction forces; measuring some of the muscle forces directly with transducers; or grouping muscles that have similar joint actions (i.e. reduction, optimisation or direct measures). We could, alternatively, increase the number of equations by using an inverse optimisation approach, as discussed later in the chapter.

Another problem raised from summing many forces and moments is that of keeping track of the pluses and minuses in your free body diagram. With regard to the direction of a force or moment, most biomechanists adhere to the right-hand rule. With the right-hand rule forces acting upward or toward the right are considered positive and those acting downward or to the left are negative. With moments we must determine the direction of the moment vector. The moment of a force about a point acts in a direction that is orthogonal to the plane defined by the point of rotation (O), the point of application of force (P) and the force vector (F) (Figure 4.2(b)). Because the moment must act orthogonal to the plane of points of interest the only options for rotation or bending are clockwise or counterclockwise to that plane. The direction of a moment is specified using the 'right-hand rule' where the fingers of the right hand are curled such that they follow the sense of rotation (if the force could rotate about the point, O), the thumb then points along the moment axis (Figure 4.2(c)). More specifically, if we direct our fingers in the direction of the moment arm r such that we can then curl them to the direction of F, then the thumb points in the direction of the moment vector. Using our examples in Figure 4.2, the moment of the diver is acting to bend the board in a counterclockwise direction. Based on the right-hand rule convention, counterclockwise moments are considered positive and clockwise moments are considered to be negative. Keeping an accurate record of positive and negative signs is of the utmost importance particularly when dealing with multi-segment systems. If you adhere to the sign conventions of your free body diagram you should not have a problem.

In the following sections we will go through several examples of inverse dynamics analyses of increasing complexity from a static single segment to more complex segment chains. We will begin by considering single body segments: first a static, and then a dynamic, single muscle example, then the same segment but with several muscles. We will progress to a two-segment kinetic chain, and then look, in principle, at how we can extend the procedure to the whole human musculoskeletal system, which contains multiple-segment chains. At all stages, the simplifications and assumptions involved will be highlighted. We will also discuss further the issues of indeterminacy and optimisation.

Example 1 – Static joint and muscle forces for a single segment with one muscle

Beginning with a static example is easiest because the system is in equilibrium. Static equilibrium defines the state in which the sum of the forces and the sum of the moments acting on the system are zero. A system in mechanical equilibrium is not accelerating linearly or rotationally but technically might still experience movement at a constant linear velocity. The example to be considered here is that of a single muscle holding a combined segment, consisting of the forearm and hand, in a steady horizontal position (Figure 4.3(a)). A free body diagram (Figure 4.3(b)) shows the biomechanical system of interest, here the forearm-hand segment, isolated from the surrounding world. The effects of those surroundings are represented on the free body diagram as force vectors. In this example these are: the weight of the forearm and hand ($F_g = m\,g$), at their centre of mass, the muscle force (F_m) and the x- and y-components of the joint force (Fj_x, Fj_y), producing the three force equations of 4.1.

$$Fj_x = F_m \cos\varphi$$
$$Fj_y = -F_m \sin\varphi + F_g \qquad (4.1)$$
$$F_m = r\,F_g\,/(r_m \sin\varphi)$$

Applying the vector equations of static force (F) and moment (M) equilibrium ($\Sigma F = 0$; $\Sigma M = 0$), produces the scalar equations of 4.2.

$$Fj_x - F_m \cos\varphi = 0$$
$$Fj_y + F_m \sin\varphi - F_g = 0 \qquad (4.2)$$
$$r_m F_m \sin\varphi - r\,F_g = 0$$

The, as yet unknown, joint force components are shown, by convention, as positive in the x- and y-component directions. As F_m has an x-component to the left (negative as $\varphi<90°$) then Fj_x is positive (to the right); as F_m will be shown in the example below to have a y-component upwards (positive) that is larger than the weight downwards (negative), then Fj_y will be downwards (negative). The forces will form a vector polygon (as in Figure 4.3(c)). The muscle force and joint force components in equations 4.2 can be calculated from kinematic measurements if the segment mass (m), the position (r) of its mass centre, the muscle moment arm (r_m), and angle of pull (φ) are known. Some of these values can be estimated experimentally and the rest obtained from standard anthropometric data (see, for example, Bartlett, 2007). Values that are known are as follows: m = 2.0 kg, r = 0.14 m, r_m = 0.05 m and $\varphi = 80°$.

If the forearm-hand segment is stationary and horizontal as in Figure 4.3(a): (i) calculate the muscle force and the components of the joint force using equations 4.1; (ii) verify the answer using a force polygon.

Figure 4.3 Static forces acting on a single segment with one muscle acting: (a) the forearm and hand segment showing centre of mass (COM); (b) the free body diagram representing the forearm and hand; (c) the vector polygon of forces acting on the segment. Note that Fj_y is acting downwards, not upwards as we predicted in our free body diagram.

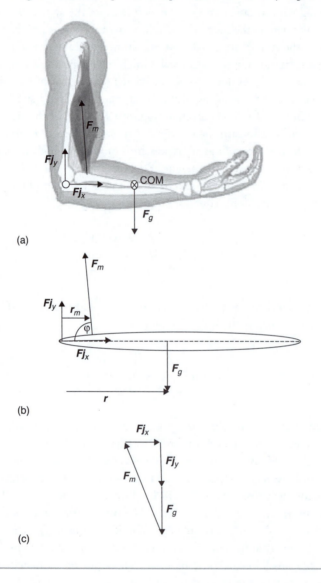

(a)

(b)

(c)

$$F_m = r \, F_g / (r_m \sin\varphi)$$

Therefore:

$$F_m = 0.14 \text{ m} \times 2 \text{ kg} \times 9.81 \text{ m/s}^2 / (0.05 \text{ m} \times \sin 80°)$$
$$= 2.75 / (0.05 \times 0.9848) \text{ N}$$
$$= 55.8 \text{ N}$$
$$Fj_x = F_m \cos\varphi$$

Therefore:

$$Fj_x = 55.8 \text{ N} \times \cos 80° = 55.8 \text{ N} \times 0.1736$$
$$= 9.69 \text{ N}$$
$$Fj_y = -F_m \sin\varphi + F_g$$

Therefore:

$$Fj_y = -55.8 \text{ N} \times \sin 80° + 2 \text{ kg} \times 9.81 \text{ m/s}^2$$
$$= (-55.8 \times 0.9848 + 2 \times 9.81) \text{ N}$$
$$= -35.2 \text{ N}$$

(Note: as this value is negative, this means that Fj_y acts downwards, not upwards as was assumed.)

The vector polygon for these forces is shown in Figure 4.3(c). This polygon is closed as the forces are in equilibrium. The polygon is a graphical expression of the vector equation:

$$0 = \Sigma F = F_m + Fj + F_g = F_m + Fj_x + Fj_y + F_g$$

Example 2 – Dynamic joint and muscle forces for a single segment with one muscle

Now we move to a more complex example where the segment is undergoing acceleration either linearly or rotationally or both. The example to be considered here is that of a single muscle holding a combined segment, consisting of the forearm and hand, in an instantaneously horizontal position as it rotates with an angular acceleration (α) and angular velocity (ω). Here, the forearm and hand are assumed to move together; that is, the two segments behave as a rigid body (this is sometimes called a quasi-rigid body; from the Latin word quasi meaning 'as if' or 'almost'). The free body diagram (Figure 4.4(a)) again shows the forearm-hand segment isolated from the surrounding world, but with the direction of its angular velocity and acceleration shown; the convention that these are positive counterclockwise is used here. The vector equations of the linear and rotational second laws of motion (see, for example, Bartlett, 2007) are: for force ($F = m\,a$), and for the moment ($M = I_o\,\alpha$), where m is the mass of the segment, a is the linear acceleration vector of the mass centre, I_o is the moment of inertia about the joint axis of rotation, assumed to be at O and α is the angular acceleration of the segment. Applying these produces the vector component equations of 4.3.

$$Fj_x - F_m \cos\theta = m\,a_x$$
$$Fj_y + F_m \sin\theta - m\,g = m\,a_y \tag{4.3}$$
$$r_m \times F_m + r \times (m\,g) = I_o\,\alpha$$

Figure 4.4 Dynamic forces on a single segment with one muscle: (a) the free body diagram; (b) including tangential and centripetal acceleration components.

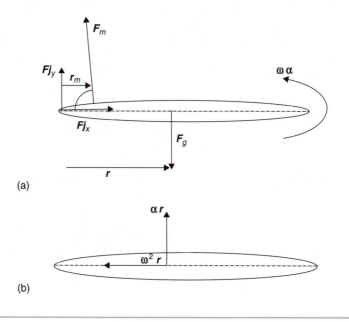

(a)

(b)

In the third of these equations, the muscle moment is the vector cross product of the muscle moment arm and the muscle force. To convert these equations into scalar equations to calculate the three unknown forces, we must use the magnitudes and directions of all forces and moment arms. The two moment arms are positive (left to right) for this example; F_m has an x-component to the left (negative) and a y-component upwards (positive); g is downwards (negative). To calculate the linear acceleration components we note (see Bartlett, 2007) that this segment rotating about a fixed axis (O) with an angular acceleration, α, and angular velocity, ω, has a tangential component of acceleration, magnitude αr, and a centripetal component, magnitude $\omega^2 r$, whose directions are as shown in Figure 4.4(b). In this case $a_x = -\omega^2 r$ and $a_y = \alpha r$. The muscle force and joint force components are then obtained from the following equations:

$$Fj_x - F_m \cos\theta = -m\,\omega^2\,r$$
$$Fj_y + F_m \sin\theta - m\,g = m\,\alpha\,r \qquad (4.4)$$
$$r_m\,F_m \sin\theta - r\,m\,g = I_0\,\alpha$$

In addition to the values needed to calculate the three forces in the previous example, we now need to know the angular velocity and acceleration (or the mass centre acceleration components), and the segment's moment of inertia about O. Values that are known are as follows: $m = 2.0$ kg, $r = 0.14$ m, $r_m = 0.05$ m, $\theta = 80$, $\alpha = 1.5$ rad/s^2, $\omega = 2.5$ rad/s and $I_0 = 0.09$ kg/m^2.

If the forearm-hand is instantaneously horizontal, as in Figure 4.4(b), calculate the muscle force and the components of the joint force using equations 4.4.

$$F_m = (r\, m\, g + I_o\, \alpha)/(r_m \sin\theta)$$

Therefore:

$$F_m = (0.14 \text{ m} \times 2 \text{ kg} \times 9.81 \text{ m/s}^2 + 0.09 \text{ kg/m}^2 \times 1.5 \text{ rad/s}^2)/(0.05 \text{ m} \times \sin 80°)$$
$$= 2.88/(0.05 \times 0.9848) \text{ N}$$
$$= 58.5 \text{ N}$$
$$Fj_x = F_m \cos\theta - m\, \omega^2\, r$$

Therefore:

$$Fj_x = 55.8 \text{ N} \times \cos 80° - 2 \text{ kg} \times (2.5 \text{ rad/s})^2 \times 0.14 \text{ m}$$
$$= 55.8 \text{ N} \times 0.1736 - 1.75 \text{ N}$$
$$= 8.41 \text{ N}$$
$$Fj_y = -F_m \sin\theta + m\, g + m\, a\, r$$

Therefore:

$$Fj_y = -55.8 \text{ N} \times \sin 80° + 2 \text{ kg} \times 9.81 \text{ m/s}^2 + 2 \text{ kg} \times 1.5 \text{ rad/s}^2 \times 0.14 \text{ m}$$
$$= (-55.8 \times 0.9848 + 2 \times 9.81 + 0.42) \text{ N}$$
$$= -34.9 \text{ N (again, note that } Fj_y \text{ acts downwards).}$$

Assumptions underlying the above models

The following assumptions were made in arriving at the representation of the forearm-hand segment model in the above examples.

- The motion is planar (two-dimensional) and the muscles exert their pull only in that (the sagittal) plane. The points of insertion and the angles of pull of the muscles are assumed to be known. The muscles are also assumed to pull in straight lines, whereas most do not, owing to bony pulleys, for example. More realistically, each muscle should be represented by a three-dimensional line or curve joining the centroids of its areas of origin and insertion. Even then, anatomical data are generally only precise to about 2 cm, which can lead to large errors in moment arms (Pierrynowski, 1995).
- An inertial (non-accelerating) frame of reference is located at the axis of rotation of the elbow joint, through O. This will not be true, for example, when the elbow is itself rotating about the shoulder, as in many sports movements.
- The combined forearm-hand segment behaves as a rigid body and has a fixed and known mass, length, centre of mass location and moment of inertia throughout the motion to be studied (forearm flexion). This would clearly not be so if the wrist joint

flexed or extended. Also, in impacts, the soft tissue movements are not the same as those of the rigid bone; in such cases, a more complex 'wobbling mass' model may be needed (e.g. Nigg, 1994).

• Only one muscle acted to cause the motion. This is a large, and generally false, assumption that was made to simplify the problem. A more reasonable assumption, made in the next section, is that only the three main elbow flexors contribute to the muscle moment at the elbow joint. Even this assumes no activity in the elbow extensors (triceps brachii and anconeus), wrist and finger extensors (extensores carpi radialis brevis and longus, extensor carpi ulnaris, extensor digitorum and extensor digiti minimi), the wrist and finger flexors (flexores carpi radialis and ulnaris, palmaris longus and flexor digitorum superficialis) and pronator teres and supinator. The validity of some, at least, of these assumptions would require electromyographic (EMG) investigation.

• The assumption that the segment was horizontal was, again, made only to simplify the resulting equations. The solution can be generalised to non-horizontal cases as well.

THE INDETERMINACY PROBLEM

As discussed earlier a problem arises when we have more unknowns than equations to solve them, n equations can only be solved if the number of unknowns does not exceed n. The first question you should be asking is when does this happen, when do we have more unknowns than equations to solve them? The answer is that there can be many instances depending on what motion is being measured and what we want to determine from the inverse dynamics analysis. But generally the problem exists when there are more sources for force production or transfer than we can account for. So, when looking at multi-segment models of gait the problem becomes indeterminate. When both feet are in contact with the ground, we cannot determine how much force can be attributed to each leg, only the total force exerted by both. We also encounter the indeterminacy problem when trying to estimate the forces acting on a single segment when we have many muscles active simultaneously. For example when we introduce a more realistic representation of the muscles acting on the forearm-hand segment in Figure 4.5(a) where we now have three flexors simultaneously active. Applying the equations of static force and moment equilibrium (that is the sum of all the forces equals zero and the sum of all the moments equals zero) now gives:

$$\Sigma F = 0 = F_g + F_p + F_j + F_{bb} + F_b + F_{br}$$
$$\Sigma M = 0 = r_g \times F_g + M_p + r_{bb} \times F_{bb} + r_b \times F_b + r_{br} \times F_{br}$$

(4.5)

where, in the second equation, the muscle moments are the cross products (×) of the muscle moment arms and muscle forces. If, as assumed above, the moment arms (r) of the three muscle forces are known, these two equations contain five independent unknowns. These are the forces in the three flexors, biceps brachii (F_{bb}), brachialis (F_b) and brachioradialis (F_{br}), and the joint contact force, F_j. The fifth force (F_p) is that due to the ligaments and capsule of the joint (and other soft tissues around the joint) and is caused by their passive elasticity; this has an associated moment (M_p). A pair of equations (such as 4.5) is said to be indeterminate as n equations can only be solved if the number of unknowns does not exceed n. In this case, we have two equations and five independent unknowns (F_p and M_p are interrelated). Assuming that the passive force and moment are negligibly small and that the force in brachioradialis is small in comparison with those in the other two agonists would not remove the indeterminacy, as we would still have three unknowns and only two equations. While the system presented is a static example we can generalise the same problem to a dynamic one as in Figure 4.5(b). There

Figure 4.5 Forces on a single segment with more than one muscle: (a) the free body diagram; (b) including tangential and centripetal acceleration components; (c) including the joint reaction forces and moment.

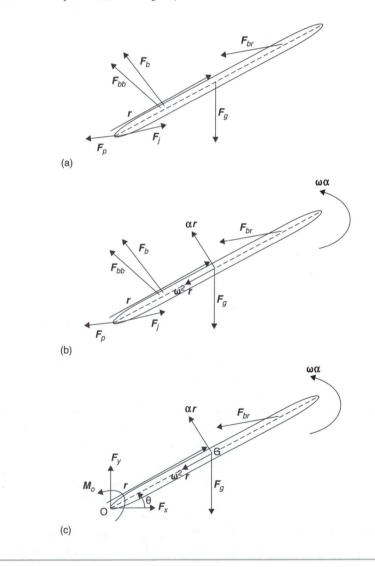

(a)

(b)

(c)

are several ways of tackling this problem of obtaining values of these forces, which are particularly important in understanding injury. We will spend the remainder of the chapter looking at ways around indeterminacy and ways to produce best estimates.

Net forces

Single body segments

One way of tackling the indeterminacy problem is to sidestep it. Instead of trying to calculate the individual muscle forces and the actual force in the joint, we calculate the so-called net forces and moments (sometimes called the joint contact forces and moments). The principle of moments, also known as Varignon's theorem, states that the moment of a force about a point is equal to the sum of the moments of the force's components about a point. Therefore, when we have two or more forces acting on the system we can simplify the calculations by summing the moments or finding the net moment. This principle is important for two-dimensional dynamics because it allows us to reduce the number of unknown variables by replacing the actual muscles by a single muscle group, which exerts a joint reaction moment, M_o (Figure 4.5(c)), equivalent to that exerted by the individual muscles, if we ignore the passive elastic tissues.

As explained earlier, segment diagrams are designed to end at a joint. We use this to our advantage so we can use the concept of joint reaction forces (Fj). The joint reaction force is the representation of the adjacent body segment's action upon the segment under investigation. Using the joint reaction force simplifies our analysis because it is derived from the net force that is transmitted from one segment to the other. The net force may represent many different forces, such as muscles, ligaments and bone-on-bone contacts. It is important to note that the joint reaction force as such is not a real occurrence and cannot be directly measured; it is a mathematical construct, that is, the sum of all the different forces exerted on the segment. We cannot tell from the net forces and moments how the load is shared between the various internal structures of the segment. Thus, this approach does not allow the direct calculation of the actual forces acting on joints and bones and within muscles and other soft tissues. However, the joint reaction forces and moments do provide important information about the dynamics of the movement.

In a two-dimensional example, the joint reaction force can be divided into two components that are normal to the surface (F_y) and a shear component (F_x), in the three-dimensional case there would be a second shear component (F_z). For a single segment example, the joint reaction force components, F_x, F_y, are the components of the force exerted by the adjoining segment (the upper arm) on this segment. Applying the equations of force and moment equilibrium produces scalar equations 4.5. In these equations, a_x and a_y are the x and y component accelerations of the mass centre (G) of the segment, which has mass m, and whose mass centre is a distance, r, from the axis of rotation (O). Please note that we are using scalar equations here because our main interest is finding the magnitude. Direction of forces is implied via subscripts x and y.

$$F_x = m\,a_x$$
$$F_y = m\,a_y + m\,g \qquad (4.6)$$
$$M_0 = m\,k_0^2\alpha + m\,g\,r\cos\theta$$

where $m\,k_o^2\alpha = m\,k_g^2\alpha + mr^2\alpha$, with k_o and k_g being, respectively, the radii of gyration of the segment about O and G respectively. The joint reaction forces and moments in equations 4.5 can be calculated from kinematic measurements of the segment angle (θ) and angular acceleration (α) and the acceleration components of its centre of mass (a_x, a_y) if the required segmental anthropometric data (k, m and r) are known.

Equations 4.6, and their extension to two or more segments and more complex segment chains, are the ones that should be used for inverse dynamics calculations. They involve fewest calculations and thus minimise the propagation of errors owing to measurement inaccuracies in the values of the kinematic and anthropometric variables. Some interesting features of the movement can, however, be revealed by resolving the accelerations in the x and y directions into ones along and tangential to the segment's longitudinal axis (Figure 4.5(b and c)). Then $a_x = -(\omega^2\cos\theta + \alpha\sin\theta)$ and $a_y = (-\omega^2\sin\theta + \alpha\cos\theta)$. Substituting these into equations 4.5 gives:

$$F_x = -\,m\,r\,(\omega^2\cos\theta + \alpha\sin\theta)$$
$$F_y = m\,r\,(-\,\omega^2\sin\theta + \alpha\cos\theta) + m\,g \qquad (4.7)$$
$$M_o = m\,k_o^2\alpha + m\,g\,r\cos\theta$$

The joint reaction force components are both seen to provide centripetal ($r\,\omega^2$) and tangential acceleration ($r\,\alpha$) of the segment, with the y-component also supporting the segment's weight ($m\,g$). The joint reaction moment provides the angular acceleration of the segment (α) and balances the gravitational moment. For a single segment motion, equations 4.7 enable, for example, the contributions of the segment's motion to ground reaction force to be assessed.

For the simplest case, of constant angular velocity, $F_y = -m\,\omega^2\sin\theta + m\,g$; the segment's rotation then causes an increase in the vertical ground reaction force (F_y) above the weight of the sports performer ($m\,g$) if the segment is below the horizontal (that is $0 > \theta > -180°$, so that $\sin\theta$ is negative). A reduction in the vertical ground reaction force occurs if the segment is above the horizontal (that is $0 < \theta < 180°$, so that $\sin\theta$ is positive). This analysis can be extended to consider movements with angular acceleration of the segments. Such an insight is useful, as appropriately timed motions of the free limbs are considered to make an important contribution to the ground contact forces acting on the sports performer, and can aid weighting and unweighting. Examples of this include take-off in the long jump (see also Chapter 6) and high jump.

Segment chains

For non-compound segment chains, such as a single limb, joint reaction forces and moments can be calculated by extending the Newtonian approach of the previous section. For a chain of two segments (Figure 4.6) the result for the joint reaction moments is as follows:

Figure 4.6 Two-segment kinetic chain.

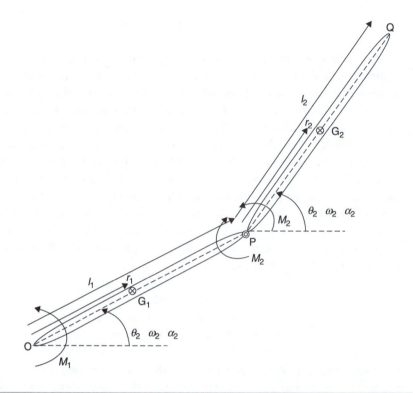

$$M_1 = c_1 \cos\theta_1 + c_2 \cos\theta_2 + c_3 \, \alpha_1 + c_4 \, \alpha_2 + c_5[(\alpha_1 + \alpha_2)\cos(\theta_1 - \theta_2) + (\omega_2^2 - \omega_1^2)\sin(\theta_1 - \theta_2)]$$
$$M_2 = c_2 \cos\theta_2 + c_4 \, \alpha_2 + c_5[\alpha_1 \cos(\theta_1 - \theta_2) - \omega_1^2 \sin(\theta_1 - \theta_2)] \tag{4.8}$$

where the coefficients c_i are combinations of various segmental anthropometric (inertial and geometrical) quantities as follows (see Figure 4.6 for nomenclature): $c_1 = m_1 \, g \, r_1$; $c_2 = m_2 \, g \, r_2$; $c_3 = I_{g1} + m_1 \, r_1^2 + m_2 \, I_1^2$; $c_4 = I_{g2} + m_2 \, r_2^2$; $c_5 = m_2 \, I_1 \, r_2$. The symbols m_1, m_2, I_{g1}, I_{g2} are the masses and moments of inertia about the centres of mass for segments 1 and 2 respectively. The use of a more elegant (but also more complex) mathematical technique, such as the Lagrange Formalism (e.g. Andrews, 1995) or Kane's method (e.g. Kane and Levinson, 1985), is often preferred in advanced biomechanics research. For further reading and examples using Kane's method see Yamaguchi (2001).

A full interpretation of equations 4.8 is much more complex than for the example in the previous section. The first terms on the right side of each equation represent the muscle moments required to raise the segments against gravity, g, as is evident from the coefficients c_1 and c_2. The α_1 and α_2 terms account for the moment required to angularly accelerate the respective segment. The ω^2 terms are components attributed to centripetal force. The exact meaning of the interactions between segmental angular velocities may seem somewhat obscure. It should, however, be obvious that, in such segment chains, statements such as 'flexors flex' or 'muscles generate angular accelerations at the joints they cross' are oversimplified. As evidenced by, for example, the square-bracketed terms in equations 4.8, the joint reaction moment at each joint in the segment chain depends on the kinematics (and some anthropometric properties) of all segments in the chain. It is also well worth noting that these equations are highly non-linear. This has led, among other factors, to many sport biomechanists adopting non-linear dynamical systems theory as a coherent underpinning of their work (see also Chapters 5–7).

Many interesting relationships have been reported between joint reaction moments and muscle action (see, for example, Zajac and Gordon, 1989). For example, in multi-joint movements, all muscles tend to accelerate all joints, not just the ones they span, and the acceleration effect at an unspanned joint can exceed that at a spanned joint (Zajac and Gordon, 1989). This is evident for the acceleration effect of the soleus on the ankle, which it spans, and the knee, which it does not (Figure 4.7(a)). For knee angles of greater than 90° the soleus acts more to accelerate the knee into extension than it does to accelerate the ankle into plantar flexion (i.e. the ratio of knee to ankle acceleration is greater than 1).

Figure 4.7 Two examples of the interesting relationships between joint reaction moments and muscle action: (a) the effect of the soleus muscle on the angular acceleration of the knee relative to ankle; (b) three possible actions of gastrocnemius related to relative moment arm ratios at the knee and ankle (adapted from Zajac and Gordon, 1989).

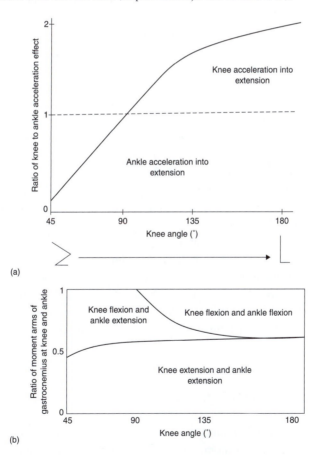

When conducting an analysis of a multi-segment chain, we typically begin with the most distal segment because it reduces the indeterminacy problem. Proximal segments tend to have contact points or joints at either end of the segment, two joints means we have two moments to solve for, which would give us more unknowns than we have equations. Recall we have just three equations maximum. Thus, we begin with the most distal segment; here we have only one joint and thus only one moment to solve for. Once the joint reaction force is calculated at the most distal segment we may then proceed to the adjacent segment. On the adjacent segment we can use our knowledge of Newton's third law to apply the negative joint reaction force of the preceding segment to the distal end of the current segment. With the distal joint force known we can then solve for the unknown joint reaction force at the proximal end. We can continue this iterative procedure up the kinetic chain.

The iterative nature of the Newtonian–Euler method means that the moment at the proximal joint of a multi-segment chain is uniquely determined by the moment at the distal joint. Specifically, the moment at the proximal end of the segment is opposed by an equal and opposite moment at the distal end of the adjacent segment. One underlying assumption when using this method is that the movement of the multi-segment chain is actuated by a series of monoarticular (single joint) muscles. Thus, the sequential approach to calculating the inter-segmental moments does not reflect the potential role of biarticular (two-joint) muscles. A two-joint muscle that applies a direct moment to accelerate joint A into flexion and joint B into extension can actually accelerate joint B into flexion or joint A into extension. This is shown in the three regions (Figure 4.7(b)) for the effects of the gastrocnemius on the knee and ankle joints in standing (Zajac and Gordon, 1989). This shows how the roles played by the gastrocnemius at the knee and ankle joints are affected by both the knee angle and the ratio of the muscle's moment arms at the two joints. The roles normally ascribed to the gastrocnemius – ankle plantar flexion and knee flexion – only apply for moment-arm ratios greater than 0.5 and, depending on this ratio, knee angles between 90° and 135°. The action of the muscle at the ankle depends on whether its plantar flexor torque at the joint exceeds the ankle dorsiflexor action produced by the muscle's knee flexor torque. In practice, the muscle is rarely a major accelerator as it works near the boundaries of the regions in Figure 4.7(b) (Zajac and Gordon, 1989). Inertial coupling (the effects of the acceleration components of one segment on another) also plays an important role in this respect during movement (as in the square-bracketed terms in equations 4.8). As inertia forces can be large in sports movements, such apparently paradoxical phenomena may be common in such movements. Nevertheless, because of the sequential nature of the traditional inverse dynamics method means that including the action of biarticular muscles leads to an indeterminacy problem (Cleather et al., 2010).

SOLVING THE INDETERMINACY PROBLEM

As was shown in the previous section, one way of side stepping the indeterminacy problem is to use net moments and forces such as the reaction forces and moments at the joints. However, as explained above this technique does not allow the researcher to estimate forces from individual structures or understand load sharing among different structures. The biggest obstacle to inverse dynamics analysis is the lack of accurate and non-invasive methods of estimating muscle and ligament forces. It represents a major obstacle to the contribution that biomechanists can make to the prevention and rehabilitation of sports injury. However, many researchers have been working on this problem and have established various other approaches to tackle the indeterminacy problem and enable us to estimate the joint contact force and the forces in the muscles and other soft tissues. Each technique comes with its own set of limitations and issues.

The problem with having multiple muscle groups acting on a joint or segment is that many may act to produce the same outcome. This synergistic function represents a degree of redundancy in the human system and a mathematically indeterminate system. Obviously the easiest way to overcome this indeterminacy problem is to measure muscle forces directly. This may be done using transducers inserted directly into the tendon (e.g. Komi, 1990; Gregor, 1993; Gregor and Abelew, 1994; Powell and Trail, 2004). The value of direct measurement of tendon force is obvious, as are its limitations. Because of calibration difficulties, the few tendons for which it is suitable, and ethical issues, its use in sport is likely to be limited. Yet, direct measures have great value for validating other methods of estimating muscle force, such as the inverse optimisation approach discussed in the following section. Other researchers have tried to estimate muscle force from EMG signals (e.g. Kernozek and Ragan, 2008). However, the use of EMG as an indicator of mechanical function is difficult because EMG directly measures the electrical signal and not the mechanical properties of the muscle contraction. But due to its non-invasiveness it does provide a nice alternative to muscle transducers.

Using the reduction method the forces of the contributing muscles to the joint moment can be estimated by functionally grouping the muscles to make the system determinate (An *et al.*, 1995). In the reduction method the number of unknowns is reduced by grouping muscles with similar functions or muscles with common anatomical insertion points and eliminating muscles that are considered to be inactive. Assumptions about muscle activity must be validated using EMG. Other assumptions might be made, for example, that the passive force is negligible. This might be acceptable for vigorous sporting activities. This model is still quite simple and represents a major limitation of underestimating of the load sharing among muscles crossing a joint. Oversimplified models of this type can lead to errors, which may be particularly problematic when conducting injury research. As an example, in the Chaffin (1969) model a single force vector representation of the back extensor muscles linking the spinous processes 5 cm from the centre of the discs was used, which predicted compressive loads exceeding vertebral end-plate failure tolerances, for lifting loads that could actually be performed with no ill-effect. Thus, an alternative method is required that can allow the researcher to maximise or minimise certain muscle actions to mimic load sharing better without an oversimplification of the functional anatomy of the system.

INVERSE OPTIMISATION

Inverse optimisation is a method of musculoskeletal modelling that resolves resultant joint moments into individual muscle forces by using a mathematical optimisation technique of cost functions and constraint equations. The inverse optimisation technique attempts to apportion the joint reaction moment among the muscles of the joint. The calculation of the joint reaction forces and moments from inverse dynamics serves as one of the inputs for inverse optimisation because the muscle force distribution arrived at must still satisfy the joint reaction moment (M) equation of inverse dynamics. This equation therefore serves as one constraint (known as an 'equality' constraint) on the force distribution. Expressed by:

$$M = \Sigma(Fm_i\, r_i) \tag{4.9}$$

where Fm_i are the muscle forces, r_i are the muscle moment arms and the passive elastic torque or moment (M_p in equation 4.5) has been neglected. If these passive (mostly ligamentous) forces and torques can be neglected, the joint reaction force equation of inverse dynamics can then be used to estimate the joint contact force.

The question now arises of how the forces are apportioned between the relevant muscles. The use of an optimisation algorithm to represent a hypothetical control of movement by the central nervous system has an intuitive appeal. Such an algorithm minimises or maximises a suitable 'cost' or 'objective' function, usually of the form shown in equation 4.10:

$$U(t) = \Sigma(Fm_i\, /\, k_i)^n \tag{4.10}$$

where $U(t)$ is the cost function, k_i are constants (for example, the muscle physiological cross-sectional areas, $pcsa_i$), and n is an index, usually a positive integer. Further constraints may also be imposed on possible muscle force distributions. These are normally in the form of 'inequality' constraints, such as:

$$Fm_i\, /\, pcsa_i < \sigma_{max} \tag{4.11}$$

where σ_{max} is the maximal muscle 'stress'. In equations 4.9 to 4.11, the muscle forces are the variables (these are called the design variables) that are systematically changed until the cost function is optimised while the constraint functions are satisfied.

Many cost functions have been proposed and tested. Some of these have predicted results that do not conform to physiological reality (An et al., 1995). These include linear functions, for which $n = 1$ in equation 4.10. These are mathematically convenient but only predict synergy if the first recruited muscle reaches an enforced inequality constraint, such as maximal tissue 'stress', equation 4.11 (Figure 4.8(a)). This example, for elbow flexion, shows the three elbow flexors to be recruited in sequence, an additional muscle being recruited only when the previous one reaches the enforced inequality constraint. Without that constraint, only one muscle would be recruited.

Different cost functions lead to different muscle activation predictions from the model. The sum of muscle forces has the constants (k_i) in the cost function (equation 4.10) equal to unity. This cost function preferentially recruits the muscle with the largest moment arm, for example the brachioradialis for elbow flexion. Whereas the sum of muscle 'stress' or 'specific tension' (force divided by physiological cross-sectional area (pcsa)), favours muscles with greater products of moment arm and pcsa (as in Figure 4.8(b)), minimising muscle energy, related to the velocity of contraction, favours muscles with lower contraction velocities because of shorter moment arms (for example the tensor fasciae lata, the smallest of the hip abductors). The muscle recruitment patterns predicted from such assumptions have generally been contradicted by EMG evidence.

Figure 4.8 Effects of two different sets of moment arm and physiological cross-sectional area (pcsa) values on muscle activation pattern or recruitment sequence.

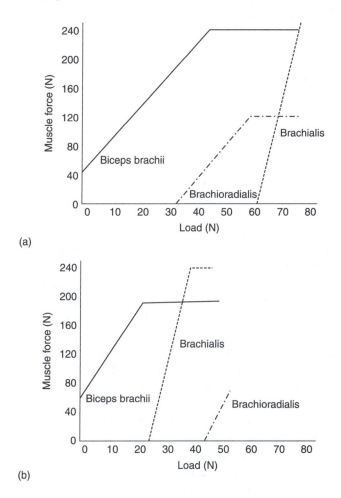

(a)

(b)

There are several energy or metabolic cost models but many require parameters that are extremely difficult to obtain or are completely unavailable and therefore are difficult to use or validate. One example of an energy cost function by Praagman *et al.* (2006) attempted to optimise muscle force by calculating force as a function of energy consumption (E_m) within the muscle. This form of cost function is based on the two major energy-consuming processes within the muscle, the re-uptake of calcium (E_a) and the detachment of the cross bridges (E_f). The metabolic cost is the summed cost over the activated sarcomeres. This calculation requires input variables related to pcsa as well as those related to muscle fibre length (l_f), muscle volume (V) and density (ρ) (equations 4.12–4.14). The re-uptake of calcium is considered to be related to the active state of the muscle and calcium concentration. It can be described by the ratio of muscle force (F_m) to maximal isometric muscle force at optimum length (F_{max0}) multiplied by the normalised force-length $(f_l\,(l_m))$ and force-velocity $(f_v\,(v_m))$ relationships where muscle force at optimal length (F_{max0}) can be described by the product of pcsa and maximal muscle stress (Praagman *et al.*, 2006).

$$\Sigma E_{mi} = \Sigma E_{fi} + E_{ai} \tag{4.12}$$

where, $E_{fi} \sim l_f F_{mi}$. Therefore,

$$E_{fi} \sim l_f F_{mi} = V\frac{F_{mi}}{pcsa_{mi}} = \frac{m}{\rho}\frac{F_{mi}}{pcsa_{mi}} \tag{4.13}$$

and

$$E_{ai} \sim V_a = \frac{m}{\rho}\frac{F_m}{F_{max0}f_l(l_m)\,f_v\,(v_m)} \tag{4.14}$$

Other cost functions have been reported, many of which have been claimed to be related to some physiological property. The first, known as the polynomial criterion, include non-linear functions of muscle force or physiological cross sectional area (pcsa) and instant muscle strength. These types of cost functions are only meaningful if equipped with additional constraints that prevent individual muscle forces from exceeding the physiological range (Rasmussen *et al.*, 2001). Other non-linear functions include the muscle force normalised to either the maximum moment the muscle can produce or the maximum force in the muscle. Siemienski (1992) used a 'soft-saturation' criterion. In this, the muscle stress limit does not have to be applied as a separate constraint, but is contained within the cost function (Figure 4.9(b)), where $U(t) = \Sigma\sqrt{(1 - (Fm_i/(\sigma_{maxi}\,pcsa_i))}$, whereas in Figure 4.9(a), $U(t) = \Sigma\,(Fm_i/pcsa_i)$ and $(Fm_i/pcsa_i) \leq \sigma_{max}$. This criterion produces somewhat more natural results, for instance muscles do not reach their maximum force production while there are other less-loaded muscles that may contribute. This approach has been extended, for example, to the activity of the lower limb muscles in sprinting (Siemienski, 1992).

Minimising neuromuscular activation (Kaufman *et al.*, 1991) has also been considered as a cost function for inverse optimisation. Gracovetsky (1985) proposed that

Figure 4.9 Non-linear cost functions for the three agonist muscles: (a) sum of stresses squared; (b) using soft-saturation point.

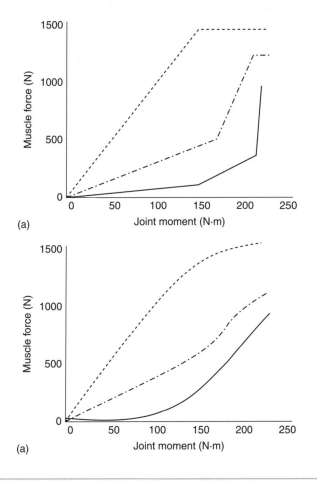

(a)

(a)

optimal locomotion dictates that the stresses at the intervertebral joints of the lumbar spine should be minimised, and that the central nervous system modulates the moments at these joints. Schultz and Anderson (1981) also minimised the compressive stresses in the lumbar spine, with a maximum stress of 1 MPa. However, it has been argued that such minimum compression schemes do not account for antagonist contractions and, therefore, may be less realistic (McGill and Norman, 1993).

The minimum–maximum criterion distributes the collaborative muscle forces in such a way that the maximum relative muscle force is as small as possible (Rasmussen *et al.*, 2001). This may be relevant in reducing muscle fatigue by maximising the muscle endurance time – the maximum duration for which an initially relaxed muscle can maintain the required output (Dul *et al.*, 1984) appears relevant for endurance sports. Crowninshield and Brand (1981a) used minimisation of the cube of muscle stress, which has since been disputed as a measure of endurance time, for example by Denoth

(1988). Dul *et al.* (1984) used a function of muscle force, its maximum value, and the percentage of slow twitch fibres. They showed that the predicted force distribution for muscles with unequal proportions of slow twitch fibres was non-linear. This non-linearity is evident for gastrocnemius (48% slow twitch fibres) and the long or short hamstrings (67% slow twitch fibres) in Figure 4.10(a). It is in clear contrast to, and more realistic than, the linear load sharing predicted even by non-linear muscle stress and normalised muscle force cost functions (see Figure 4.10(a and b)). Dul *et al.* (1984) reported good agreement between their force distribution predictions and tendon transducer experiments (Figure 4.10(b)), although this has been questioned. It would appear that a cost function based on maximising endurance time would have little relevance to explosive athletic activities such as throwing and jumping.

Figure 4.10 (a) Muscle force distribution during knee flexion for different non-linear criteria: *MF* minimum fatigue; *C* sum of cubes of muscle stresses; *Q1*, *Q2* sums, respectively, of normalised and non-normalised muscle forces. Note that only *MF* gives a non-linear distribution. (b) Range of more than 95% of experimental results (between dashed lines) and predicted load sharing for two cat muscles: 1, minimum fatigue; 2, quadratic sum of muscle forces; 3, quadratic sum of normalised muscle forces; 4, sum of cubes of muscle stresses; 5, linear criteria.

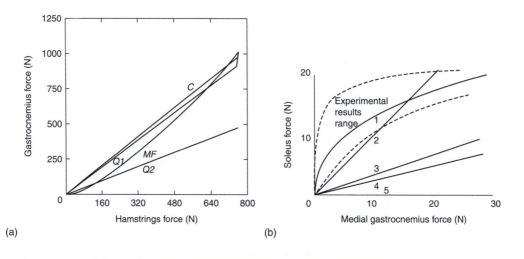

(a)   (b)

The cost function used should relate to some relevant physiological process, although it is unclear what, if anything, the central nervous system does optimise. Furthermore, the physiological data to substantiate the choice of cost function are not, in general, yet available. The cost function is likely to depend on the specific sports movement, for example maximising speed in sprinting and minimising energy expenditure in long distance running. It could vary for different performers and during an event, for example as speed changes (Herzog and Leonard, 1991) or at the onset of fatigue. Possibly the cost function needs to include weighted criteria, such as muscle, ligament and joint forces (Crowninshield and Brand, 1981a). Alternatively, the cost function may need to be implemented in stages – for example minimise the upper band of muscle stress then the sum of muscle forces using the optimal muscle stress (Bean *et al.*, 1988).

The results from the cost function chosen should be evaluated, as little evidence exists that the muscle forces are estimated accurately (e.g. Herzog and Leonard, 1991). The need remains to refine and develop experimental techniques to do this, particularly as small changes in assumptions can markedly influence the estimated forces (as in Figure 4.8). The solution to the force distribution problem is predetermined by the choice of cost function (e.g. An *et al.*, 1995). It is sensitive to small changes in the anatomical data used, such as moment arm and physiological cross-sectional area (Figure 4.8(a and b)) and maximal muscle stress. Comparisons that have been made of force distributions using different cost functions have shown differences between them. Solutions to the force distribution problem have generally ignored any contribution of ligament and joint contact forces to the cost function and the net muscle force. This may represent a significant simplification for joints such as the knee and it ignores any peripheral or central neuromotor role (Buchanan *et al.*, 2004).

The difficulty of solving inverse optimisations analytically relates directly to the number of design variables and constraints. Because muscle forces are zero or positive (tensile), linear cost functions offer simple solutions, as do cases where the cost function is 'convex' (e.g. n is even in equation 4.9). The cost function of Crowninshield and Brand (1981a):

$$U(t) = \Sigma (Fm_i/\text{pcsa}_i)^3 \tag{4.15}$$

reduces to a convex one for a one joint planar movement with two muscles. In this case:

$$Fm_1 = Fm_2 \, (r_1/r_2) \, (\text{pcsa}_1/\text{pcsa}_2)^{3/2} \tag{4.16}$$

The solution is shown in Figure 4.11. The reader interested in a mathematical consideration of the general inverse optimisation problem is referred to Herzog and Binding (1994).

Figure 4.11 Schematic diagram of optimal force distribution between muscles for a single degree of freedom joint.

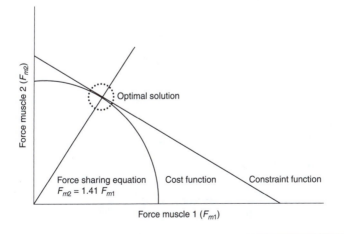

The optimisation approaches discussed above are either static (and hence solved only once) or solved independently for each sample interval during a movement; these have been called, respectively, inverse static and inverse dynamic optimisation (Winters, 1995). They have not often been used for the fast movements that occur in sports activities (but see McLaughlin and Miller, 1980). An inverse dynamics integrated optimisation approach, where the cost function is defined over the time course of the activity (Winters, 1995), may prove more appropriate for such movements. Also, while nonlinear optimisation can predict co-contraction of pairs of antagonist two-joint muscles, it does not account for co-contraction of antagonist pairs of single-joint muscles. Such co-contractions have been measured using EMG, for example by Crowninshield (1978) in the brachialis and triceps brachii (medial head) in forced elbow extension. Furthermore, inverse optimisation has failed, to date, to predict the loops in muscle force curves that are frequently reported from force transducer studies (e.g. Prilutsky *et al.*, 1994). For example, the predicted (lines 1–5) and measured (loop E) forces reported by Herzog and Leonard (1991) did not agree (Figure 4.12). This occurred because the changes in force sharing during the step cycle and at different locomotor speeds were ignored in the optimisation models (also compare Figure 4.12 with Figure 4.10(b)).

Figure 4.12 Measured loops in muscle force curves (E) at increasing locomotion speeds ((a)–(c)) compared with predictions using various cost functions (1–5).

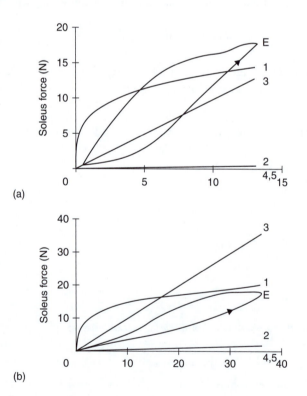

(a)

(b)

Figure 4.12 (*continued*)

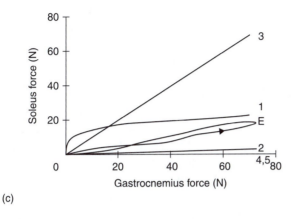

(c)

Comparisons of the results of studies that do and do not incorporate muscle dynamics (Herzog, 1987(a and b)) suggest that, for the high contractile velocities and large ranges of movement that occur in sport, muscle dynamics and activation possibly cannot be ignored. These effects have been incorporated in the inequality constraints (e.g. Happee, 1994; Kaufman *et al.*, 1991) or in the cost functions (e.g. Herzog, 1987(a and b)). In the former case, the inequality constraint then incorporates the physiology of the muscle based on its length–tension and force–velocity characteristics. This will be, for example, in the form:

$$0 \leq Fm_i \leq (\alpha\ Fm^a_i + Fm^p_i)\ \mathrm{pcsa}_i\ \sigma_{\mathrm{max}} \tag{4.17}$$

where Fm^a_i is the normalised muscle active force, Fm^p_i is the normalised muscle passive force and a represents the upper bound of the activation of the muscle. A unique solution can be obtained by minimising α (Kaufman *et al.*, 1991).

The solution of the force distribution problem has been hampered by a lack of reported quantitative musculoskeletal anatomy and analyses of the estimation of individual participant data by suitable scaling (e.g. Crowninshield and Brand, 1981b). This has been partially rectified by, for example, Pierrynowski (1995), but the precise muscle models needed and the difficulties of obtaining data *in vivo* on muscle properties of sportsmen and sportswomen remain to be resolved.

The equations of forward dynamics can also be used to determine muscle and joint forces. For example, Nubar and Contini (1961) proposed the minimum energy principle for static muscular effort, which was developed to an optimal control model by Chow and Jacobson (1971). The complexity of forward dynamics optimisation is, however, great, particularly for three-dimensional models of multiple-segment systems, such as the sports performer.

THE USE OF EMG TO IMPROVE MUSCLE FORCE ESTIMATES

Inverse optimisation models that use EMG as an index of muscle activation have some similarities with other approaches that incorporate the use of EMG records. In both these approaches, the EMG signal is usually normalised to that for a maximum voluntary contraction (MVC) to partition the joint reaction moment. Allowance is also usually made for instantaneous muscle length and velocity, contraction type and passive elasticity (e.g. Caldwell and Chapman, 1991; McGill and Norman, 1993). This approach allows for co-contraction, and some success with validation has been reported (for example, see Gregor and Abelew, 1994). Force estimations from EMG are difficult for deep muscles, and the approach rarely predicts moments about the three axes that equal those measured (McGill and Norman, 1993). Limitations exist in the use of the MVC as a valid and reliable criterion of maximal force for normalisation (summarised by Enoka and Fuglevand, 1993). These include the standardisation, in an MVC, of the neural control of muscle coordination and the mechanical factors of joint angle and its rate of change, which could confound interpretation of the results. Furthermore, reported motor unit discharge rates of 20–40 Hz during an MVC are inconsistent with those needed to elicit the maximal tetanic force in all motor units of a muscle (80–100 Hz for a fast twitch motor unit). The inability of some high threshold motor units to sustain activity also suggests caution in interpreting motor unit activity in the MVC as maximal. Obviously more research is needed into why the central nervous system apparently cannot fully activate muscle in an MVC (Enoka and Fuglevand, 1993). Practical difficulties – of pain, fear of re-injury and motivation – also arise in eliciting MVCs from previously injured individuals. To overcome these, Frazer *et al.* (1995) devised a scaling method that does not require an MVC. This method estimates the active muscle force as the product of the EMG signal, muscle length and force factors and the slope of the muscle force–EMG relationship between 60% and 70% maximal efforts.

Many of the above limitations also apply to the use of EMG to predict muscle tension. Although important strides have been made in this respect for isometric and some voluntary dynamic contractions (e.g. Hof *et al.*, 1987), no successful EMG-to-muscle tension predictions have yet been reported for a fast sporting activity. Furthermore, the substantial EMG variations at constant maximal force suggest (Enoka and Fuglevand, 1993) that the EMG is not a direct index of the magnitude of the neural drive to muscles at the high forces that occur in much sporting activity. Difficulties also arise from reported variability in the electromechanical delay with movement pattern and speed (Gregor and Abelew, 1994). Further difficulties are evident, for example, in the different shapes of the 'loops' in the muscle force and EMG curves for the soleus plotted against the gastrocnemius (Prilutsky *et al.*, 1994), shown in Figure 4.13.

When calculating muscle force distribution, the EMG signal has also been used to validate the predicted temporal pattern of muscle activation. In this approach, a predicted muscle force is compared with the existence or otherwise of an EMG signal for that muscle. For example, the continuous synergy of all agonists predicted by non-linear cost functions (Denoth, 1988) can be evaluated. Although such information may

Figure 4.13 (a) Muscle force loops compared with (b) integrated EMG (IEMG) loops.

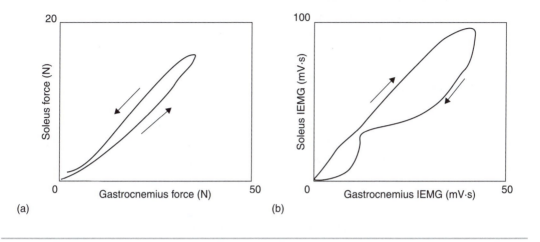

(a)   (b)

appear to provide some subjective validation of the force distribution solution, limitations arise because of some of the factors discussed earlier in this section.

If muscle forces can be estimated accurately, then the inverse dynamics equation for forces (e.g. equations 4.4) can be used to calculate the joint contact force (F_j) if an assumption is made about the passive, ligamentous forces (F_p). One such assumption might be that no force was present in the ligament during its slack period (Morrison, 1968). Alternatively, the ligament force could be calculated from stiffness values assigned to that ligament when not slack (Wismans *et al.*, 1980). To investigate further the effect of the joint contact force on the stress distribution in the bone, finite element modelling is often used (see, e.g. Beaupré and Carter, 1992; Ranu, 1989). The assumptions of some finite element bone models, such as bone is isotropic and homogeneous, are suspect and the validity of many model results have not been assessed (King, 1984). This is mainly because of a lack of data on material properties of biological material, which has limited the use of such modelling methods in sports injury.

SUMMARY

In this chapter we examined the method of two-dimensional inverse dynamics. The equations for planar force and moment calculations from inverse dynamics, for single segments or for a segment chain, were explained, along with how the procedures can be extended to multiple-segment systems. We also highlighted the difficulties of calculating the forces in muscles and ligaments arising from the indeterminacy problem, including typical simplifications made in inverse dynamics modelling. The various approaches to overcoming the indeterminacy (or redundancy) problem were described.

We covered the method of inverse optimisation, and attempted to evaluate some of the various cost functions used in research. The uses and limitations of EMG in estimating muscle force were outlined.

STUDY TASKS

1 We presented a list of assumptions that were made when presenting the static and dynamic examples to arrive at an inverse dynamics model of forearm flexion. Can you list and describe any other simplifications that you consider the model to contain?

2 (a) Draw a free body diagram of a static non-horizontal single-body segment (e.g. the combined forearm-hand segment flexing about the elbow as in Figure 4.5(a)) with one muscle, with an angle of pull of 90°.

(b) Show that the force and moment equations for this segment are:

$$Fj_x - F_m \sin\theta = 0$$
$$Fj_y + F_m \cos\theta - m\,g = 0$$
$$r_m\,F_m - (r\cos\theta)\,m\,g = 0$$

where θ is the angle of the segment to the horizontal.

(c) The mass of the forearm-hand segment of an athlete is 2 kg and the centre of mass of the combined segment is 14 cm (0.14 m) from the elbow joint. Flexion is assumed to be performed by a single muscle that inserts 5 cm (0.05 m) from the joint with an angle of insertion, or angle of pull, of 90°. If the forearm-hand segment is stationary and at an angle (θ) of 30° to the horizontal: (i) calculate the muscle force and the components of the joint force; (ii) verify the answer using a force polygon, using Figure 4.3(c) as a model.

(d) Draw another free body diagram of a non-horizontal single body segment similar to that in (a) but showing the centripetal and tangential accelerations during a movement with angular acceleration and velocity as in Figure 4.3(a). Show that the force and moment equations for that segment are:

$$Fj_x - F_m \sin\theta + m\,r\,(\omega^2 \cos\theta + \alpha \sin\theta) = 0$$
$$Fj_y + F_m \cos\theta - m\,g - m\,r\,(\omega^2 \sin\theta + \alpha \cos\theta) = 0$$
$$r_m\,F_m - (r\cos\theta)\,m\,g - I_o\,\alpha = 0$$

(e) The mass of the forearm-hand segment of an athlete is 2 kg and the centre of mass of the combined segment is 14 cm (0.14 m) from the elbow joint. Flexion is assumed to be performed by a single muscle that inserts 5 cm (0.05 m) from the joint with an angle of insertion of 90°. If the forearm-hand is instantaneously at an angle (θ) of 30° to the horizontal, with a positive angular acceleration of

1.5 rad/s² and angular velocity of 2.5 rad/s, calculate the muscle force and the components of the joint force using the equations in part (d). The moment of inertia of the combined forearm-hand segment about the elbow joint is 0.09 kg·m².

3　Draw the joint reaction force and moment equivalents of your figures from Study Task 2. In each case, calculate the joint reaction moment and force components. Explain any differences between the joint reaction force components and the actual joint force components in Study Task 2.

4　Draw a free body diagram of a two-segment kinetic chain. Write the moment equations for both segments. Explain the physical meaning of each of the terms in these equations.

5　Draw a sagittal plane view of a runner during ground contact. Explain, with the use of clear diagrams, a procedure for calculating the forces and moments at each joint in this planar representation of the runner, if ground reaction forces were not measured. A frontal plane view of this activity might use rigid triangular models of the pectoral and pelvic girdles: explain the limitations of these models of the pelvic and pectoral girdles.

6　After consulting the relevant Further Reading, describe, compare and evaluate the methods for overcoming the indeterminacy (redundancy) problem.

7　Explain the uses of inverse optimisation. Summarise the limitations for sports movements of the following cost functions: linear functions; quadratic functions; the 'soft-saturation' criterion; functions supposedly relating to muscle energy, muscle fatigue or minimum compression; and functions incorporating muscle dynamics. Comment on some of the general difficulties with the inverse optimisation approach. You will probably find van den Bogert (1994) or Herzog (1996) useful for answering this question.

8　Describe the limitations on the use of EMG to estimate muscle force.

GLOSSARY OF IMPORTANT TERMS

Centripetal force Force directed toward the centre of rotation in a rotating body.

Cost function A function used to constrain the optimisation model; a feasible solution to the cost function that minimises or maximises, if that is the goal, the cost function is called an optimal solution. The minimisation of the cost functions is an attempt to imitate the body's criteria for deciding which muscles to recruit and the order of recruitment. We can also define the level of activation that will produce appropriate motion or posture for a specific task. The selection of the most appropriate criterion to use in the optimisation process resides upon several aspects such as the type of motion under analysis, the objectives to achieve or the presence of any type of pathology (Ambrósio and Kecskeméthy, 2007).

Finite element modelling Used to visualise stresses and strains in a structure. It uses a numerical technique called 'finite element analysis' for finding approximate solutions of partial differential equations as well as of integral equations.

Inertial reference frame A 'frame of reference' is a standard relative to which motion and rest may be measured. An inertial reference frame is relative to motions that have distinguished dynamical properties. An inertial frame is a spatial reference frame together with some means of measuring time, so that uniform motions can be distinguished from accelerated motions. In Newtonian dynamics, an inertial frame is a reference frame with a time scale, relative to which the motion of a body (disregarding external forces) is always rectilinear and uniform, accelerations are always proportional to and in the direction of applied forces, and applied forces are always met with equal and opposite reactions.

Indeterminate system A system of simultaneous equations that has infinitely many solutions or no solutions at all. If there are fewer unique equations than variables, then the system must be indeterminate.

Inequality constraints A restriction that limits the value of a dependent or independent variable. An inequality constraint is used to apply a limitation to a feature that may vary, such as joint movement, speed and torque.

Inverse dynamics A method for computing forces and moments of force based on the kinematics of a body and the body's inertial properties.

Inverse optimisation An optimisation technique in which the ideal solution or outcome (i.e. movement) is known. We use the technique to optimise the muscle recruitment or muscle forces involved so as to simulate the known movement criteria.

Mathematically indeterminate A problem that has an infinite number of solutions, or one in which there are fewer imposed conditions than there are unknowns.

Maximum tetanic force Maximum force produced by a muscle in a state of sustained maximal tension.

Maximum voluntary contraction A measure of strength that can be expressed as a maximal exertion of force, reported either as a force or as a moment (or torque) around a joint.

Optimisation A procedure or set of procedures that are used to make a system as functional as possible.

Physiological cross sectional area The cross sectional area of a muscle perpendicular to the muscle fibres.

Right-hand rule A procedure for identifying the direction of an angular motion vector.

Varignon's theorem Also called the 'principle of moments' and states that the moment of any force is equal to the algebraic sum of the moments of the components of that force.

Wobbling mass model One of the assumptions of linear inverse dynamics is that the body being studied is a series of rigid segments. However, we can see from high-speed recordings of impacts, the soft parts of each segment of the human body are shifted relative to the bony parts and start to 'wobble' in a complex damped manner. Therefore, some researchers have developed ways of modelling the essential properties of the human body as 'wobbling masses', which are coupled quasi-elastically and strongly damped to each rigid bony part. The wobbling mass model allows the researcher to study the effects of the different mechanical behaviour of the soft tissues and the rigid bony parts of the human body.

REFERENCES

Ambrósio, J.A.C. and Kecskeméthy, A. (2007) 'Multibody dynamics of biomechanical models for human motion via optimization', in J.C. García Orden, J.M. Goicolea and J. Cuadrado (eds) *Multibody Dynamics: Computational Methods and Applications, Vol. 4*, Amsterdam: Springer, pp. 245–272.

An, K.N., Kaufman, K.R. and Chao, E.Y.S. (1995) 'Estimation of muscle and joint forces', in P. Allard, I.A.F. Stokes and J.P. Blanchi (eds) *Three-Dimensional Analysis of Human Movement*, Champaign, IL: Human Kinetics, pp. 201–214.

Andrews, J.G. (1995) 'Euler's and Lagrange's equations for linked rigid-body models of three-dimensional human motion', in P. Allard, I.A.F. Stokes and J.P. Blanchi (eds) *Three-Dimensional Analysis of Human Movement*, Champaign, IL: Human Kinetics, pp. 145–175.

Bartlett, R.M. (2007) *Introduction to Sports Biomechanics: Analysing Human Movement Patterns*, London: Routledge.

Bean, J.C., Chaffin, D.B. and Schultz, A.B. (1988) Biomechanical model calculations of muscle contraction forces: a double linear programming method. *Journal of Biomechanics, 21*, 59–66.

Beaupré, G.S. and Carter, D.R. (1992) 'Finite element analysis in biomechanics', in A.A. Biewener (ed.) *Biomechanics Structures and Systems: A Practical Approach*, Oxford: Oxford University Press, pp. 149–174.

Buchanan, T.S., Lloyd, D.G., Manal, K. and Besier, T.F. (2004) Neuromusculoskeletal modeling: estimation of muscle forces and joint moments and movements from measurements of neural command. *Journal of Applied Biomechanics, 20*, 367–395.

Caldwell, G.E. and Chapman, A.E. (1991) The general distribution problem: a physiological solution which includes antagonism. *Human Movement Science, 10*, 355–392.

Chaffin, D.B. (1969) Computerized biomechanical models: development of and use in studying gross body actions. *Journal of Biomechanics, 2*, 429–441.

Chow, C.K. and Jacobson, D.H. (1971) Studies of human locomotion via optimal programming. *Mathematical Biosciences, 10*, 239–306.

Cleather, D., Goodwin, J. and Bull, A. (2010) An optimisation approach to inverse dynamics provides insight as to the function of the biarticular muscles during vertical jumping. *Annals of Biomedical Engineering, 39*, 147–160.

Crowninshield, R.D. (1978) Use of optimisation techniques to predict muscle forces. *Journal of Biomechanical Engineering, 100*, 88–92.

Crowninshield, R.D. and Brand, R.A. (1981a) A physiologically based criterion of muscle force prediction in locomotion. *Journal of Biomechanics, 14*, 793–801.

Crowninshield, R.D. and Brand, R.A. (1981b) 'The prediction of forces in joint structures: distribution of intersegmental resultants', in D.I. Miller (ed.) *Exercise and Sport Sciences Reviews, Vol. 9*, Washington, DC: Franklin Institute, pp. 159–181.

Denoth, J. (1988) 'Methodological problems in prediction of muscle forces', in G. de Groot, A.P. Hollander, P.A. Huijing and J.G. van Ingen Schenau (eds) *Biomechanics XI – A*, Amsterdam: Free University Press, pp. 82–87.

Dul, J., Johnson, G.E., Shiavi, R. and Townsend, M.A. (1984) Muscular synergy – II. A minimum fatigue criterion for load-sharing between synergistic muscles. *Journal of Biomechanics, 17*, 675–684.

Enoka, R.M. and Fuglevand, A.J. (1993) 'Neuromuscular basis of the maximum voluntary force capacity of muscle', in M.D. Grabiner (ed.) *Current Issues in Biomechanics*, Champaign, IL: Human Kinetics, pp. 215–235.

Frazer, M.B., Norman, R.W. and McGill, S.M. (1995) 'EMG to muscle force calibration in dynamic movements', in K. Häkkinen, K.L. Keskinen, P.V. Komi and A. Mero (eds) *XVth*

Congress of the International Society of Biomechanics Book of Abstracts, Jyväskylä: University of Finland, pp. 284–285.

Gracovetsky, S. (1985) An hypothesis for the role of the spine in human locomotion: a challenge to current thinking. *Journal of Biomedical Engineering*, *7*, 205–216.

Gregor, R.J. (1993) 'Skeletal muscle mechanics and movement', in M.D. Grabiner (ed.) *Current Issues in Biomechanics*, Champaign, IL: Human Kinetics, pp. 195–199.

Gregor, R.J. and Abelew, T.A. (1994) Tendon force measurements in musculoskeletal biomechanics. *Sport Science Review*, *3*, 8–33.

Happee, R. (1994) Inverse dynamic optimisation including muscular dynamics, a new simulation method applied to goal directed movements. *Journal of Biomechanics*, *27*, 953–960.

Herzog, W. (1987a) Individual muscle force optimisations using a non-linear optimal design. *Journal of Neuroscience Methods*, *21*, 167–179.

Herzog, W. (1987b) Considerations for predicting individual muscle forces in athletic movements. *International Journal of Sport Biomechanics*, *3*, 128–141.

Herzog, W. (1996) 'Force-sharing among synergistic muscles: theoretical considerations and experimental approaches', in J.O. Holloszy (ed.) *Exercise and Sport Sciences Reviews, Vol. 24*, Baltimore: Williams & Wilkins, pp. 173–202.

Herzog, W. and Binding, P. (1994) 'Mathematically indeterminate solutions', in B.M. Nigg and W. Herzog (eds) *Biomechanics of the Musculoskeletal System*, Chichester: John Wiley, pp. 472–491.

Herzog, W. and Leonard, T.R. (1991) Validation of optimisation models that estimate the forces exerted by synergistic models. *Journal of Biomechanics*, *24*(Suppl 1), 31–39.

Hof, A.L., Pronk, C.N.A. and van Best, J.A. (1987) A physiologically based criterion of muscle force prediction in locomotion. *Journal of Biomechanics*, *14*, 793–801.

Kane, T.R. and Levinson, D.A. (1985) *Dynamics: Theory and Applications*, New York: McGraw-Hill.

Kaufman, K.R., An, K.-N., Litchy, W.J. and Chao, E.Y. (1991) Physiological prediction of muscle forces – I. Theoretical prediction. *Neuroscience*, *40*, 781–792.

Kernozek, T.W. and Ragan, R.J. (2008) Estimation of anterior cruciate ligament tension from inverse dynamics data and electromyography in females during drop landing. *Clinical Biomechanics*, *23*, 1279–1286.

King, A.I. (1984) A review of biomechanical models. *Journal of Biomechanical Engineering*, *106*, 97–104.

Komi, P.V. (1990) Relevance of in vivo force measurements to human biomechanics. *Journal of Biomechanics*, 23(Suppl 1), 23–34.

McGill, S.M. and Norman, R.W. (1993) 'Low back biomechanics in industry: the prevention of injury through safer lifting', in M.D. Grabiner (ed.) *Current Issues in Biomechanics*, Champaign, IL: Human Kinetics, pp. 69–120.

McLaughlin, T.M. and Miller, N.R. (1980) Techniques for the evaluation of loads on the forearm prior to impact in tennis strokes. *Journal of Mechanical Design*, *102*, 701–710.

Morrison, J.B. (1968) Bioengineering analysis of force actions transmitted by the knee joint. *Bio-Medicine Engineering*, *3*, 164–170.

Nigg, B.M. (1994) 'Mathematically determinate systems', in B.M. Nigg and W. Herzog (eds) *Biomechanics of the Musculoskeletal System*, Chichester: John Wiley, pp. 392–471.

Nubar, Y. and Contini, R. (1961) A minimum principle in biomechanics. *Bulletin of Mathematical Biophysics*, *23*, 377–391.

Pierrynowski, M.R. (1995) 'Analytical representation of muscle line of action and geometry', in P. Allard, I.A.F. Stokes and J.P. Blanchi (eds) *Three-Dimensional Analysis of Human Movement*, Champaign, IL: Human Kinetics, pp. 215–256.

Powell, E.S. and Trail, I.A. (2004) Forces transmitted along human flexor tendons during passive and active movements of the fingers. *Journal of Hand Surgery (British and European Volume)*, *29*, 386–389.

Praagman, M., Chadwick, E.K.J., van der Helm, F.C.T. and Veeger, H.E.J. (2006) The relationship between two different mechanical cost functions and muscle oxygen consumption. *Journal of Biomechanics, 39*, 758–765.

Prilutsky, B.I., Herzog, W. and Allinger, T.L. (1994) Force-sharing between cat soleus and gastrocnemius muscles during walking: explanations based on electrical activity, properties and kinematics. *Journal of Biomechanics, 27*, 1223–1235.

Ranu, H.S. (1989) 'The role of finite element modelling in biomechanics', in A.L. Yettram (ed) *Material Properties and Stress Analysis in Biomechanics*, Manchester: Manchester University Press, pp. 163–186.

Rasmussen, J., Damsgaard, M. and Voigt, M. (2001) Muscle recruitment by the min/max criterion – a comparative numerical study. *Journal of Biomechanics, 34*, 409–415.

Robertson, D.G.E., Cladwell, G.E., Hamill, J., Kamen, G. and Whittlesey, S.N. (2004) *Research Methods in Biomechanics*, Champaign, IL: Human Kinetics.

Schultz, A.B. and Anderson, G.B.J. (1981) Analysis of loads on the spine. *Spine, 6*, 76–82.

Siegler, S. and Wen, L. (1997) 'Inverse dynamics in human locomotion', in P. Allard, A. Cappozzo, A. Lundberg and C. Vaughan (eds) *Three-Dimensional Analysis of Human Locomotion, Vol. 2*, Chichester: John Wiley & Sons, pp. 191–209.

Siemienski, A. (1992) 'Soft saturation, an idea for load sharing between muscles. Application to the study of human locomotion', in A. Cappozzo, M. Marchetti and V. Tosi (eds) *Biolocomotion: A Century of Research Using Moving Pictures*, Rome: Promograph, pp. 293–303.

van den Bogert, A.J. (1994) 'Analysis and simulation of mechanical loads on the human musculoskeletal system: a methodological overview', in J.L. Holloszy (ed.) *Exercise and Sport Sciences Reviews*, Vol. 22, Baltimore: Williams & Wilkins, pp. 23–51.

Winter, D. A. (2005) *Biomechanics and Motor Control of Human Movement* (3rd edn), Hoboken, NJ: John Wiley & Sons.

Winters, J. (1995) 'Concepts in neuromuscular modelling', in P. Allard, I.A.F. Stokes and J.P. Blanchi (eds) *Three-Dimensional Analysis of Human Movement*, Champaign, IL: Human Kinetics, pp. 257–292.

Wismans, J., Veldpaus, F., Janssen, J., Huson, A. and Struben, P. (1980) A three-dimensional mathematical model of the knee joint. *Journal of Biomechanics, 13*, 677–686.

Zajac, F.E. and Gordon, M.E. (1989) 'Determining muscle's force and action in multi-articular movement', in. K.B. Pandolf (ed.) *Exercise and Sport Sciences Reviews, Vol. 17*, Baltimore: Williams & Wilkins, pp. 187–230.

FURTHER READING

Herzog, W. and Binding, P. (1994) 'Mathematically indeterminate solutions', in B.M. Nigg and W. Herzog (eds), *Biomechanics of the Musculoskeletal System*, Chichester: John Wiley, pp. 472–491. This is a good explanation of inverse dynamics modelling, providing the reader has enough mathematical background.

Robertson, D.G.E., Caldwell, G.E., Hamill, J., Kamen, G. and Whittlesey, S.N. (2004) *Research Methods in Biomechanics*, Champaign, IL: Human Kinetics. Of particular interest are Chapters 5 and 7. Chapter 5 (Whittlesey and Robertson) provides another overview of planar inverse dynamics with more examples and models. This chapter focuses on the lower limb and is thus a nice compliment to the chapter presented in the present text. Chapter 7, by Hamill and Selbie, provides a look at the three-dimensional case, with information about data collection as well as model development.

Winter, D. A. (2005) *Biomechanics and Motor Control of Human Movement* (3rd edn), Hoboken, NJ: John Wiley & Sons. Chapter 4 provides an overview of kinetics including link-segment model development and optimisation techniques.

Yamaguchi, G.T. (2001) *Dynamic Modeling of Musculoskeletal Motion: A Vectorized Approach for Biomechanical Analysis in Three Dimensions*, Boston: Kluwer Academic Publishers. Chapter 1 of this text introduces Kane's method and compares the outcome measures to those of the Newton–Euler approach using a planar example.

5 Performance analysis

Roger Bartlett

Knowledge assumed
Familiarity with human
movement in sport
Ability to undertake simple
analysis of videos of sports
movements
Understanding of basic sports
biomechanics (Bartlett, R.M.,
2007, *Introduction to Sports
Biomechanics: Analysing
Human Movement Patterns*,
London: Routledge,
particularly Chapters 1–3).

INTRODUCTION – WHAT IS PERFORMANCE ANALYSIS?

BOX 5.1 LEARNING OUTCOMES

After reading this chapter you should be able to:

- understand and explain what performance analysis is
- outline the main features of each of the four stages of the structured performance analysis process
- explain the differences between, and the value of, qualitative and quantitative movement analysis
- list the four key core elements of a notational analysis system
- appreciate the factors underlying design of notational analysis systems
- understand the use of notational systems, such as frequency charts, scatter diagrams and sequential systems
- be familiar with the essentials of a computerised notational analysis system
- carry out a notational analysis of netball using frequency analysis charts
- define and evaluate critically the biomechanical principles of sports movements and their applicability to various sports movements
- undertake a phase analysis of a ballistic movement of your choice and describe the functions of each phase in terms of the biomechanical principles of coordinated movement
- understand how phase analysis can be applied to other sports movements.

This chapter is designed to provide an understanding of various aspects of performance analysis, focusing on notational analysis of team sports and the biomechanical analysis of individual sports skills or 'techniques'. The terminology involved around the concepts of movement analysis, performance analysis and sports biomechanics can be a shade confusing. Figure 5.1 attempts to summarise the relationship between these and other related terms, without involving other disciplines, such as motor learning and control.

It is unclear when the term 'performance analysis' first started to be used in the context of this chapter. In the late 1990s, the British Olympic Association set up its Performance Analysis Steering Group (PASG), which initially brought together biomechanists and notational analysts, as well as coaches and athletes. For some time, there was scepticism as to whether these two groups of sport scientists had enough in common to make the group meaningful. After all, sports biomechanics is concerned with the fine detail of individual sports techniques while notational analysts are generally more concerned with gross movements or movement patterns in games or teams. Furthermore, notational analysts are more concerned with strategic and tactical issues in sport than with technique analysis and the two disciplines do not share a common

Figure 5.1 Schematic representation of the relationship between some of the terms used in performance analysis and sports biomechanics. Sports biomechanics is bounded by the rectangle with continuous lines; movement analysis by the rectangle with dashed lines; performance analysis by the oval with dash-dot lines; technique analysis by the oval with dash-double dot lines; notational analysis by the oval with longer dashed lines; and gait analysis by the oval with shorter dashed lines. The overlaps should be obvious.

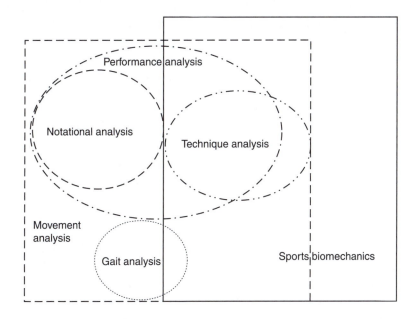

historical background. Later, the PASG expanded to include motor learning and sports technology specialists.

The similarities between notational analysis and sports biomechanics are far more marked than the differences. A crucial similarity is evident when we look at the other sport science disciplines: sports psychology and physiology (including nutrition) essentially focus on preparing the athlete for competition. Performance analysts, in contrast, focus on the performance in competition to draw lessons for improving performance; this is true of both notational and biomechanical analysis. Both are fundamentally concerned with the analysis and improvement of performance. Both are rooted in the analysis of human movement. Both make extensive use of video analysis and video-based technology. Although both evolved from manual systems, they now rely heavily on computerised analysis systems. Both have a strong focus on data collection and processing. Both sports biomechanics and notational analysis produce vast amounts of information. This is sometimes claimed to be a strength of both types of analysis; however, it often requires careful information management when providing feedback to athletes and coaches. Many of these important topics were covered in a special issue of the *Journal of Sports Sciences on Performance Analysis* in 2002 (Hughes and Bartlett, 2002).

In addition, biomechanists and notational analysts both emphasise the development of systematic techniques of observation (see the next section). This is more obvious in notational analysis and, perhaps, in the qualitative analysis approach of biomechanics than in quantitative biomechanical analysis. Both have a strong focus on the provision of feedback to the coach and performer to improve performance (see Chapter 8) and each group is now learning and adopting best practice from the other.

Sports biomechanics and notational analysis were, in the past, sometimes accused by other sports scientists of lacking theoretical foundations and being over-concerned with methodology. Although this accusation might have had some justification, this practical focus and relevance might partially explain the attraction of performance analysis to coaches. However, theoretical models do exist in both biomechanics and notational analysis. These models can also be effectively represented graphically – by flowcharts for notational analysis and 'deterministic' or 'hierarchical' models for biomechanics. Both disciplines have 'key events' as important features of their theoretical foundations. These models and a focus on key events help to present information clearly and simply to coaches and sports performers, as evidenced by the current popularity of 'coach-friendly' biomechanical analysis packages, such as Siliconcoach (http://www.siliconcoach.com) and Dartfish (http://www.dartfish.com) and notational analysis packages, such as Focus (www.elitesportsanalysis.com) and SportsCode (www.sportstec.com). These theoretical models can, at least in principle, be mapped onto the sophisticated approaches of artificial intelligence, such as expert systems and artificial neural networks (see Chapter 7), hopefully offering exciting future developments in improving sports performance. The theoretical models are highly sport, or movement, specific, although there are general principles, particularly across groups of similar sports. Both sports biomechanics and notational analysis have strong theoretical and conceptual links with other areas of sport science and information technology, particularly the dynamical systems approach of ecological motor control (see also Hughes and Bartlett, 2008).

Many practical issues, which impinge strongly on performance improvement, are common to sports biomechanics and notational analysis. These include optimising feedback to coaches and athletes, the management of information complexity, reliability and validity of data, and the future exploitation of the methods of artificial intelligence. Sharing of approaches and ideas has already begun to have mutual benefit.

But, you might ask, is performance analysis really helpful in improving performance? Many sports teams and clubs now employ performance analysts, who often carry out both notational analyses and qualitative biomechanical analyses. As to their value for the coach, sports biomechanics identifies the features of performance that relate to good and poor movement techniques, thereby helping to identify how techniques can be improved. It also facilitates comparative analysis of individual performers and helps to identify injurious techniques. The latter is well exemplified by the contribution made by biomechanists to establishing the link between low back injury and the mixed technique in cricket fast bowling discussed in Chapter 8. Notational analysis identifies the performance indicators that relate to good and poor team performance and identifies good and poor performances of team members. It, therefore, facilitates comparative analysis of teams and players. In addition, it helps to assess the physiological and psychological demands of various games.

FOUR-STAGE APPROACH TO STRUCTURED PERFORMANCE ANALYSIS

The approach outlined in this section, and developed further in Chapter 6, focuses on the systematic observation and introspective judgement of sports movements to provide the best intervention to improve performance. This approach is necessarily interdisciplinary and integrated, involving motor development, motor learning and performance analysis.

The approach here is largely based on that outlined for qualitative biomechanical analysis by Knudson and Morrison (2002) (Figure 5.2) but is also used, often implicitly rather than explicitly, in notational analysis and should be used, more frequently than it is, in quantitative biomechanical analysis too.

Stage 1 – Preparation

For qualitative biomechanical analysts and notational analysts, the preparation stage will often begin by conducting a 'needs analysis' with the people commissioning the study to ascertain what they want from it. This stage of the process involves gathering knowledge of the sport and the performers involved (describe the sport from the general to the specific). The most important aspect of the preparation stage is in identifying the performance indications (the key factors of performance) that are to be observed, recorded or measured (see Hughes and Bartlett, 2004). In qualitative biomechanical analysis, this means establishing the 'critical features' of the movement and, possibly, their range of correctness (Chapter 6). In this stage we also develop a systematic observation (or measurement) strategy for the observation stage; for notational analysts, this

Figure 5.2 The four-stage structured analysis process (adapted from Knudson and Morrison, 2002).

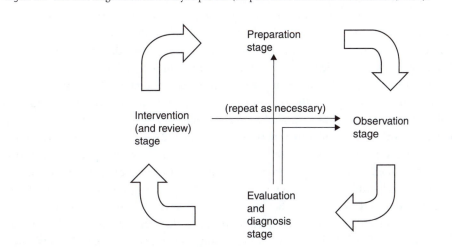

will also involve devising a recording method that is efficient and easy to learn (Hughes, 2008a). For sports biomechanists, it will sometimes include deciding on other qualitative presentations of movement or coordination patterns to be used (Chapter 6) and considering effective instruction, including cue words and phrases or task sheets, for the intervention stage.

Stage 2 – Observation (recording or measurement)

The observation stage primarily involves implementing the systematic observation strategy developed in the preparation stage. We may gather information about the movement technique or sport that is being studied from the senses as well as from video recordings. We need to decide, particularly in notational analysis, on the focus of observation, for example, on an individual player (for time-motion analysis) or on the 'play' if we are logging actions (see below). Where to observe is another consideration, but for studies seeking to improve performance this will usually be 'in the field' – an ecologically valid environment not a controlled one. We need to decide from where to observe movement – usually where to place our video cameras. We need to decide on the number of observations to be made; how many games or trails are to be recorded – there is no such thing as a representative game or a representative trial. In a quantitative biomechanical analysis, measurement issues predominate (see, for example, Payton and Bartlett, 2008).

Stage 3 – Evaluation and diagnosis (the analysis stage)

In the evaluation and diagnosis stage of the overall movement analysis process, we evaluate the strengths and weaknesses of the performance, primarily using the video footage we have recorded or observations made during a 'live' performance. In sports biomechanics, we may use other qualitative movement patterns in addition to video images (Chapter 6). We then need to select the best intervention to improve performance; this involves judgement of causes of poor performance. In notational analysis, where we are often trying to improve the performance of a team, we may need, for example, to look at sequences of actions that led to critical incidents, such as turnovers or scoring opportunities. Errors will often need to be related to previous actions. In sports biomechanics, poor technique often arises from errors in the earlier phases (see below) of the movement, which only become apparent later. Other approaches to prioritising interventions include focusing on what promises the greatest improvement in performance, proceeding in order of difficulty of changing critical features – from easiest to hardest, or working from the base of support up. In this stage, we also need to address the validity and reliability of our observations (or measurements). In qualitative analysis, the reliability (repeatability) of observations is generally poor to moderate for a single analyst and poor across analysts; increased training of the analyst and analysing more trials both help.

Stage 4 – Intervention

In the intervention stage, we try to 'put things right' so as to improve performance of the individual athlete or the team. This stage of the process emphasises feedback to performers to improve technique and performance, although there is more to it than that (see Chapter 8). In this stage, we should also conduct the main review of the overall analysis process in the context of the needs analysis in the preparation stage – this does not preclude reviews at other stages of the process as implied by the straight line arrows in Figure 5.2. Many issues arise about how, when and where to provide feedback. This stage also raises issues about practice, which need to address motor control models, and about training. Some of these issues are addressed in depth in Chapter 8.

QUANTITATIVE AND QUALITATIVE ANALYSIS

The analysis of sports movements – whether biomechanical or notational – can be categorised as follows. It should be noted that these three levels of analysis fall on a continuum on which the boundaries are not always obvious (for further details, see Bartlett, 2007).

Qualitative analysis

Qualitative analysis is based on observation, either in real time or, far more frequently, from video, the latter often in slow motion. This analysis involves an observational assessment of the movement technique and is usually conducted to determine if the technique is being performed correctly. That is, is the technique in accordance with relevant movement principles? Until recently, qualitative analysis was mainly used in sports biomechanics, usually in conjunction with a deterministic performance model. Qualitative biomechanical analysis should uncover the major faults in an unsuccessful performance; this is the approach used by most coaches and teachers. Developments in notational analysis software packages over the last decade now allow the tagging of all of the actions performed by a team – such as turnovers or tackles – or by an individual player. In the latter context, this now allows the performance analyst to put together a sequence of all the passes, shots on goal, or whatever by one player (see the examples on the book's website); this enables the qualitative analysis of those skills to identify strengths and weaknesses and what the outcomes were. In this capacity, the performance analyst is now carrying out qualitative biomechanical analyses, neatly combining the two roles of notational analyst and biomechanical analyst: the performance analyst has become a very marketable package!

Semi-quantitative analysis

Semi-quantitative analysis tends to be the predominant type of analysis used in notational analysis. The focus is often on the number of actions that occur, where on the playing surface various actions took place, and which players were involved in different actions. Alternatively, there may be a combined focus on actions and positions, such as smashes from the mid-court in badminton, or scoring shots played behind the wicket on the leg side in cricket. These basic data can then be 'normalised' to other data, for example, goals divided by shots on goal, turnovers per number of possessions. In sports biomechanics, semi-quantitative analysis is used when only simple, but good, estimates of a few selected performance indicators are required. The simple measurements usually include the timings of the phases of the movement (see below). Other simple measurements may include the range of movement of a joint. For the purpose of the rest of this book, semi-quantitative analysis is subsumed into qualitative analysis. For both types of performance analysis, this combined category comprises the analyses normally carried out by coaches, teachers and performance analysts working with sports practitioners. In this important respect, it is more directly used to improve performance than is quantitative analysis.

Quantitative analysis

Quantitative analysis usually involves detailed measurements, mathematics and modelling. In a quantitative biomechanical analysis, a full temporal and kinematic and, often, kinetic specification of the movement is obtained, usually from video or from an automatic marker-tracking system and computer analysis (see also Payton and Bartlett, 2008). Quantitative analysis can be used to make a detailed, numerical assessment of the technique and to conduct objective comparisons. A quantitative analysis also enables us to quantify the critical features of the movement and can help to define optimum performance parameters, such as the best angle of release for a javelin thrower. With the relevant body segment inertia parameters, the method of inverse dynamics can be used to calculate the net joint reaction forces and moments (see Chapter 4). Quantitative notational analysis often involves some mathematical modelling of the actions or other aspects of the game, using techniques such as Markov chains, perturbation analysis, and movement trajectory analysis (see, for example, McGarry, 2008; O'Donoghue, 2008; Bourbousson *et al.*, 2010). Although quantitative analysis can be (and is) used in the direct improvement of sports performance, it is more often a research tool that gives us a better insight into a specific skill on which we can later draw for use in performance improvement.

NOTATIONAL ANALYSIS

What notational analysis can achieve

The definition of tactical patterns of play in sport has been a profitable source of work for notational analysts. The maturation of tactics can be analysed at different stages of development of a specific sport, usually by means of a cross-sectional design. The different tactics used at each stage of development within a sport will inevitably depend upon technical development, physical maturation and other variables. 'Maturation models' have very important implications for coaching methods and directions at different stages of development, for example, in each of the racket sports. Empirical modelling of tactical profiles is also important in notational analysis. Comparing the patterns of play of successful and unsuccessful teams or players in elite competitions enables the definition of those performance indicators that differentiate between the two groups. This research template has been used in several sports to highlight the tactical parameters that determine success; it has been extended, for example, in tennis to compare the patterns of play that are successful on the different surfaces on which the major tournaments are played. An interesting theme that has emerged, from some recent research, is that tactical models change with time, as players become fitter, stronger, and faster (consider, for example, the changes in rugby union since profession-alisation in 1996), and as sports equipment changes – for example, all rackets have become lighter and more powerful. As an example, over a period of less than 15 years the length of rallies in squash, for elite players, has decreased from about 20 shots to about 12 shots per rally (see also Hughes and Bartlett, 2008).

To define quantitatively where movement technique fails or excels has very practical uses not only for coaches but also for sports scientists aiming to analyse performance at different stages of development of athletes. Technique analysis is a crucial part of sports biomechanics (see also Chapter 6) and, therefore, it is an important aspect of the work of performance analysts. For example, winners and errors are powerful indicators of technical competence in racket sports and have often been used in research in notational analysis of net-wall games. It has been found that, for all standards of play in squash, if the winner : error ratio for a particular player in a match was greater than one, then that player usually won. However, in-depth technique analysis (usually quali-tative) is necessary to establish strengths and weaknesses in the movement techniques for the various strokes that lead to winners and errors. As noted earlier, an error may be due to an earlier badly executed stroke rather than the one immediately before the error.

Time–motion analysis can be used to establish the fitness profiles of players (see O'Donoghue, 2008). By so doing, for example, it is possible to determine the physio-logical 'work-rates' of the different positions in a soccer team, from the distances covered in a game and the percentage time spent walking, jogging, running and sprinting. To do this, as we noted above, it is essential to focus on individual players, rather than 'following the ball'. This requires the use of multiple observers, multiple cameras or observation of multiple games. Modern player tracking systems have taken much of the chore out of gathering player positional data and have made the development of player databases and data modelling in notational analysis much easier. The systems mostly used in player tracking in competition are video-based, such as Prozone® (www. prozonesports.com) and TRACAB™ (www.tracab.com). The systems are widely used in elite professional soccer and use multiple cameras to track the trajectories of all the players and the ball (see, for example, Figure 5.3) at sampling rates of 25 Hz or less. These video-based systems are essentially semi-automatic, as human intervention is needed to identify each player and the ball at the start of the game, and sometimes to verify player two-dimensional trajectories during the game, if trajectory occlusion occurs. Player tracking systems in which players wear a device of some kind are not currently allowed in most competitive sports games, but are widely used in training by many top teams, for example, in soccer and both rugby codes. These systems are usually based on the global positioning system (GPS), for example GPSports (www.gpsports.com), and provide completely automatic tracking as each player is uniquely identified, at sampling rates of 15 Hz or less. They require players to wear a receiver about the size of a match box and cannot be used indoors. For a review of player-tracking systems, see Barris and Button (2008). For further details of data modelling and analytical techniques in notational analysis, see Hughes and Franks (2008) and O'Donoghue (2010).

Figure 5.3 Player tracking in Prozone.

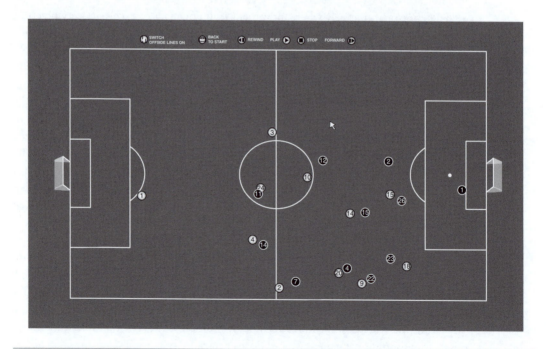

Notational analysis systems

As noted in an earlier section, one of the important considerations of a notational analysis is devising a notation system that is efficient and easy to learn. In this sub-section, we look at how to do this. For a more in-depth treatment, the reader is again referred to Hughes and Franks (2008).

The essentials of a notational analysis system

Although, in principle, any sports activity, including running, golf and boxing, can be notationally analysed, most notational analyses have been conducted on team or racket sports. The key elements of a notational analysis system for such sports are:

- **Player**. The player is often identified by a code, such as their shirt number in soccer or rugby, or letters in netball.
- **Position**. To specify the position, we divide the playing surface into coded cells, noting that a compromise is often needed between accuracy and meaningfulness in deciding on these. In competition, the analyst will rarely be able to add surface markings to those already marked on the playing surface. Trying to 'interpolate' cells between physical markings adds to the unreliability of positional data.
- **Action**. The actions that are recorded depend on what we are trying to find out (see, for example, Study Task 4). We try to capture the logic of the game (for which we often use flowcharts and action–outcome logic tables, as in the next sub-section) and use simple codes for each action.
- **Time**. The final element is time, which is very difficult to incorporate if the notating is being done 'in-event', but is automatically coded in video-based computerised notation systems.

Not all four of these elements will be present in every notation system, as in two of the examples that follow later. Analysts are often tempted to add a fifth element–outcome. However, all four of the elements above are present at each 'event', which involves an action, a player, a position and which occurs at a particular time in the game. Outcomes only arise from some 'events'. I prefer to code outcomes as part of the action category, either as a separate action, such as 'goal' in soccer, or by having two actions, such as 'successful shot' and 'unsuccessful shot'.

Capturing the logic of the game

As we noted above, notational analysts often use flowcharts and action–outcome logic tables to capture the logic of the game they wish to notate. The first step is often to represent the four key elements of the system as a hierarchical structural model of the sport. An example for a possession-dominated game is shown in Figure 5.4.

Figure 5.4 A hierarchical structural model of a possession-dominated game (adapted from Hughes, 2008a).

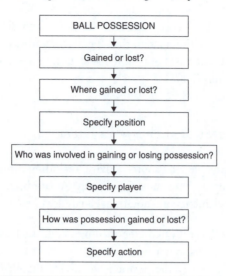

Table 5.1 Action–outcome logic table for soccer (simplified; not all possible actions are included here)

ACTION	OUTCOME	EFFECT ON POSSESSION
Pass	Successful	Retained
	Unsuccessful	Lost
Shot (including penalty)	Wide or high	Lost
	Saved	Lost
	Goal	Lost
	Blocked	Retained or lost
Tackle	Successful	Gained
	Unsuccessful	Not gained
Cross	Successful	Retained
	Unsuccessful	Lost
Corner	Successful	Retained
	Unsuccessful	Lost
Goal kick	Successful	Retained
	Unsuccessful	Lost
Throw-in	Successful	Retained
	Unsuccessful	Lost
Goalkeeper's throw	Successful	Retained
	Unsuccessful	Lost
Goalkeeper's kick	Successful	Retained
	Unsuccessful	Lost

This can then be supplemented by an action–outcome table; a simplified example for soccer is shown in Table 5.1. The many different actions that can be included in such a table can be appreciated by visiting the soccer analysis website http://www.capelloindex.com.

A hierarchical structural model and action–outcome logic table can then be combined to give a schematic flowchart. A simple example, focusing on the badminton serve, is shown in Figure 5.5. For further examples, you should see, for instance, Hughes (2008a).

Examples of notational analysis systems

In this sub-section, we introduce some examples of notational analysis systems, and touch on their uses and drawbacks.

Scatter diagrams

Scatter diagrams are used to represent the playing area, with actions notated where they took place and, if required, the player involved. For example, in Figure 5.6, we have shown the positions (x) on a soccer pitch where one team lost possession, what action (Cl = clear, Cr = cross, D = dribble, K = kick by goalkeeper, P = pass, S = shot) led to loss of possession, and which player (shirt number) was involved (the x is somewhat redundant as the action letter and player number can indicate the position). Simple scatter diagrams, such as Figure 5.6, can show a coach where his or her team lost the ball, which player lost the ball, and what action resulted in a lost ball. Clearly, more than one such diagram would be needed to record lost possessions during a whole game. Scatter diagrams are simple and quick to use; they can provide accurate records with practice. They can be used in-event and provide immediate feedback. However, they do not record the sequence of actions, except in the sense that consecutive diagrams throughout a game can be numbered.

Frequency tables

The summary information from frequency tables is routinely used on television to summarise the events in, for example, the first half of a rugby match or the first quarter of a netball match (see also Study Task 4). They can be used to log actions relevant to the information the coach requires about the team as a whole (as in Study Task 4) or about individual team players, as in Table 5.2. Frequency tables are simple and quick to use. They can provide accurate records with practice. They can be used 'in-event' and can provide immediate feedback. There is usually no need to process the data further. However, they provide no sequence of events nor do they show where on the playing surface the actions occurred, both of which can lead to misinterpretation of these simple data.

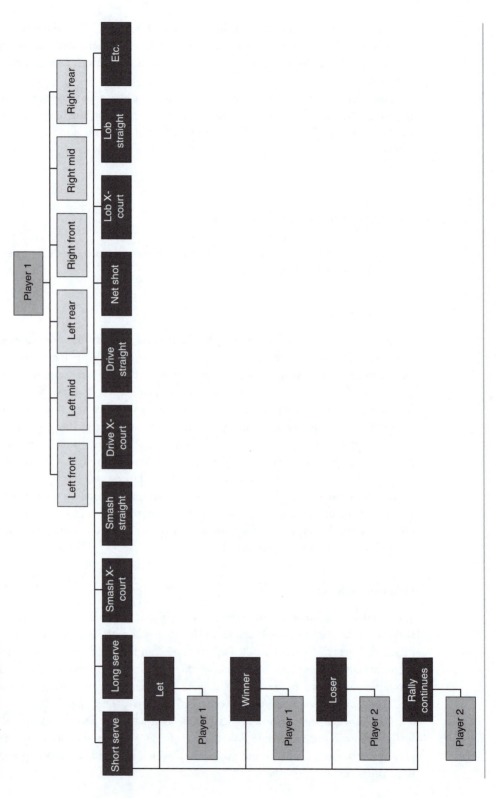

Figure 5.5 A simplified schematic flowchart for badminton. All six positions on the court are shown – front court is between the service line and the net, mid and rear court are the front and rear halves respectively of the rest of the court; however, actions are shown only for the left mid court, and the logic of action–outcomes on possession is shown only for the short serve.

Figure 5.6 Scatter diagram for one team during 15 minutes play of a 2010 FIFA World Cup soccer match; X marks the position on the pitch where possession was lost, the number is that of the player who lost possession, and the letters represent the action that resulted in lost possession: Cl = clear, Cr = cross, D = dribble (run with ball), F = foul, FK = free kick, H = header, P = pass, S = shot on goal. It is worth noting how few losses of possession resulted from actions in the team's own half (the vertical arrow on the right of the figure indicates the attacking direction for the team).

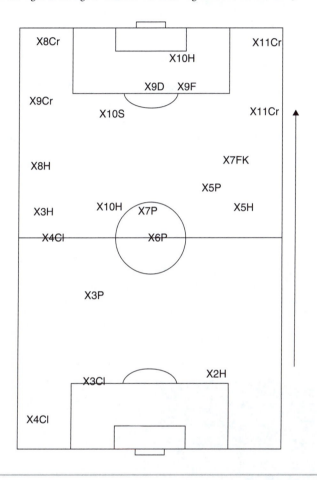

Sequential systems

Sequential systems, which log when actions took place and can include the players and positions as well, were occasionally used with in-event hand notation in the early days of notational analysis (see, for example, Hughes, 2008b). However, sequential analyses are usually performed using video-based computerised systems, in which time is automatically coded. The example shown in Figure 5.7 is taken from the notational analysis package, Focus, for a netball match between Australia and New Zealand in 2009. A frequency table of different types of passes in each position on the netball court is shown in the top right of this figure. Such frequency tables are easily constructed from the log of teams, players, actions and so on that is shown below the table (under Events). Here, we

Table 5.2 Frequency table for rugby union (not all actions included; 'group' actions, such as scrums and mauls, omitted for simplicity). Data taken from 15 minutes play of a 2010 Tri-Nations game for one of the two teams. The o in the 'Penalty goal' category indicates a missed penalty kick

ACTION	1	2	3	4	5	6	7	8	9	10	11	12	13	14	15
Try															
Conversion															
Penalty goal										ox					
Drop goal															
Tackle		X		X		X	XX	X	X	XX	X	X	X		
Pass			XXX						XXXXXX XXXXXX	XXX		XXX	XX	X	XXX
Run with ball		XX	X	X		XX	X	X	XX	XX	X	XXX	XXXX	XXXX	XX
Kick to touch															
Kick in field									X	XXXXX					X
Lineout catch															
Lineout assist															
Knock on					X							X			

Figure 5.7 Screen from the Focus notational analysis package for the analysis of a netball match between New Zealand Silver Ferns and Australian Diamonds in 2009. The video is shown on the left half of the screen, with its controls and time code at the bottom left. A pass by position frequency table is shown at the top right with a log of events below it. The sets of five category buttons (team, player, action, pass, position) are shown at the bottom right. Players: GK = goalkeeper; GD = goal defence; WD = wing defence; C = centre; WA = wing attack; GA = goal attack; GS = goal shooter. Positions: 1 = attacking goal circle for New Zealand (NZ); 2 = attacking goal third for NZ outside of position 1; 3 = centre third; 4 = defensive goal third for NZ outside of position 5; 5 = defensive goal circle for NZ. See the text for further elaboration.

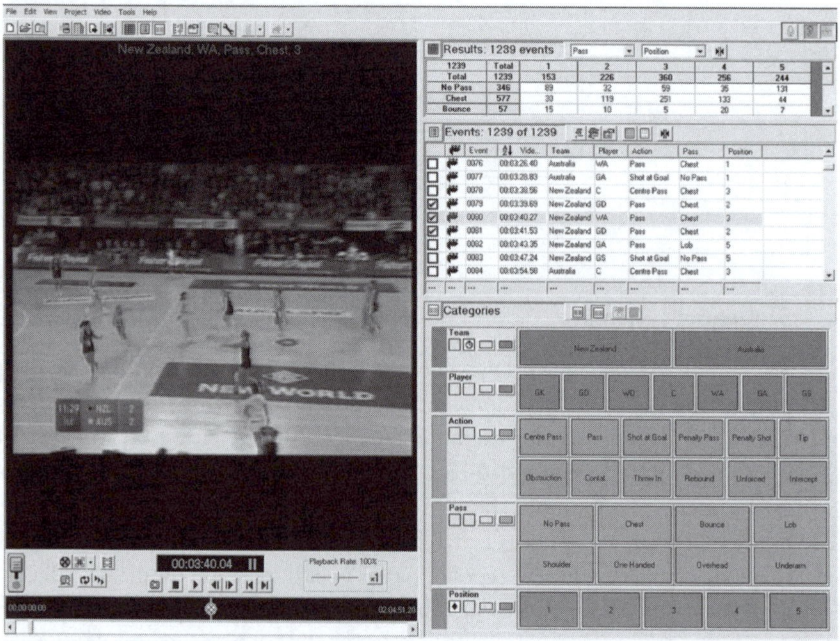

can see in the first column the number of the event; the second column is the time code, showing the time at which the event occurred. The third column shows which team was involved and the fourth column the individual player involved, by the letters worn. The fifth column shows the type of action and the sixth column the type of pass (if the action was not a pass, then No Pass is indicated). The seventh column shows where on the court the action occurred. Columns three to seven correspond to the five category sets at the bottom right of the figure (Team and Pass – the latter the focus of this study – have been added to the standard Player, Action and Position categories). Furthermore, the software allows the analyst and coach to group together similar events for sequential viewing with user-selected 'pre-roll' and 'post-roll' times before and after the selected event; in this example, all chest passes by New Zealand has been chosen (ticks in the boxes on the left of the Events log). In the figure, event 0080 – a chest pass from the New Zealand wing attack (WA) from the centre third of the court (position 3) is highlighted in light grey and appears in the video screen on the left of the figure. We could have chosen to look at all of the actions performed by the New Zealand wing attack, or any other combination of categories, depending on what the analyst or coach wished to focus on. Such collated action sequences allow the analyst and coach to focus on the skills involved in those actions. Tagging, and subsequent viewing, of similar actions was a great step forward in performance analysis: it was arguably the most important development in bringing together in a practical context sports biomechanics and notational analysis.

BIOMECHANICAL ANALYSIS

Sports biomechanics predominantly involves the study of sports skills, also known as movement techniques. At highly skilled standards of performance, we are concerned with the study of coordinated movement patterns, whereas for less skilful movements, the learning of coordinated movements is involved. Sports biomechanics can be described as the observation, measurement and analysis of human movement patterns, which also involves other sport science disciplines, such as motor learning and notational analysis. Noting that the analysis may be qualitative or quantitative, as discussed above, we identify different measuring techniques needed to carry out various analytical focuses in sports biomechanics (Table 5.3).

Table 5.3 Biomechanical analysis focus and recording techniques (see also Payton and Bartlett, 2008)

FOCUS OF ANALYSIS	RECORDING TECHNIQUE
Purely qualitative	Videography
Temporal, movement phases	Timing from any image-based motion analysis system (usually from videography)
Kinematics	Any image-based motion analysis system or accelerometry
Kinetics	Force or pressure plates, force or pressure transducers, image-based motion analysis system and inverse dynamics

Biomechanical movement principles

We can describe the biomechanical principles of coordinated movement as being made up of the general laws – based mostly on physics and biology – that determine human motion. These principles may be subdivided into:

- **Universal principles**, which are valid for all sports movements.
- **Principles of partial generality**, which are valid for large groups of sports activities, for example, force, speed, endurance, accuracy, or balance tasks.
- **Specific principles**, which are valid for specific sports activities.

These principles need to take into account the constraints on any movement (Figure 5.8). These constraints are generally grouped as follows.

- **Organismic constraints**. These are internal to the individual, such as anatomical-anthropometric characteristics, strength, flexibility, and fitness.
- **Task constraints**. These are the specific constraints of the task, such as the forces, torques (moments of force), inertia, accuracy and speed that are needed to perform the task. This grouping also includes the rules of the sports task.
- **Environmental constraints**. These are external to the individual – the spatial and temporal constraints. Environmental constraints can also be considered to include equipment.

Figure 5.8 Diagrammatic representation of the constraints model.

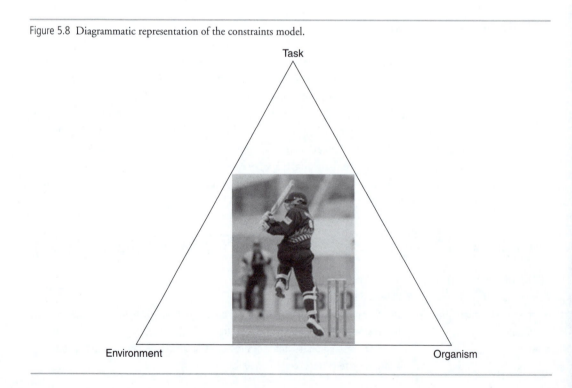

It should be noted that, although the coordination of joint and muscle actions is often considered to be crucial to the successful execution of sports movements, too few of the underlying assumptions have been rigorously tested. For example, the transfer of angular momentum from proximal to distal segments (e.g. trunk to upper arm to forearm) is often considered to be a feature of vigorous sports movements. However, in kicking, the principle of angular momentum transfer from the upper leg (thigh) to the lower leg (calf) does not explain correctly why the thigh decelerates because of the interaction between the two segments. Instead, the angular deceleration of the thigh is caused by the motion of the calf, through inertia coupling between the two segments (as illustrated by the equations for two-segment motion in Chapter 4). The performance of the kick would be improved if the thigh did not decelerate, rather than the deceleration of the thigh facilitating angular momentum transfer to enhance performance. The reader should bear in mind the relative shortage of systematic research into the applicability in sports movements of the principles of coordinated movement.

Universal movement principles

Use of pre-stretch or the stretch–shortening cycle of muscular contraction

In performing many activities, a segment often moves in the opposite direction to the one intended: this is considered further in phase analysis below. This initial counter movement is often necessary simply to allow the subsequent movement to occur. Other benefits arise from: the increased acceleration path; initiation of the stretch reflex; storage of elastic energy; and stretching the muscle to optimal length for forceful contraction, which relates to the muscle's length–tension curve. The underlying mechanisms of the stretch–shortening cycle were considered in Chapter 2.

Minimisation of energy used to perform a specific task

There is some evidence to support this minimisation of energy principle as an adaptive mechanism in skill acquisition; for example, the reduction in unnecessary movements during the learning of throwing skills. The large number of multi-joint muscles in the body supports the importance of energy efficiency as an evolutionary principle.

Principle of minimum task complexity – or control of redundant degrees of freedom in the kinetic chain

The kinetic chain proceeds from the most proximal to the most distal segment. Coordination of that complex chain of body segments becomes more complex as the number of degrees of freedom – the possible axes of rotation plus directions of linear motion at each joint – increases. A simple kinetic chain from shoulder girdle to fingers contains at least 17 degrees of rotational freedom. Obviously, many of these need to be 'controlled' to permit the movement to achieve its goal; for example, in a basketball set shot the player keeps the elbow well into the body to reduce the redundant degrees of freedom. The forces need to be applied in the required direction of motion. This principle explains why skilled movements look so simple. The temporal and spatial characteristics of the relevant kinetic chains are often the main focus of many quantitative biomechanical analyses.

Principles of partial generality

Sequential action of muscles – or transfer of angular momentum along the kinetic chain

This principle is most important in activities requiring speed or force, such as discus throwing. It involves the recruitment of body segments into the movement at the correct time. In throwing, movements are generally initiated by the large muscle groups of the legs, which are usually pennate and which produce force to overcome the inertia of the whole body plus the object to be thrown. The sequence is continued by the faster muscles of the arms, which have not only a larger range of movement and greater speed but also improved accuracy owing to the smaller number of muscle fibres innervated by each motor neuron (the innervation ratio). In correct sequencing, proximal segments move ahead of distal ones, which ensures that muscles are stretched to develop tension when they contract.

Minimisation of inertia – or increasing acceleration of motion

This is most important in endurance and speed activities. Movements at any joint should be initiated with the distal joints in a position that minimises the moment of inertia, to maximise rotational acceleration. For example, in the recovery phase of sprinting, the hip is flexed with the knee also flexed; this configuration has a far lower moment of inertia than an extended or semi-flexed knee. This principle relates to the generation and transfer of angular momentum, which are affected by changes in the moment of inertia.

Principle of impulse generation–absorption

This principle is mainly important in force and speed activities. It relates to the impulse–momentum relationship: impulse = change of momentum = mean force multiplied by the time over which the force acts. This shows that a large impulse is needed to produce a large change of momentum; this requires a large mean force or a long time of action. In impulse generation, the former must predominate because of the explosive short duration of many sports movements, such as a high jump take-off, which requires power – the rapid performance of work (see below). In absorbing momentum, as when catching a cricket ball, the time is increased by 'giving' with the ball to reduce the mean impact force, preventing bruising or fracture and increasing success.

Maximising the acceleration path

This principle arises from the work–energy relationship (change in mechanical energy = work done = mean force multiplied by the distance over which the force acts). This relationship shows that a large change in mechanical energy requires a large mean force or the maximising of the distance over which force is applied, often referred to as the effective acceleration path. This is an important principle in events requiring speed and force, for example, a shot-putter making full use of the width of the throwing circle.

Stability

A wide base of support is needed for stability; this applies not only for static activities but also for dynamic ones in which sudden changes in the momentum vector occur, such as Olympic weightlifting.

Movement phase analysis

The first step in the biomechanical analysis of a sports skill is often the timing of the duration of the phases of the movement, as in the phase analyses of the following subsections. The division of a movement into separate, but linked, phases is helpful in developing a qualitative analysis of a technique, because of the sheer complexity of many sports techniques. The phases of the movement should be selected so that they have a biomechanically distinct role in the overall movement which is different from that of preceding and succeeding phases. Each phase then has a clearly defined biomechanical function and easily identified phase boundaries, often called key moments or key events. Although phase analysis can help the understanding of complex movements in sport, the essential feature of these movements is their wholeness; this should always be borne in mind when undertaking any phase analysis of sports movements.

Phase analysis of ballistic movements

Many 'ballistic' sports movements, such as hitting, throwing and kicking, can be subdivided into three phases:

- Preparation (backswing).
- Action (hitting).
- Recovery (follow-through).

Each of these phases has specific biomechanical functions. The later phases depend upon the previous phase or phases. It should be noted that, when recording the durations of these phases, a suitable definition of the phase boundaries needs to be chosen. For example, in a tennis serve the end of the backward movement of the racket might be chosen as defining the end of the preparation phase and the start of the action phase.

However, at that instant, the legs and trunk will be in their action phase while the distal joints of the racket arm will not yet have reached the end of their preparation phase. This is reflected in the principle of sequential action of muscles (see above). This indicates one drawback of phase analysis – the selection of the key events can be somewhat arbitrary.

Preparation phase

This phase has the following biomechanical functions.

- It puts the body into an advantageous position for the action phase.
- It maximises the range of movement of the performer's centre of mass (and the object being thrown in throwing skills); that is, it increases the acceleration path.
- It allows the larger segments to initiate the movement (sequential action of muscles).
- It makes use of the length–tension relationship of the agonist muscles by increasing the muscle length to that at which maximum tension is developed (about 1.2 times the resting length).
- It allows the storage of elastic energy in the series elastic and parallel elastic elements of the agonist muscles. This energy can then be 'repaid' during the action phase.
- Contraction of the antagonist muscles in this phase provides Golgi tendon organ facilitation for the agonists in the action phase.
- It puts the agonist muscles on stretch (the stretch–shortening cycle), thus increasing the output of the muscle spindle to reinforce the gamma discharge and increase the neural impulse through afferent neurons to the motor pools of the active muscles.

If the requirement of the movement is force or speed, then a fast backswing will gain the advantage of an increased phasic (speed-dependent) muscle spindle discharge, while a long backswing will increase the tonic (position-dependent) response. A fast backswing will promote a greater rise in spindle frequency leading to a stronger action, while a minimum hesitation between the preparation and action phases will allow full use of the phasic response. If the movement requires force or speed but the preparatory position must be held, as in a discus throw, then the phasic response cannot be used. To make full use of the tonic response, it is then necessary to use the longest possible backswing consistent with other requirements. If accuracy is the main goal, then a short and slow preparation is needed to control both the phasic and tonic spindle output so as to produce only the small forces needed. A short hesitation at the end of the preparation allows the phasic response to subside to the tonic level and aids accuracy; this is evident in the cueing techniques of skilful snooker players.

Action phase

Many of the biomechanical principles of coordinated movement (see above) become evident here. In skilful performers, we observe the sequential action of muscles, as body segments are recruited into the movement pattern at the correct time. Movements are initiated by the large muscle groups and continued by the faster, smaller and more distal muscles of the limbs, increasing the speed throughout the movement as the segmental ranges of movement increase. The accuracy of movement also increases through the recruitment of muscles with a progressively decreasing innervation ratio. The segmental forces are applied in the direction of movement and movements are initiated with minimum inertia as the movement proceeds along the kinetic chain. Finally, redundant degrees of freedom are controlled. The movements should be in accordance with these biomechanical features if the movement pattern is to be deemed as 'correct'. In ballistic movements, where speed is usually the predominant requirement, all these principles should be evident, whereas in force, accuracy or endurance movements, one or more principles may be of lesser importance.

Recovery phase

This involves the controlled deceleration of the movement by eccentric contraction of the appropriate muscles. A position of temporary balance (stability) may be achieved, as at the end of a golf swing. For a learner, the follow-through may require a conscious effort to overcome the Golgi tendon organ inhibition, which is reinforced by antagonistic muscle spindle activity.

Phase analysis of running

The obvious division of running into support and non-support phases does not provide an adequate biomechanical description of this activity. A better, more specific one divides each of these phases into three sub-phases.

Support phase

- **Foot strike**. The function of this sub-phase is impact absorption; this has often been described as the amortisation phase for some jumping activities.
- **Mid-support**. This serves to maintain forward momentum and to support the body's weight. It is characterised by a relative shortening of the overall limb length towards the lowest position of the whole body centre of mass.
- **Take-off**. This sub-phase has the function of accelerating the body forwards and upwards by a relative increase in the limb length (leg extension). Effort is transferred from the powerful muscles of the trunk and thigh to the faster muscles of the calf.

Non-support (recovery) phase

- **Follow-through**. This is functionally a decelerating sub-phase, characterised by a slowing of hip extension followed by the start of thigh flexion, both accompanied by, and the latter assisting, knee flexion.
- **Forward swing**. Although a preparation for foot descent, the main biomechanical function of this sub-phase is the enhancement of the forward and upward ground

reaction thrust. The sub-phase begins as the foot moves forwards; this forward swing of the recovery leg coincides with the take-off sub-phase of the opposite leg.

- **Foot descent**. This sub-phase begins with the arresting of the forward motion of the leg and foot, by the hamstrings, and continues until the foot contacts the ground. Its main biomechanical function is to have the foot strike the ground with a backward speed relative to the body's centre of mass as near in magnitude as possible to the speed of the mass centre relative to the ground. Such an 'active landing' is desirable to reduce 'braking' and to allow a smooth transition to foot strike.

Phase analysis of other activities

Examples exist in the literature of attempts to force the preparation–action–recovery pattern on techniques to which it is not strictly applicable. It is far preferable to treat each technique on its own merits, as in the two brief examples below.

Volleyball spike

- Run-in: generating controllable speed.
- Landing: impact absorption.
- Impulse drive: horizontal to vertical momentum transfer.
- Airborne phase of preparation.
- Hitting phase.
- Airborne phase to landing (airborne recovery).
- Landing: to control deceleration; preparation for the next move.

Javelin throw

- Run-up: generation of controllable speed.
- Withdrawal: increase of acceleration path of javelin.
- Cross-over steps: change from front-on run-up to side-on delivery stride.
- Delivery stride: the action phase.
- Recovery.

Both the above techniques involve the ballistic preparation–action–recovery sequence as part of a more complex movement pattern. In some sports a phase–sub-phase analysis is more appropriate. An example for swimming is provided in Table 5.4. It is left to the reader to identify the biomechanical functions of each of the sub-phases of this activity (see Study Task 8).

Concluding comments on movement phase analysis

By splitting a complex movement into its temporal components (phases), it is easier to conduct a qualitative analysis of the skill, which can then be used to identify incorrect

MAIN PHASE	SUB-PHASES
Start	Impulse generation
	Flight
	Glide
Stroking	Initial press
	Outward scull
	Inward scull
	Recovery
Turning	Preparation for turn
	Contact phase
	Glide from turn

Table 5.4 Main phases and sub-phases in swimming

features of the technique analysed. This will usually be facilitated by some quantitative analysis of the technique. It has already been mentioned that the selection of the key events that form the phase boundaries can be somewhat arbitrary. Also, it is not clear that the phases represent any important temporal events of motor behaviour. For example, as noted above, foot strike (foot contact with the ground) is often used as a key event in the running cycle. However, muscle activation, which is related to movement control, usually precedes foot strike by as much as 100 ms. This observation suggests that, in future, techniques could be developed for subdividing movements into phases that are more meaningful for motor behaviour. It should also be recognised, in technique analysis, that, as the phases blend into a coordinated whole, an apparent deficiency in technique in one phase may often be caused by an error in an earlier phase. For example, in a gymnastics vault, problems in the post-flight may be traced back to a poor generation of vertical or angular momentum during contact with the vaulting horse. This may, in turn, result from errors even earlier in the vault.

SUMMARY

In this chapter we explored the meaning of performance analysis, and how it evolved. The main features of each of the four stages of the structured analysis process were outlined and the differences between qualitative, quantitative (and semi-quantitative) analysis were explained, along with the value of each. We then considered what constitutes notational analysis and looked at the four key elements of a notational analysis system. An appreciation was provided of the factors underlying the design of a notational analysis system, and examples were given of the uses of scatter diagrams and frequency charts. We also considered the essentials of a computerised notational analysis system and its use in sequential analysis. Various aspects of biomechanical analysis of the movements of the sports performer were covered. The biomechanical principles of coordinated movement – both universal and partially general – were covered, along with their applicability to various sports movements. The importance of the phase analysis of sports movements was emphasised and illustrated with reference to ballistic movements and running; other sports movements were touched on briefly. The functions of movement phases in terms of the biomechanical principles of coordinated movement were considered.

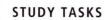

STUDY TASKS

1   List the similarities and differences between notational analysis and biomechanical analysis of sports.

2   Explain the circumstances in which qualitative analysis, semi-quantitative analysis and quantitative analysis would be used. Give examples for both notational and biomechanical analysis.

3   Carry out a simple notational analysis of a team sport of your choice for at least 15 minutes of play:

    (a) using a scatter diagram
    (b) using a frequency table.

    Focus on only one team but consider each player in that team. You will find this much easier to do from video than in-event.

4   Notate a quarter (15 minutes) of a netball match, using the frequency table for netball (Figure 5.9). The coach has asked for basic information about what actions (including different types of turnover) lead to goals (you will not notate passes between other actions and goals nor actions leading to penalty throws, free throws or penalty shots). Log and count up the frequency of each action and when they lead (directly or via passes) to goals. You need to obtain a video of a quarter's play in a netball match for this purpose. Play the video through once to familiarise yourself with the various actions and then complete the frequency table without pausing the video, to simulate doing the analysis in-event. Repeat the analysis a few days later, to check your consistency. Finally, repeat the analysis once more, but this time pausing and, when necessary, 'rewinding' the video to ensure you have logged each action correctly. Explain any differences between the numbers of actions you logged on the three occasions.

5   Make a list of the biomechanical principles of coordinated movement, both universal and partially general. Then describe the meaning of each of the principles, giving examples from sports of your choice. For the principles of partial generality, state whether they are relevant or not for groups of movements in which, respectively, speed, force and accuracy are the dominant factors.

6   Using a good quality 50 Hz video camera, make a recording of a good runner, running reasonably fast. From your recording, try to measure the duration of each of the six sub-phases of running described above. By qualitative analysis, determine

Figure 5.9 Simplified frequency table for netball, to be used in conjunction with Study Task 4. The actions to be logged are shown, and briefly explained, in the centre column. Log the number of times each team performs each of these actions in the 'Number of each action' columns and the number of times each of these actions leads to a goal, directly or via passes, in the 'Number of goals' columns.

Team A (left to right)		Action	Team B (right to left)	
Number of goals	Number of each action		Number of each action	Number of goals
		Centre passes (to start the game and after each goal)		
		Interceptions (include bad passes but not touches with no loss of possession)		
		Throws in (after ball has gone out of court)		
		Defensive rebounds (defence gathers failed shot)		
		Free or penalty passes (log all even when no change of possession)		
		Penalty shots (log all even when no change of possession)		

whether the descriptions of those sub-phases apply to your runner: account for any discrepancies. If possible, repeat for a range of running speeds or runners of varying ability.

7 Perform a full phase analysis (including the durations of each phase) from your own or commercially available video recordings of any ballistic sports movement. Be very careful to define sensible and meaningful phase boundaries.

8 Identify the biomechanical functions of each of the sub-phases of the three main phases of swimming (see Table 5.4) for any of the four competitive strokes.

GLOSSARY OF IMPORTANT TERMS

Artificial intelligence The branch of computer science that deals, loosely speaking, with 'intelligent machines' – machines (computers) that do things that would require intelligence if done by a human. The two most important branches to date for performance analysts are expert systems and artificial neural networks (see also Chapter 7).

Ballistic movements Movements that are initiated by muscle activity in one muscle group, continue with a period (sometimes called coasting) of no muscle activity, and end by deceleration by the antagonistic muscle group or by passive tissues, such as ligaments.

Cross-sectional designs The term is used to refer to research designs taken at a specific time (a 'snapshot'). As an example, one or more trials by each finalist in the javelin throw at an international championship would be studied (see also Chapter 7).

Deterministic (or hierarchical) performance models These are models of the factors that influence sports performance in which the factors in the lower levels of the model completely determine (hence, deterministic) those in the higher levels. The top level is the factor by which performance is assessed, called the performance criterion – such as the time of a race or distance of a throw or jump. They resemble hierarchical models, for example in Microsoft Word, hence the alternative name (see also Chapter 6).

Empirical modelling This involves devising mathematical models, usually statistical ones, using experimental data. It is used widely in sports biomechanics and notational analysis.

Golgi tendon organs These are small stretch receptors located at the junction of a muscle and its tendon. Their discharge causes inhibition of the muscle in which they are located (which helps to protect the muscle) and facilitation of the antagonist muscle.

Innervation ratio The number of muscle fibres that are stimulated, or innervated, by a single motor neuron; the number of muscle fibres in a particular motor unit. This ratio varies from as few as 10 for muscles requiring very fine control to over 1000 for the weight-bearing muscles of the lower extremities.

Markov chains Named after A. A. Markov, a Markov chain is a random process in which one state depends only on the previous state. Markov chains are useful as tools for statistical modelling, particularly, in the context of this book, in modelling the outcomes of games, such as squash.

Movement trajectory analysis A term normally used to refer to the analysis of the two-dimensional paths (or trajectories) taken by players over time across the surface of a sports pitch or court.

Net-wall games Games involving a net or a wall. Table tennis, tennis, badminton and volleyball are net games and squash and fives are wall games. One of the three common categories of formal games, the others being striking and fielding games (such as cricket and baseball) and invasion games (such as rugby, basketball, soccer and netball).

Pennate muscles The class of muscles, accounting for 75% of the body's musculature, with relatively short fibres angled away from the tendon. The arrangement allows more fibres to be recruited, which provides a stronger, more powerful movement at the expense of range and speed of movement. The class includes the tibialis anterior (a unipennate muscle), flexor hallucis longus (a bipennate muscle) and the deltoid (a multipennate muscle).

Perturbation analysis Used in notational analysis of sports (particularly, to date, squash) to refer to disruptions to steady rhythms of play, through critical incidents or perturbations. These perturbations may then lead to the end of a rally or be smoothed out, resulting in the establishment of a new steady rhythm of play. They can often be seen by experienced observers as well as measured.

Stretch reflex The contraction of a muscle in response to a sudden stretching of that muscle. It occurs in the stretch–shortening cycle.

REFERENCES

Barris, S. and Button, C. (2008) A review of vision-based motion analysis in sport. *Sports Medicine, 38*, 1025–1043.

Bartlett, R.M. (2007) *Introduction to Sports Biomechanics: Analysing Human Movement Patterns*, London: Routledge.

Bourbousson, J., Séve, C. and McGarry, T. (2010) Space–time coordination dynamics in basketball (in two parts). *Journal of Sports Sciences, 28*, 339–358.

Hughes, M.D. (2008a) 'Sports analysis', in M.D. Hughes and I.M. Franks (eds) *The Essentials of Performance Analysis: An Introduction*, London: Routledge, pp. 85–97.

Hughes, M.D. (2008b) 'An overview of the development of notational analysis', in M.D. Hughes and I.M. Franks (eds) *The Essentials of Performance Analysis: An Introduction*, London: Routledge, pp. 51–84.

Hughes, M.D. and Bartlett, R.M. (eds) (2002) *Journal of Sports Sciences, 20(10)*, Special Issue on Performance Analysis.

Hughes, M.D. and Bartlett, R.M. (2004) 'The use of performance indicators in performance analysis', in M.D. Hughes and I.M. Franks (eds) *Notational Analysis of Sport: Systems for Better Coaching and Performance in Sport*, London: Routledge, pp. 166–188.

Hughes, M.D. and Bartlett, R.M. (2008) 'What is performance analysis?', in M.D. Hughes and I.M. Franks (eds) *The Essentials of Performance Analysis: An Introduction*, London: Routledge, pp. 8–20.

Hughes, M.D. and Franks, I.M. (eds) (2008) *The Essentials of Performance Analysis: An Introduction*, London: Routledge.

Knudson, D.V. and Morrison, C.S. (2002) *Qualitative Analysis of Human Movement*, Champaign, IL: Human Kinetics.

McGarry, T. (2008) 'Probability analysis of notated events in sports contests: skill and chance', in M.D. Hughes and I.M. Franks (eds) *The Essentials of Performance Analysis: An Introduction*, London: Routledge, pp. 206–225.

O'Donoghue, P. (2008) 'Time–motion analysis', in M.D. Hughes and I.M. Franks (eds) *The Essentials of Performance Analysis: An Introduction*, London: Routledge, pp. 180–205.

O'Donoghue, P. (2010) *Research Methods in Sports Performance Analysis*, London: Routledge.

Payton, C.J and Bartlett, R.M. (eds) (2008) *Biomechanical Evaluation of Movement in Sport and Exercise: The British Association of Sport and Exercise Sciences Guide*, London: Routledge.

FURTHER READING

Bartlett, R.M. (2007) *Introduction to Sports Biomechanics: Analysing Human Movement Patterns*, London: Routledge. This book should be particularly useful if you have struggled with any of the biomechanics material in this chapter, and will help to prepare you for later chapters. For the purposes of this chapter, you should focus on Chapters 1 and 2 of this further reading material.

Hughes, M.D. and Franks, I.M. (eds) (2008) *The Essentials of Performance Analysis: An Introduction*, London: Routledge. This textbook develops many themes on notational analysis that have only been touched on in this chapter. Chapters 2, 5–8 and 11 should be particularly useful.

6 Performance improvement through qualitative biomechanical analysis

Roger Bartlett

Knowledge assumed
Ability to undertake simple
descriptive analysis of videos
of sports movements
Understanding of the basics
of performance analysis
(Chapter 5)
Familiarity with movement
phase analysis and
biomechanical movement
principles (Chapter 5)
Familiarity with graphs of
one variable plotted as a
function of a second variable,
often time

▮ INTRODUCTION

BOX 6.1 LEARNING OUTCOMES ▮

After reading this chapter you should be able to:

- plan and undertake a qualitative video analysis of a sports technique of your choice
- develop a critical insight into qualitative biomechanical analysis of movement in sport
- appreciate the need for a structured approach to qualitative movement analysis and understand the tasks of the four stages of the structured approach to qualitative analysis
- outline the principles of deterministic modelling and perform a qualitative analysis of a sports skill in detail, using a deterministic (or hierarchical) model
- appreciate how use of a deterministic model can avoid some of the pitfalls of qualitative analysis
- explain the various forms of movement pattern that are important for any movement analyst
- be able to interpret graphical patterns of angle as a function of time in terms of angular velocity and angular acceleration from the shape of the angle–time patterns
- understand the basic patterns used to study joint coordination.

In the previous chapter, we discussed what performance analysis is and how performance analysts in general use notational analysis and biomechanical analysis to try to improve the performance of teams and individual athletes respectively. We also noted that performance analysts often use qualitative and semi-quantitative analysis in their work with coaches and athletes, rather than quantitative analysis. The increasing demand from the real world of sports performance – coaches, athletes and other practitioners – outside of academia has generated an increasing demand for good qualitative movement analysts; this is our main focus in this chapter. We also consider further the structured approach to qualitative biomechanical analysis that was touched on in Chapter 5 (see also Bartlett, 2007; Knudson and Morrison, 2002; Knudson, 2007). This approach is very similar to that recommended by some professional agencies that represent sports biomechanists, or by agencies that hire sports biomechanists, such as the New Zealand Academy of Sport. Although the approach outlined here is used more by qualitative biomechanical analysts than by quantitative analysts, it could – and should – be adopted by the latter group to provide a structure for their work.

An important part of the focus on seeking to improve sports performance throughout the second half of this book involves the use of models of performance; in this chapter, we consider the use of deterministic models of performance in qualitative analysis, and some alternatives. Nearly all of these approaches focus on qualitative analysis based on identifying errors in the movement and how to correct them. Whichever approach has been used, the tendency has been to focus on instantaneous events, such as a leg, arm, or trunk angle at release of an implement – after all, for the qualitative analyst, these 'critical features' need to be observable. However, such 'discrete parameters' often miss information about the overall movement, the distinctive features of which are its whole-ness and the coordination of the skill. One of the aims of this book is to help to rectify this lack of focus on movement wholeness and coordination. Therefore, in this chapter we also focus on other 'tools' that are available to qualitative movement analysts, through the study of the qualitative features of graphical representations of movement patterns as time series graphs or coordination patterns. These deserve far more attention from, and use by, qualitative movement analysts.

PREPARATION STAGE – IDENTIFYING CRITICAL FEATURES

As noted in Chapter 5, the preparation stage of the structured qualitative analysis process involves gathering of knowledge, including the undertaking of a needs analysis, identi-fying critical features of the performance, and preparing for the later stages of the anal-ysis process. We will focus here mainly on the second of these – identifying the critical features of the movement.

Gathering knowledge

The gathering of relevant knowledge is dynamic and on going. A successful movement analyst needs knowledge, first and foremost, of the activity or movement, from which he or she will then develop the critical features of performance. Second, knowledge is needed of the performers; this includes the performers', and coaches' or therapists', needs, which should be identified through a 'needs analysis'. Although the preparation for later stages of the qualitative analysis process takes place, at least in gathering relevant knowledge, in the preparation stage, these will be dealt with under later stages. Developing a systematic observation strategy is covered in the next section and developing an intervention strategy is dealt with in Chapter 8 and only touched on in this chapter. Later in the chapter, we will discuss the qualitative representations of movement and coordination patterns, in addition to video analysis, which can be used in the evaluation and diagnosis stage.

Your knowledge of the activity, as a movement analyst, should draw on many sport and exercise science disciplines. For example, as a primary physical education teacher, you would source knowledge mainly from the discipline of motor development: a secondary physical education teacher, by contrast, would focus more on an analysis of individual skills and techniques using, primarily, sports biomechanics. As a movement analyst working with novices, motor learning and practice would be major sources of information for you. On the other hand, a movement analyst working with good club-standard performers would probably focus on a biomechanically-derived identification of critical features, and a movement analyst working with elite performers would concentrate on the critical features at that standard, and might use a more quantitative approach.

In all of our work as movement analysts, whether qualitative or quantitative, we should always seek to adhere to 'evidence-based' practice, which raises the question as to what evidence to gather and from where. A movement analyst has, in general, access to various sources of knowledge about the sports activity being studied. Some issues arise in using these sources, including the fragmentary nature of some sources and weighing conflicting evidence from various sources. Experience also influences success in using source material, and helps to deal with anecdotal evidence and, with care, personal bias. The gathering of valid knowledge of the activity under consideration is invaluable if done systematically, and one needs to keep practising developing critical features based on the knowledge gathered. A warning here is appropriate; although the Internet is a fruitful source of information, in general there is little, if any, quality control over what appears there. There are exceptions to this warning, particularly peer-reviewed websites such as the Coaches' Information Services site (http://coachesinfo.com/) run by the International Society of Biomechanics in Sports (ISBS; www.isbs.org). Valid information is best sourced from such expert opinion, which can also be found in professional journals such as the *Sport and Exercise Scientist* (British Association of Sport and Exercise Sciences, UK: www.bases.org.uk) and sport-specific coaching journals (such as *Swimming Technique*, now an integral part of Swimming World Magazine: www.swimmingworldmagazine. com) – many of these sources are accessible though the Internet. The sports performers and their support staff included in any 'real-world' study are also a potential source of knowledge about their sport, as may be other coaches and performers involved; not all of their knowledge will normally be evidence-based and some may be biased, so care is needed in using it. Problems associated with synthesising all of this knowledge include conflicts of opinion, a reliance on the 'elite-athlete template' – what the most successful do must also be right for others – and incorrect notions about critical features.

Scientific research should provide the most valid and accurate sources of information. Movement analysts need some research training, however, to interpret research findings: applied BScs or MScs should provide such training in an applied context, while research PhDs often focus on quantitative biomechanical analysis, which we will discuss in the next chapter. The best sources of relevant, applied research are applied sports science research journals, such as *Sports Biomechanics* (www.tandf.co.uk/journals/rspb) published on behalf of the ISBS, and the best coaching journals, such as *New Studies in Athletics* (www.iaaf.org/development/studies/index.html). Sports-specific scientific review papers draw together knowledge from many sources and provide a valuable source of information for movement analysts, providing the reviews have an applied rather than a fundamental research focus. A fruitful source for such review papers has been the *Journal of Sports Sciences* (www.tandf.co.uk/journals/titles/02640414.asp). The major problem with scientific research as a source of information for the qualitative movement analyst might be called the validity conflict between internal (research) validity and ecological (real-world) validity – in the laboratory or in the field.

It is not sufficient just to gather knowledge of the activity; it must also be theoretically focused and practically synthesised. Adopting a 'fundamental movement pattern' approach is now seen as flawed, because of its over-reliance on the motor programme concept of cognitive motor control. The constraints-led approach, introduced briefly in Chapter 1, considers the movement 'space' (the set of all possible solutions to the specific movement task) as constrained by the task, environment and organism; this is the approach of ecological motor control, which is still evolving (see Davids *et al.*, 2008). The critical features approach, adopted in the next sub-section, is the most widely-used by movement analysts from a sports biomechanics perspective. The analyst needs to keep practising this practical approach, whose points are widely used in teaching and coaching. The movement criterion might be injury risk, movement effectiveness – defined as achievement of the movement goal – or efficiency, the economical use of metabolic energy; our focus here will be on improved performance. Analysts often specify a range of correctness of critical features, this range must be observable. One common error is not focusing sufficiently on devising cue words for use in correcting technique errors; error correction should be seen as the responsibility of the movement analysis team, which includes the coach and the movement analyst, not the coach alone.

Relevant knowledge of the performers will include their age, sex, and standard of performance; physical abilities, such as fitness, strength, and flexibility; injury status and history; and cognitive development, which relates to the feedback to be provided in the intervention stage. Also relevant here is knowledge of the particular activity as related to a specific performer, which may require knowledge from motor development and motor learning. An extremely important knowledge source is the 'needs' of the performers and their coaches or therapists; to address this properly requires a 'needs analysis' led by the movement analyst, based on the foregoing points and knowledge of the sports activity. This needs analysis (including in the real world, a project costing to deliver what is needed) then has to be approved by your 'clients', before leading into the acquisition of other relevant knowledge, being translated into a systematic observation strategy, driving the evaluation and diagnosis, and providing the structure for the intervention.

The requisite knowledge for development of a systematic observation strategy (see also the next section) includes how to observe, based on the overall movement or its phases, the best observation (or vantage) points, and how many observations are needed. Aids to the development of this strategy include the use of videography and rating scales. It is advisable for all movement analysts to practise observation even when using video, particularly if movements are fast and complex, as in notating games. Furthermore, the analyst should develop pre-pilot and pilot protocols to ensure all problems are overcome before the 'big day'. The advice 'pilot, pilot, then pilot some more' is well founded.

Knowledge of effective instruction, feedback and intervention provide the appropriate information to translate critical features into intervention cues, couched in behavioural terms, which are appropriate to one's 'clients'. These should not be verbose – no more than six words, and figurative not literal. Remember that analogies must be meaningful; advising that the backhand clear in badminton is like 'swiping a fly off the ceiling with a towel' has no meaning to someone who has never performed such an action or seen another person do it. The cues to be devised can be verbal, visual, aural or kinaesthetic, and may differ for various phases of a movement; for example, a javelin coach may see value in attending to the aural cues of footfall during the run-up, but would switch to other cues for the delivery phase. The movement analyst needs, therefore, to derive relevant cues for each movement phase, and should attend to: the cue structure (what the action is); its content (what does the action – the doers); and cue qualification (how to gauge success). Special conditions may be added if more information is needed. Examples include: rotate (action) the hip and trunk (the doers); swing (action) the racket (doer) forwards (qualification).

Identifying critical features of a movement

Much of our work as movement analysts involves the study and evaluation of how sports skills are performed. To analyse the observed movement 'technique', we need to identify 'critical features' of the movement. These features should be crucial to improving perform-ance of a certain skill or reducing the injury risk in performing that skill, sometimes both. For a qualitative biomechanical analyst, this means being able to observe those features of the movement; for the quantitative analyst, this requires measuring those features and, often, further mathematical analysis (Chapter 7). Identification of these critical features is probably the most important task facing a qualitative biomechanical analyst, and we will look at several approaches to this task in this section. None is foolproof but all are better in identifying these crucial elements of a skill than an unstructured approach. Sometimes it can be helpful to define a 'scale of correctness' for critical features, for example, poor = 1 to perfect = 5, or a 'range of correctness', such as 'wrist above elbow but below shoulder'; an example is given in the section below on 'Qualitative Movement Analysis Packages'.

The 'ideal performance' or 'elite athlete template' approach

This approach involves devising a set of critical features identified from an 'ideal' – sometimes called a 'model' – performance, often that of an elite performer, hence the alternative name. This approach has nothing to recommend it except, for a lazy analyst, its minimal need for creative thought. It assumes that the ideal or elite performance is applicable to the person or persons for whom the analyst is performing his or her anal-ysis. There is now wide agreement among movement analysts that there is no universal 'optimal performance model' for any sports movement pattern. Each performer brings a unique set of organismic constraints to a movement task; these determine which movements, out of the many possible solutions for the task under those constraints, are best for him or her. You are advised to avoid this approach.

Movement principles approach

Categorising principles as general, partially general, or specific (Chapter 5), while it does conform to the constraints-led approach (see below), does not provide a suitable 'recipe' approach to modelling and identifying the critical features of a movement. We would caution against a mechanistic application of the movement principles approach. We would advise instead that you develop an awareness of the important movement principles (Chapter 5) that need to be used in devising a deterministic model of a given sports movement. The principles used should be specific to the sport, the performer and the constraints on the movement.

Deterministic modelling

Principles of deterministic modelling

Deterministic models of sports activities, also known as hierarchical models as they descend a hierarchical pyramid, can be easily drawn using SmartArt hierarchical models in Microsoft Word. They work best with sports that have an objective 'performance criterion' – the outcome or result. This is often, for example in track and field athletics, to go faster, higher or further. In such cases, we have a clear and objective performance criterion, such as race time, which we seek to minimise, or distance jumped or thrown, which we seek to maximise. Splitting a movement into phases, as we have done below for the long jump (see also Chapter 5), can not only aid the establishment of a deterministic model but also help the identification of critical features for each phase.

The next stage is to sub-divide the performance criterion, where possible, as in the examples below (see also Figure 6.1). The crucial stage of identifying critical features then follows. Once this is done, and the model has been developed to the necessary stage – which should arrive at observable critical features in a qualitative analysis (or measurable ones for a quantitative analysis, Chapter 7) – it needs to be evaluated and its limitations noted. Generally, the critical features highlighted in the model will be biomechanical features or variables such as joint angles, or body segment parameters such as a skater's moment of inertia. Generally, it is advisable not to use ambiguities, such as 'timing' or 'flexibility' or even, perhaps, 'coordination'. If critical, these should be identified more precisely, such as specifying why hamstring flexibility is important because it improves the joint range of movement, or which joint movements need to be coordinated and how.

A model entry at one 'level' should be completely defined by those associated with it at the next level down, for example, those at the top level 1 – this would be the performance criterion – by those at level 2. This association should either be a division – as in the link between levels 1 and 2 in the simple examples of a throw model and a swimming model of

Figure 6.1 The various levels of a general deterministic model.

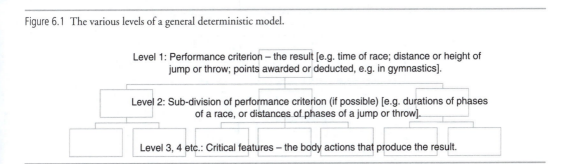

Level 1: Performance criterion – the result [e.g. time of race; distance or height of jump or throw; points awarded or deducted, e.g. in gymnastics].

Level 2: Sub-division of performance criterion (if possible) [e.g. durations of phases of a race, or distances of phases of a jump or throw].

Level 3, 4 etc.: Critical features – the body actions that produce the result.

Figures 6.2 and 6.3 respectively – or a biomechanical relationship, as in the links between levels 2 and 3 in those two models. In the simple throw model, Figure 6.2, the principle (or equations if you prefer) of projectile motion (this could be considered as a specific movement principle) link flight distance and the release parameters of the throw. In the swimming model, Figure 6.3, the swimming time (level 2) is linked to distance swum and swimming speed (level 3) by the simple movement relationship: average speed = distance swum ÷ time taken. A further movement relationship is found between levels 3 and 4, for which average speed = average stroke length × stroke rate, a specific movement principle.

Figure 6.2 Levels 1, 2 and 3 of a deterministic model of a throw. The release distance is the distance that the centre of mass of the thrown object is ahead of (or behind, negative value) the point from which the throw is measured, such as the stop board in a shot, discus or hammer throw. The landing distance is the distance the object lands ahead of its centre of mass; this will normally be zero – however, for a javelin throw it will be the distance that the point of the javelin (to which the throw is measured) lands ahead of its centre of mass.

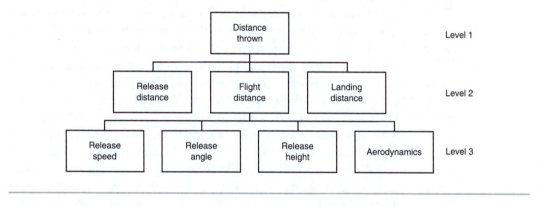

Figure 6.3 Levels 1 to 4 of a deterministic model of swimming.

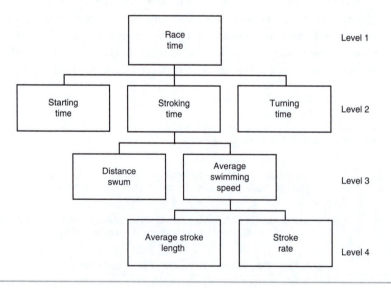

The difference between the use of movement principles within a deterministic model and simply using a list of movement principles is that, in the former approach, the principle flows from the model rather than being slavishly adopted from a list of these things. In addition, this modelling approach is easily adapted to alternative ways of identifying critical features, for example, through a constraints-led approach. Another advantage of hierarchical models over lists of principles is that they help the movement analyst to spot 'blind alleys'; this is again illustrated in the following example.

A deterministic model for qualitative analysis of the long jump
The first step in developing a full deterministic model for qualitative analysis of the long jump is to define the performance criterion, which is very simple for this task, being the distance jumped. We will ignore here compliance with the rules of the event, which are task constraints in their own right, assuming the jumper analysed is able to conform to the rules. The next step – level two of our model, as in Figure 6.4 – is to ask if we can divide the distance jumped into other distances, which might relate to the phases of the movement. Here, it can be subdivided into the take-off distance, the flight distance and the landing distance (these are explained in Figure 6.5).

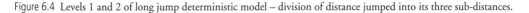

Figure 6.4 Levels 1 and 2 of long jump deterministic model – division of distance jumped into its three sub-distances.

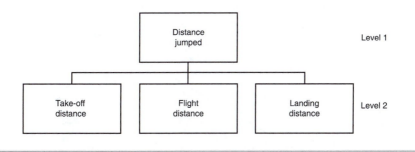

Figure 6.5 Diagrammatic explanation of the three sub-distances of the long jump model: TOD = take-off distance; LD = landing distance. White circles denote the positions of the whole body centre of mass of the jumper at take-off and landing.

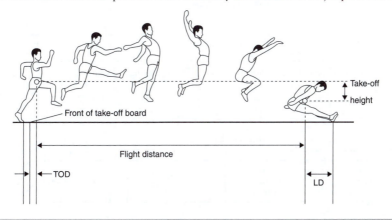

We have now completed level 2 of our long jump model and now need to prioritise further development according to which of the three sub-distances is most important. Clearly, from Figure 6.5, the flight distance is by far the most important and is the distance the jumper's centre of mass travels during the airborne, or flight, phase. This distance can be specified by a biomechanical relationship as it fits the principles of projectile motion.

We have to make a choice at this stage. Do we represent the take-off parameters for the long jump similarly to those for the simple throw model of Figure 6.2; here, these would become the take-off speed, take-off angle and take-off height? Or do we use the alternative approach represented in Figure 6.6, in which we view the take-off velocity as being specified not by the take-off speed and angle but by the take-off horizontal and vertical velocity components? The latter approach is preferable for two reasons in this case. First, while on the take-off board, a long jumper needs to generate vertical velocity while minimising the loss of horizontal velocity from the run-up; for the horizontal component, there tends to be an initial 'braking' force followed by an accelerating force. Second, muscles generate force, hence acceleration and velocity, not angle; take-off angle is the consequence of the ratio of the two velocity components not the other way around. Level 3 of our deterministic model for the flight distance (Figure 6.7) also shows that this distance is affected by the aerodynamics of the jumper – the air resistance. This can be neglected for the long jump.

Figure 6.6 Take-off velocity components for long jump.

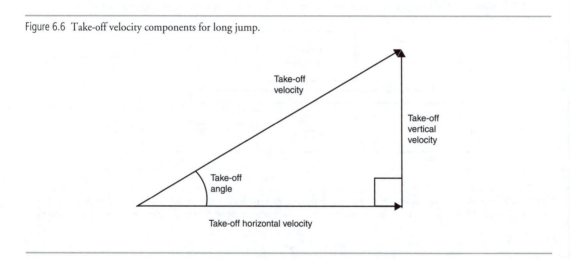

Take-off velocity

Take-off vertical velocity

Take-off angle

Take-off horizontal velocity

Figure 6.7 Level 3 of long jump deterministic model – factors affecting the flight distance.

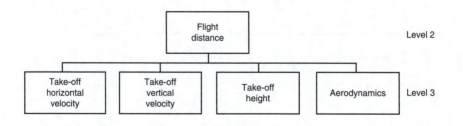

Flight distance — Level 2

Take-off horizontal velocity | Take-off vertical velocity | Take-off height | Aerodynamics | Level 3

We now need to prioritise the development of level 3 of the model. Which of the take-off parameters is most important? We will choose to develop our model for the take-off horizontal velocity before that for the take-off vertical velocity, if for no other reason than that the horizontal component is about 2.5 times greater than the vertical one. Level 4 for the take-off horizontal velocity is shown in Figure 6.8, in which the take-off horizontal velocity has been divided into the touchdown horizontal velocity (the horizontal velocity at board contact, or the run-up speed) and the horizontal velocity added (or lost) on the take-off board. The first of these gives us our first critical feature – the jumper must have a fast run-up; we need to develop an 'eye' for this as qualitative analysts, whereas a quantitative analyst would need to devise the best way of measuring this speed. The second component – horizontal velocity added on the board – is of little direct use, being unobservable (although measurable), so we need to develop it further into level 5 using the appropriate biomechanical relationship.

The one relationship that springs to mind – because it is the simplest – is the impulse–momentum relationship (see Chapter 5 under 'Impulse generation or absorption'). This would then be represented graphically by developing horizontal velocity added on the board (level 4a) as the take-off impulse and the athlete's body mass (at level 4b of the model). Take-off impulse, in turn, would depend at the next level down (level 4c) on the mean force and the time spent on the take-off board. However, for the long jump, this 'branch' of the model would be a blind alley. The reason is that it would suggest that the jumper needs to maximise both the mean force and the time on the board to improve performance. Given the fast run-up of good long jumpers, trying to extend the

Figure 6.8 Level 4 of long jump deterministic model – factors affecting take-off horizontal velocity using work–energy relationship. See text for further explanation. CoM = whole body centre of mass of jumper.

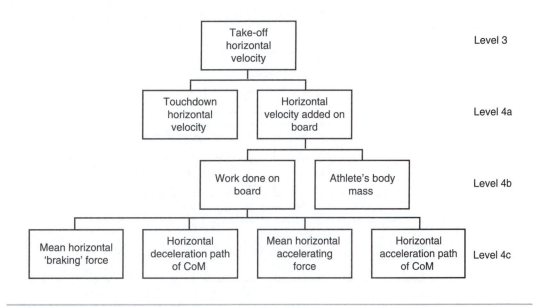

board contact time (about 120 ms) would be difficult at best; if feasible, it would have a deleterious effect on the mean force. Fortunately, we would have escaped from this blind alley simply by being unable to observe the critical features based on the impulse–momentum relationship – impulse, mean force and time on board; that is not always the case.

A better approach altogether for the long jump example is to use the work–energy relationship (see under 'Maximising the acceleration path' in Chapter 5). Here, the work done (mean force × distance over which the force acts) is approximately (ignoring changes in potential energy) the change in the jumper's kinetic energy, which relates to the jumper's mass and change of velocity. This is shown in levels 4a–c of our model for take-off horizontal velocity in Figure 6.8. Although the mean force and the acceleration path of the jumper's centre of mass (CoM) will not yet appear to be observable, we do have the right relationship, as the jumper correctly needs to try to maximise both of these factors. You should note the deceleration and acceleration sub-phases of the board contact phase implied in this model. The first sub-phase involves the mean horizontal 'braking' force and horizontal deceleration path of the whole body centre of mass: the jumper should strive to minimise this sub-phase. This is followed by an acceleration sub-phase, in which the jumper should strive to maximise the mean horizontal accelerating force and horizontal acceleration path of the whole body centre of mass. The model for the take-off vertical velocity (Figure 6.9) is simpler as it only involves an acceleration phase, assuming the vertical velocity at touchdown on the board is zero, which is very nearly the case.

Now all we have to do is develop observable features that capture these biomechanical entities. At this stage, to remove what are now superfluous details, so as to clarify the model,

Figure 6.9 Level 4 of long jump deterministic model – factors affecting take-off vertical velocity using work–energy relationship. CoM = whole body centre of mass of jumper.

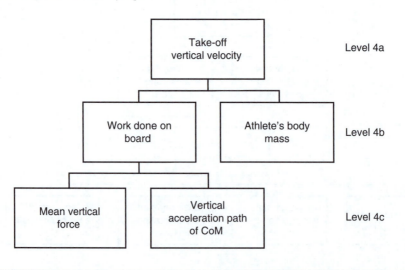

we have deleted level 4a (take-off horizontal velocity = horizontal velocity and touchdown + horizontal velocity added on take-off board). We have also removed level 4b – the 'work done on board' boxes of our long jump model, as these are completely specified by the level below, and omitted the 'athlete's body mass' box, as this is rather trivial. As the take-off velocity is made up of the take-off horizontal and vertical velocities, we can combine these simplified figures, from Figures 6.8 and 6.9 into the final branch of our long jump model for take-off velocity (take-off vertical and horizontal velocity) of Figure 6.10.

We now need to consider what observable, critical features of the movement contribute to the lowest level of each branch of this model. We depart slightly from slavish adherence to the principles of deterministic modelling at this stage but we must ensure that we can propose biomechanical, physiological or other scientific principles to justify these lower levels of the model. We have already identified 'fast run-up speed' as a critical feature (CF1) for this event. We have also noted that maximising the mean force and the acceleration path are desirable to maximise take-off velocity (but see below), so we now need only to translate these terms into things that can be observed. The mean forces are maximised by the jumper maximising force generation (Figure 6.10). This can be done in three ways: directly, by a fast and full extension of the take-off leg (CF2) increasing the force on the take-off board; and, indirectly, by a fast, high, and coordinated swing of the free leg (CF3) and the two arms (CF4). These are demonstrated clearly by the diagram of the jumper in Figure 6.5.

Figure 6.10 Levels 4–6 of long jump deterministic model for combined take-off horizontal and vertical velocity showing derivation of critical features CF1–7. See text for further details. CoM = whole body centre of mass of jumper.

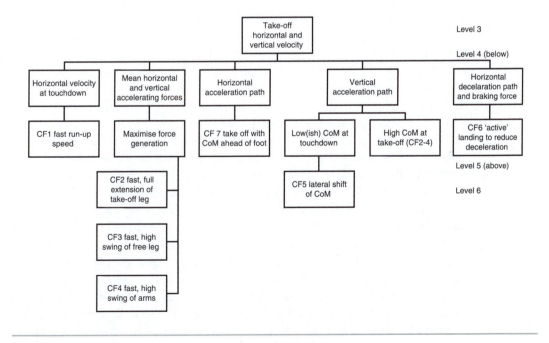

Moving on to maximising the vertical acceleration path, we first note that this is expressed as the difference between the heights of the athlete's centre of mass at take-off and touchdown. The jumper can achieve a high centre of mass at take-off by a combination of critical features 2 to 4 (CF2–4). A lowish centre of mass at touchdown might suggest a pronounced flexing of the knee at touchdown. Although knee flexion will occur to some extent and this will reduce impact forces and, thereby, injury risk, it would be a mistake for the jumper to try to increase this flexion – it would lower the centre of mass height at touchdown but have far more important and deleterious effects on the take-off speed. A mechanism that many good long jumpers tend to use to lower slightly the centre of mass at touchdown is a lateral pelvic tilt towards the take-off leg. This is clearly evident from a front-on view and illustrates two important points for a successful qualitative movement analysis: know your sport or event inside out and never view a sporting activity just from the side, even when it seems two-dimensional.

Now let us consider the horizontal acceleration path. This is more tricky since, in the first part of board contact until the centre of mass has passed forward of the support foot, the horizontal velocity will be decelerating not accelerating. The last thing the jumper would want to do is to plant the take-off foot too far ahead of the centre of mass, which would increase the deceleration of the centre of mass, yet another blind alley. Instead, the jumper minimises this distance by seeking an 'active' landing – one in which the foot of the take-off leg would be moving backwards relative to the take-off board at touchdown – to reduce the horizontal deceleration (CF6). Then, once the centre of mass has passed over the take-off foot, the jumper needs to lengthen, within reason, the acceleration path of the centre of mass up to take-off, which can be done by taking off with the centre of mass ahead of the foot (CF7). This also serves to minimise any tendency for the take-off distance (Figure 6.4) to be negative. This is also excellently illustrated by the diagram of the jumper in Figure 6.5.

Well, we have finished with take-off velocity. The take-off height is the height of the whole body centre of mass at take-off minus the height of the whole body centre of mass at landing in the sandpit. The height at take-off (level 3 of the model, see Figure 6.4) depends mainly on critical features 2–4 (CF2–4, Figure 6.10). We still need to look at the landing component of the take-off height, which we will do in the next paragraph – leaving us with the take-off and landing distances.

From Figure 6.5, it should be obvious that the take-off distance is the distance of the centre of mass in front of the take-off foot at take-off minus the distance of the take-off foot behind the front of the take-off board, from which the jump distance is measured. We have already considered how to increase the first of these distances (CF7, Figure 6.10), so we now note the need to plant the take-off foot as close to the front of the take-off board as possible (CF8, Figure 6.11) – this has implications for the control of the run-up, so we might wish to amend our first critical feature (CF1) to 'fast and controlled run-up'. The landing distance (Figure 6.5) is the distance of the centre of mass behind the feet at landing minus the distance that the point of contact of the jumper's body closest to the take-off board is behind where the feet land. That leads to Figure 6.12, which contains our last four critical features. First, from the observation that the athlete should land with his or her centre of mass behind their feet and low to

Figure 6.11 Level 3 of long jump deterministic model for take-off distance, showing derivation of critical features CF7 and 8. CoM = whole body centre of mass of jumper.

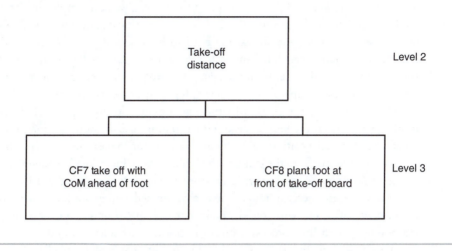

Figure 6.12 Levels 3 to 5 of long jump deterministic model for landing distance, showing derivation of critical features CF9–11. See text for further details. CoM = whole body centre of mass of jumper.

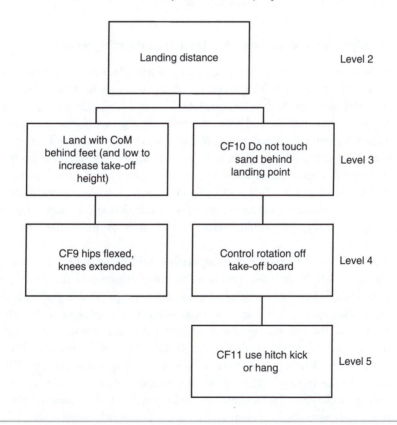

increase take-off height, we derive the need to land with 'hips flexed and knees extended' (CF9), which is evident from Figure 6.5. To reduce any loss of landing distance from touching the sand behind the landing point for the feet, we note simply 'don't touch the sand behind the landing point' (CF10). The final critical feature is less obvious and emphasises two important points: the need to be aware of the movement principles relevant to the activity analysed and to have a thorough knowledge of that activity. The forces acting on the jumper from the take-off board generate 'angular momentum' that tends to rotate the jumper forwards during flight. If uncontrolled, this would cause an early landing in the pit, which is why tucking or piking during flight would be counter-productive. Instead, the jumper needs either to minimise forward rotation by adopting an extended 'hang' position, as in Figure 6.5, or, for longer jumpers to transfer this angular momentum from the trunk to the limbs using a 'hitch-kick' technique ('running in the air'), leading to our last critical feature 'use hitch kick or hang' (CF11).

Well, we've got there, although it may have seemed a long journey. It is worthwhile, because we finish up with confidence in our critical features from the rigour of the deterministic modelling process, which is impossible to achieve from the copying of an 'ideal' or 'model' performance, very difficult to achieve merely from a list of movement principles, and not always clear from other approaches. Also, as already noted, the process highlights blind alleys, helping us to avoid them, and provides a well-structured approach for identifying critical features.

Identifying critical features when there is a subjective performance criterion

In sports involving a subjective judgement, such as gymnastics, diving and figure skating, we may approach identifying a performance criterion differently, although a deterministic modelling approach is still possible (Hay and Reid, 1982). The score awarded by the judges will not depend upon a single performance factor, whether objective or subjective, but on guidelines established by the sport. Consider a women's artistic gymnastics vault. What is the performance criterion? Clearly, it is the judges' score. Can we model this deterministically: can the score be subdivided? Yes, first into the scores by the 'A' Judges and 'B' Judges. A Judges mostly look at the vault difficulty and related aspects. B Judges address technical faults – execution and artistry – and apply deductions. Generally, we would focus on the latter as they relate more to vaulting technique.

On the other hand, a better approach would be to use the judging guidelines of that sport, which are based mainly on technical elements of the skills involved. These should largely have been developed from movement principles applicable to movements within that sport, so this approach has much to recommend it. In other words, we would use the criteria for awarding and deducting points: here Article 8 of the International Gymnastics Federation (FIG) Code of Points for Women's Artistic Gymnastics (WAG) (on the FIG website: www.fig-gymnastics.com); Table 6.1 shows some score deductions. We then have a movement phase approach. It is relevant to ask, are these technical points observable – for judges, clearly the answer is YES. Furthermore, in the context of the next chapter, they are also generally measureable.

Table 6.1 Part of faults table and points deductions (0.1, 0.3 or 0.5) for women's artistic gymnastics vault (see www.fig-gymnastics.com)

FAULTS	POINTS DEDUCTED		
	0.1	0.3	0.5
First flight phase			
Incomplete longitudinal (LA) turn	≤45°	≤90°	>90°
Poor technique			
− Hip angle	X	X	
− Arch	X	X	
− Legs separated	X	X	
− Knees bent	X	X	X
Repulsion phase			
Poor technique			
− Staggered/alternate hand placement	X	X	
− Shoulder angle	X	X	
− Failure to pass through vertical	X	X	
Bent arms	X	X	X
Prescribed LA turn begun too early	X	X	X
Second flight phase			
Height	X	X	X
and so on			

Some sports, such as ski jumping, combine objective (distance) and subjective (style) criteria – the former lends itself to being modelled deterministically, unlike the latter. So how do we proceed when the performance criterion is:

- A combination of objective and subjective criteria, as for ski jumping? Model each separately, emphasising the most important first; here this would be the distance jumped.
- A combination of subjective criteria, as in gymnastics – A Judges specific score, B Judges specific score, and General points? Look at each separately, choosing the most critical first.
- A combination of objective criteria – e.g. fast bowling in cricket – speed and accuracy (the latter can be modelled as angle off line). Model each separately, emphasising the most important first.

OBSERVATION STAGE

The observation stage primarily involves implementing the observation strategy devised in the preparation stage, and videographing the performers involved in the study. We use the term 'videographing', or video recording, the performers advisedly; first, considerable skill is needed to observe fast movements in sport reliably by eye alone and, second, good high-definition digital video cameras are now readily available and inexpensive. We need to record sports movements as they are fast, and the human eye cannot resolve movements that occur in less than 0.25 s. Two important benefits of videography are that the performers can observe their own movements in slow motion and frame by frame, and that it makes qualitative analysis much easier. However, there are some potential drawbacks. Performers might be aware of the cameras and, consciously or subconsciously, change movement patterns (the Hawthorne effect). Also, there are ethical considerations about video recording, particularly with minors and the intellectually disadvantaged. Our systematic observation strategy should have addressed both what to focus on and how to record, and observe, the movements of interest. Clearly, we should focus on the critical features of the movement identified in the preparation stage, but these need to be prioritised. We also need to decide on the environment in which to videograph, the best camera locations within that environment and how many trials of the movement to record for analysis.

Prioritising critical features can vary with the skill of the performer, the activity being analysed, and whether a movement-phase approach is used, as in the long jump example in the previous section. Our prioritising strategy might, for example, put the critical features in descending order of importance for the performance outcome; or work from the general to the specific, for example, from the whole skill to the role of the trunk and the limbs; or focus on balance, in skills in gymnastics.

The other main issues in videography for qualitative analysis are as follows. We need to attend to the choice of camera shutter speed, where to conduct the study, the camera locations and whether the cameras are to be stationary (usually mounted on tripods) or moved (panned or tilted) to follow the analysed movements. We need to decide how many trials to record, when relevant. Do we need to use additional lighting, which must be adequate for shutter speed and frame rate? The frame rate is normally fixed, for 'domestic-quality' video cameras at 50 fields per second in Europe and 60 in North America, or 25 frames per second in Europe and 30 in North America (the unit hertz, Hz, is normally used for events per second). The background should be plain and uncluttered to help objective observation, but this is not always feasible, particularly when videographing in competitions. Participant preparation needs careful attention – briefing, clothing, habituation, and debriefing. We need to optimise the size of the performer on the image – the bigger the better, but this might require zooming the camera lens (assuming that your camera has a zoom lens) while also panning and tilting it during filming. Finally, we need to consider checks for reliability (within, or intra-, observer) and objectivity (among, or inter-, observers) in any study.

So, let us now look at these points in a little more detail. The shutter speed is the time that the camera shutter stays open for each 'picture' that the camera records. If too slow the picture will blur; if too fast for the lighting conditions, the picture may be too dark. A guide to the slowest satisfactory shutter speeds is given in Table 6.2; not all digital video cameras for the domestic market will have the fastest of these shutter speeds. Treat

Table 6.2 Recommended slowest camera shutter speeds for various activities	
ACTIVITY	SLOWEST SHUTTER SPEED (S)
Walking	1/50
Sit to stand	1/50
Bowling	1/50
Basketball	1/100
Vertical jump	1/100
Jogging	1/100 to 1/200
Sprinting	1/200 to 1/500
Baseball pitching	1/500 to 1/1000
Cricket fast bowling	1/500 to 1/1000
Batting (baseball or cricket)	1/500 to 1/1000
Soccer kicking	1/500 to 1/1000
Tennis	1/500 to 1/1000
Golf	1/1000 or faster

with caution the 'sports' option that some cheaper cameras tend to offer rather than providing a range of specified shutter speeds. We should also note that field rates, also known as sampling rates, of 50 or 60 Hz are far from ideal for the fastest activities in Table 6.2. However, most movement analysts do not have routine access to high-speed video cameras with sampling rates of up to thousands of pictures per second. If your needs analysis shows a clear requirement for such cameras, then this should be factored into the project costing in the preparation stage.

When deciding where to conduct the study, we have to balance an environment in which we have control over extraneous factors, such as lighting and background, and one that is similar to that in which the movement is normally performed; the latter ensures ecological validity. Normally, the latter dominates, but the decision may be affected by the skill of the performers, whether the activities being recorded are open or closed skills, and videographic issues. When selecting camera vantage points, the movement analyst has to address from where he or she would want to view these activities for qualitative analysis, with how many cameras, and whether the cameras need to be stationary.

The decision of how many trials, or performances, to record is very important for the reliability of qualitative analysis. However, that decision is not always made by the movement analyst. For example, if you were recording from a game, say of football, for notational analysis, you only have control over how many games you will record. If recording for technique analysis in competition, the number of recordable trials is probably fixed, for example, at six throws in the finals of a discus competition, the heats plus the finals of swimming events, and as many attempts as the jumper needs in the high jump until three failures. If recording out of competition, we need to decide how many observations we need; generally, within reason, the more the better. Because of movement variability (see Appendix 6.1), there is no such thing as a representative trial even for stereotyped closed skills. The more trials we record, the more likely are our results to be valid. Various rules of thumb have proposed between five and 20 trials as a minimum requirement; ten, if you can record that many, is often highly satisfactory. A very important consideration is the number of trials you can reasonably expect your sports performer to undertake in the time available. For maximal effort activities, fatigue and injury risk need to be carefully evaluated.

Finally, we need to ensure that, in this stage, we attend to issues that affect our ability to assess, and improve, intra- and inter-analyst reliability. Reliability is consistency in ratings by one analyst; so we need to be able to check this over several days. Objectivity is consistency in ratings across several analysts; so we need enough analysts to be able to check this; clearly, this will be affected by how well trained the analysts are. Our assessments of objectivity and reliability can be improved by identifying critical features and how, and in which order, they will be evaluated; developing specific rating scales; analyst training and practice; and increasing the number of analysts or trials.

EVALUATION AND DIAGNOSIS STAGE – WHAT IS WRONG?

The hard work for this stage should already have been completed during the preparation stage – the identification of the critical features of the movement. The observation stage should then have allowed us to collect the video 'footage' that is needed, as qualitative movement analysts, to evaluate these critical features in the performances that you have recorded. This stage also prepares us for the intervention stage. Often, in the evaluation and diagnosis stage – probably the most intellectually difficult of the four-stage process – you will start by describing the movement and progress to analysing it; trying to analyse a movement before you have thoroughly and scientifically described it can be fraught with difficulties. In this context, it should be noted that the work we do in this stage can do more harm than good; that is, we could reduce performance or increase injury risk, particularly if we have not identified and prioritised the correct critical features. This overall stage could be called the 'Analysis' stage; however, there are two separate aspects to this stage (although they often overlap). The first task is to evaluate strengths and weaknesses of performance – to establish what the symptoms are. The second aspect is to diagnose what weaknesses to tackle and how – to diagnose the symptoms and prepare to treat the condition.

Evaluation of performance

To evaluate performance we effectively need to compare the observed performances with some model of good form. However, as there is no general optimal performance model, we need a model that is appropriate for the performers being evaluated –

the model needs 'individual specificity'. For most good qualitative analysis, this clearly requires prior identification of the movement's critical features in the preparation stage, probably by the use of a deterministic model. Furthermore, a ranking of the 'correctness' of the identified critical features on some scale or within some band of correctness can be very helpful; for example, 'joint range of motion: inadequate; within good range; excessive'; or 'excellent 5 .... OK 3 .... poor 1'. As well as needing a 'model' that is individual specific, other difficulties arise in the evaluation of performance. The first of these relates to within-performer movement and performance variability (see also Appendix 6.1); as we noted in the observation stage above, this can only be accounted for by recording multiple trials. Identifying the source of movement errors can also be problematic as they can arise from: body position or movement timing (biomechanical); conditioning (physiological); the performer evaluating environmental cues (perceptual-motor); or motivational factors (psychological). All of these factors could be important, for example, in a run-out in cricket (see Study Task 4). These factors support the need for movement analysts to be able to draw on a range of disciplinary skills and knowledge. In the real world of sport, movement analysts are usually most effective when they work as part of a multi-disciplinary team of experts; this is often financially prohibitive. Analyst bias, reliability and objectivity also present problems. Bias can be reduced by the use of 'correctness' criteria. Assessing reliability and objectivity requires multiple trials or analysts respectively; the latter is often a luxury, the former is vital.

Diagnosis of movement errors

Perhaps the major issues in the evaluation and diagnosis stage relate to the lack of a consistent rationale for diagnosing movement errors: our 'critical features' approach is best, providing that we can identify and prioritise the correct critical features. As only one intervention, in the intervention stage, at any time is best, we need to focus on one correction at a time. This raises the question of how to prioritise the order in which to tackle movement errors in the intervention stage if we have identified that more than one aspect of the movement requires correction. One of the five following approaches is generally used, depending on the activity and circumstances.

The first approach focuses on 'what came before'; here, we try to establish if an error in a particular action arose from previous actions. This is most often used in sports in which actions follow in sequence (those sports most usually dealt with in notational analysis). For example, an error leading to a volley played out of court or into the net by the server in tennis may be traced back to a poor serve rather than a poor volley; we would then focus our attention on the serve rather than the volley. The second approach, somewhat related to the first conceptually, looks at the sequence of actions through the phases of a movement, focusing on earlier phases first, as in the long jump example above. For example, in our long jump model, landing problems are often due to poor generation of rotation on the take-off board or control of it in the air, so our first focus would be on what went wrong on take-off or in the air. These two approaches are conceptually attractive, as problems usually arise before they are spotted. We would normally recommend starting with one of these two approaches.

The third, and perhaps the most obvious, approach involves prioritising for attention in the intervention stage those critical features that maximise performance improvement. To use the long jump model again, if a long jumper is not jumping far, speed is overwhelmingly the most important factor; so what critical feature would we prioritise to maximise performance? Run-up speed, obviously. However, in many cases, it is not at all easy to know what will maximise improvement; furthermore, we often need also to balance short-term and long-term considerations.

A fourth, and seemingly attractive, approach, in terms of successful outcomes, is to seek to make the easiest corrections first. In other words, if several movement faults have been identified, we first tackle the one that will be easiest for the athlete to correct. This approach is impeccably logical from a motor skills viewpoint if movement errors seem unrelated and cannot be ranked. However, there is little, if any, clear support for its efficacy in improving performance.

Finally, for activities in which balance is crucial, such as gymnastics and weight lifting, we might prioritise from the base of support upwards – in other words, we look for errors close to the point of balance contact with the environment. This would be the ground in weight lifting and could be the ground or, say, the beam or vaulting box in gymnastics. You might like to consider whether this approach would work best, for example, in a sport such as target shooting.

INTERVENTION STAGE – PUTTING THINGS RIGHT

We come now to the final stage of our four-stage process of qualitative analysis – the intervention stage – in which we have the chance to correct movement errors, or put things right. Before getting this far, the movement analyst must have conducted a means analysis with the performer and his or her coach, identified the critical features relevant to the question to be answered, and prepared how feedback will be provided including, for example, keywords. Second, the movement analyst will have obtained relevant video footage and any other movement patterns (see next two sections). Finally, the movement analyst will have analysed the video and movement patterns and prioritised the critical features to be addressed. The focus in this final stage is on feedback of information to address the requirements of the needs analysis. If the previous three stages have been done badly, nothing in the intervention stage will sort matters out. On the other hand, provision of inappropriate feedback can jeopardise even good work done in the previous stages. The intervention stage is considered in detail in Chapter 8.

QUALITATIVE ANALYSIS OF MOVEMENT AND COORDINATION PATTERNS

Introduction

Although qualitative movement analysts, particularly coaches, teachers and those working as performance analysts with sports clubs or teams, mainly use qualitative analysis of video records, other movement representations are available to them to supplement this work, if they are able to measure joint angles. Joint angles can be easily measured from qualitative biomechanical analysis packages, such as Siliconcoach (see later section on 'Qualitative Movement Analysis Packages'), which most qualitative biomechanical analysts will use in their work. The angles measured in such packages are usually planar, so the focus in this section will be on the qualitative (including semi-quantitative) interpretation of sagittal plane angles. In the earlier part of this chapter, we focused on video sequences as the basic representation of movement patterns in sport. We noted, however, that these sequences are complex, because they contain so much information. It can be beneficial for the qualitative analyst to look at simpler, if less familiar, representations of movement patterns. In this and the next section, we will explore the various patterns of movement that a movement analyst can use, at his or her discretion, to supplement, though not to replace, qualitative video analysis. The patterns we will look at are all far simpler than video recordings because they focus on specific aspects of a movement; this simplicity underpins their usefulness. The additional movement representations (see also Bartlett, 2007) that we will look at are all graphs and are particularly relevant when we ask the question 'How are these movements coordinated to produce the desired outcome, and how can they be modified to improve performance?'

Graphs can be of several types, of which the most useful for the movement analyst are time series graphs and coordination patterns – angle–angle diagrams, phase planes and continuous relative phase, and cross-correlation functions. Time series are simply graphs of one movement variable, such as joint angle, as it changes over time during the course of the movement. We will first summarise how angle–time graphs can be analysed qualitatively – focusing on their geometry, or shape, not on the numerical values (for a more detailed explanation, see Bartlett, 2007). Several time series can be plotted on the same graph. Both movement and coordination graphs can add substantially to our understanding of a movement and help us to assess ways in which changes might be made to improve performance. Because different individuals find unique solutions to the demands of a sports task, under the various constraints of that task, the environment and their own organism, intra-individual studies are usually more productive than inter-individual ones. We might, for example, compare successful with unsuccessful basketball free throws, different modes of gait, or different stroke rates in rowing, or track an athlete recovering from injury. This approach deserves far more attention from qualitative biomechanical analysts rather than just from researchers.

Qualitative analysis of angular movement patterns

An understanding of angular motion is crucial for the movement analyst seeking to understand, and improve, an athlete's performance. For a consideration of the qualitative analysis of linear motion, see Bartlett (2007). The movement variables in angular motion are as follows. Angular displacement is the change in the orientation of a line segment. In two-dimensional motion, also known as planar motion as it takes place in a two-dimensional plane, this will be the angle between the initial and final orientations regardless of the path taken. Angular velocity and acceleration are, respectively, the rates of change with time of angular displacement and angular velocity. Joint angles are the most important examples of angular motion, first, as in this sub-section, when we look at the change of the angle over time and then, in this next section, for other combinations of variables in coordination patterns.

The angle–time pattern of Figure 6.13(a), a time series pattern, shows how the flexion-extension angle of the knee changes with time over one stride of treadmill running. We can learn a lot about this pattern by studying its geometry – the gradients or slopes (the two terms are essentially the same in this context) and curvatures of the graph – as we move through time from left to right. As this analysis focuses on the qualitative aspects, rather than the numbers, you need to be aware of the joint angle convention used. Here we adopt the convention normally used by sports biomechanists in two-dimensional analysis: a fully extended knee would be a larger angle (about 180°) than with the knee flexed – the angle increases upwards in the figure. Different conventions are usual in clinical biomechanics and in most three-dimensional motion analyses, so be wary!

Before you read on, satisfy yourself that you can identify where the knee is flexing and where it is extending in Figure 6.13(a). Also, in each region of the graph, what is the gradient of the curve; clue – would you be going uphill or downhill walking along the pattern? The gradient is important as it gives the knee angular velocity, which with our angle convention is positive for extension and negative for flexion. Then, identify the curvatures of the various regions of the pattern – are they positive (which I call 'valley-type' curvature) or negative ('hill-type') curvature. The curvature of the angle time series is important as it gives us the angular acceleration. Then check your answers with Figures 6.13(b and c). The gradient changes at the vertical continuous lines in Figure 6.13(b), from positive to negative or from negative to positive; the gradient (and angular velocity) is instantaneously zero at the vertical lines. The curvature changes, again from positive to negative or vice versa, at the dashed vertical lines in Figure 6.13(c); the curvature (and angular acceleration) is instantaneously zero at these vertical lines. The regions of flexion and extension (Figure 6.13(b)) and those of positive and negative curvature (Figure 6.13(c)) are also shown. Study these patterns very carefully and ensure that you understand them fully before carrying on. If you were wrong, go back to Figure 6.13(a) and try to ascertain where and why you went wrong.

Figure 6.14 is a combination of Figures 6.13(a–c), to which I have added the angular velocity (chain-dotted curve) and acceleration (dashed curve) patterns. Angular velocity – the chain-dotted pattern – is positive when the knee is extending and negative when

Figure 6.13 Variation of knee angle with time for a specific individual in treadmill running: (a) angle time series only; (b) regions of flexion and extension (negative and positive gradient); (c) regions of positive and negative curvature. Note that these patterns will vary somewhat with running speed and between individuals.

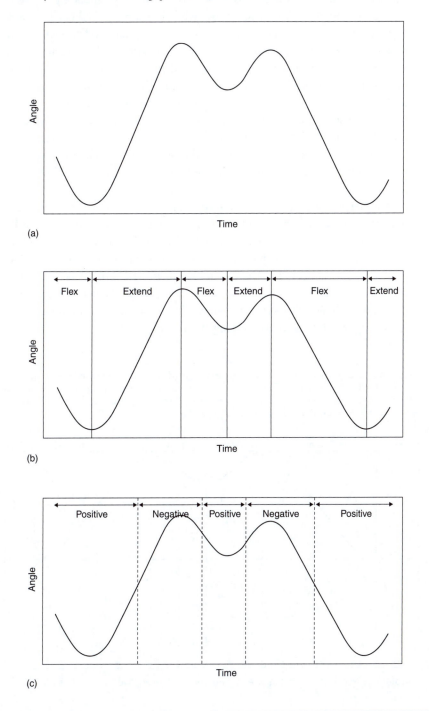

it is flexing. The horizontal line marked 0 shows where the angular velocity or acceleration is zero; values below this line are negative, those above are positive. The angular acceleration – the dashed curve – is positive, corresponding to positive (valley-type) curvature of the knee angle curve, when it is driving the knee from a flexed to an extended position; we can call this an extending acceleration. The angular acceleration is negative, corresponding to negative (hill-type) curvature of the knee angle curve, when it is driving the knee from an extended to a flexed position; we can call this a flexing acceleration. Trace through the entire patterns of Figure 6.14 until you thoroughly understand them and can explain them to your fellow students; this is a very important step towards becoming a successful movement analyst. If you are still having difficulties, see Bartlett (2007), Chapter 3. You should note that the angular velocity and angular acceleration curves in Figure 6.14 have been calculated from the angle data; however, with experience it is possible to sketch their shape quite accurately from qualitative analysis of the angle–time curve.

Another noteworthy geometric feature of Figure 6.14 is the sequence of the three movement patterns: an extending (positive) angular acceleration, caused by muscle tension, occurs before the angular velocity changes from flexing (negative) to extending (positive). The resulting sequence of peaks (or troughs) is: angular acceleration; angular velocity; angle. Also notable is the inverse phase relationship between the angle and angular acceleration patterns: one is increasing while the other is decreasing. This is typical of cyclic joint movements, but not always so apparent in movement patterns in discrete sports skills, such as jumping and throwing.

Figure 6.14 Variation of knee angle (continuous curve), angular velocity (chain-dotted curve) and angular acceleration (dashed curve) with time in treadmill running obtained from Figure 6.13. Vertical continuous lines separate positive (extension) and negative (flexion) angular velocity (gradient) and vertical dashed lines separate positive and negative angular acceleration (curvature). The data have been 'normalised' to fit the range –1 to +1.

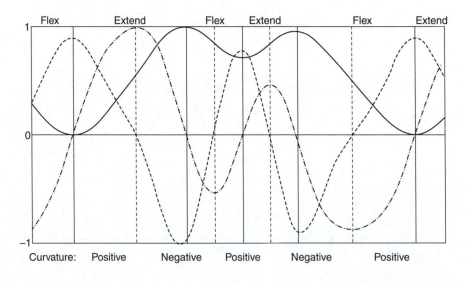

Qualitative analysis of coordination patterns

Before looking at how we interpret graphical representations of coordination, let us begin by considering what we mean by this important term. In Chapter 5, when considering movement principles, one of the universal principles we noted was 'Mastering the many degrees of freedom involved in a movement'. This is one statement of what movement coordination involves. A rather longer definition, which elaborates on the one in the previous sentence, introduces the idea of 'coordinative structures'. This viewpoint sees the acquisition of coordination as constraining the degrees of freedom into coordinative structures, which are functional relationships between important anatomical parts of a performer's body, to perform a specific activity. An example would be groups of muscles or joints temporarily functioning as coherent units to achieve a specific goal, such as hitting or catching a ball. As muscles act around joints, this explanation leads us to look at joints and their inter-relationships to gain an initial insight into how sports movements are coordinated (see also Davids *et al.*, 2008).

In the following sub-sections we will look at the qualitative analysis of several different coordination patterns. Angle–angle diagrams are graphs of one joint angle as a function of another. The focus is on how one angle changes with changes in a second angle; in other words we focus on how the two angles 'co-vary' rather than how they each evolve with time. Angle–angle diagrams are used extensively in the study of movement coordination. The phase planes used in movement analysis are normally graphs of the angular velocity of one joint as a function of the angle of that same joint. The focus is on the so called 'coordination dynamics' of that joint. Phase planes are also used extensively in the study of movement coordination and from them we can derive graphs of continuous relative phase as a function of time. Cross-correlation functions look at how the correlation coefficient between two time series, such as joint angles, changes as one time series lags behind the other. All of these graphs will be discussed in detail in the following sub-sections. The focus is on interpreting these graphs qualitatively (and semi-quantitatively); developing such interpretive skills is important to appreciate how coordination patterns can then be used to try to improve sports performance.

Angle–angle diagrams

In a previous sub-section, we looked at joint angles as a function of time – a 'time series'. However, multiple times series involving several angles can be difficult to interpret for coordination. An alternative is to plot angles against each other – these are called angle–angle diagrams; we could, in principle, show how three angles co-vary using a three-dimensional plot, but this is rarely done. Coordination in actual human movements is often more complex than the basic patterns discussed in Bartlett (2007), as for the hip–knee angle–angle diagram for one running stride in Figure 6.15(a). We do, however, distinguish 'in-phase' coordination, as when the hip and knee joints flex together or extend together, and 'anti-phase' (or out of phase) coordination, as when the hip flexes while the knee extends, or vice versa. Please note that the angle–angle diagram of Figure 6.15(a) has been slightly 'massaged' so that it forms a continuous loop, which is rarely the case owing to movement variability (see Appendix 6.1) and measurement errors. Please also be careful to distinguish between the use of the word 'phase' in 'phases' of a movement, here of a running stride, and its use in 'in-phase' and 'anti-phase' coordination.

Figure 6.15 Angle–angle diagrams for one 'ideal' treadmill running stride: (a) hip–knee coupling; (b) ankle–knee coupling; (c) ankle–hip coupling.

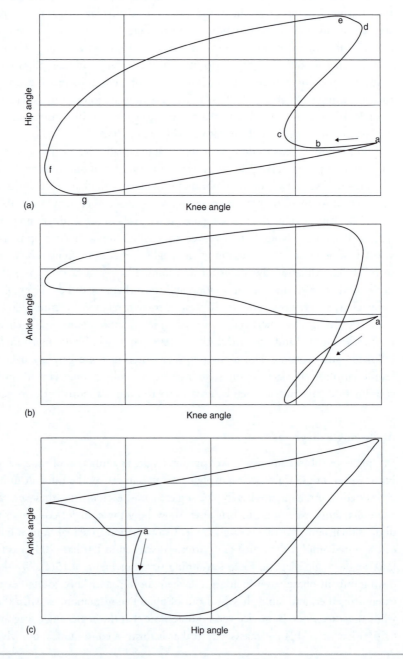

Reading around Figure 6.15(a), starting at the lower right hand spike at 'a', which corresponds roughly to touchdown, or heel strike, and progressing anticlockwise, the pattern is as follows. At the start of the stance phase of the running stride, the hip and knee flex 'in-phase' until 'b'; then, briefly, the knee continues to flex while the hip extends to 'c'; from 'b' to 'c' the two joints are 'anti-phase'. From 'c' to 'd' the two joints extend in-phase. From 'd', which is roughly at toe-off, another brief period until 'e' sees the knee flex while the hip extends, anti-phase, at the start of the swing phase of the running stride. From 'e' until 'f' the joints flex in-phase during the next part of the swing phase of the stride, after which the knee extends while the hip continues to flex, anti-phase until 'g'; both joints then extend in-phase until around touchdown. Note that there are seven changes of coordination between the two joints during this one running stride; all but one (at 'a' at which in-phase extension changes to in-phase flexion) are from in-phase to anti-phase coordination or vice versa. You should now try to repeat this description of joint movements for the same running stride but looking at the ankle–knee and ankle–hip joint couplings, in Figures 6.15(b and c) (see Study Task 6).

The study of movement coordination is crucial for the movement analyst; one method uses angle–angle diagrams, which have both advantages and disadvantages. Their advantages include that we do not have to flip between angle–time graphs and that we can pair joint angles of interest easily to show how they co-vary. These graphs show coordination patterns qualitatively, which can facilitate comparisons, for example, between individuals and for one individual during rehabilitation from an injury. We can also compare patterns between, for example, running and walking; most of these comparisons have been based on methods to quantify angle–angle diagrams. Such a reduction of a rich qualitative pattern to a few numbers seems bizarre to me and ignores the saying 'a picture is worth a thousand words'. Few attempts have been made to distinguish patterns qualitatively; one of the very few is known as 'topological equivalence'. Two shapes are topologically equivalent if one can just be stretched – albeit by different amounts in different places – to form the other; two shapes are not topologically equivalent if one has to be 'folded' rather than just stretched to form the other. Simplistically, this means that if the shapes have different numbers of loops, they are not topologically equivalent; they are then qualitatively rather than just quantitatively different, as for the ankle–knee, but not the hip–knee or ankle–hip couplings when comparing the running angle–angle diagrams in Figure 6.15 with those for walking in Figure 6.16.

An important point to make here, and it applies to other coordination patterns too, is that of inter-individual differences. Consider, for example, Figure 6.17, which shows hip–knee angle–angle diagrams for four rowers. Figures 6.17(a and b) are for two club standard rowers and c and d for two high performance rowers. It should be perfectly clear that there is no 'club' or 'elite' template here. The patterns for the two club rowers clearly differ, with one (club rower 1) having the broader part of the loop at the top right of the curve, the finish of the drive (Figure 6.17(a)), while the other (club rower 2) has the broader part of the loop at the bottom left, the start of the drive, or the 'catch' (Figure 6.17(b)). Both have two loops in their pattern, although these may not be immediately obvious from the figures; Figure 6.17(a) has a small second loop at bottom

Figure 6.16 Angle–angle diagrams for one treadmill walking stride: (a) hip–knee coupling; (b) ankle–knee coupling; (c) ankle–hip coupling.

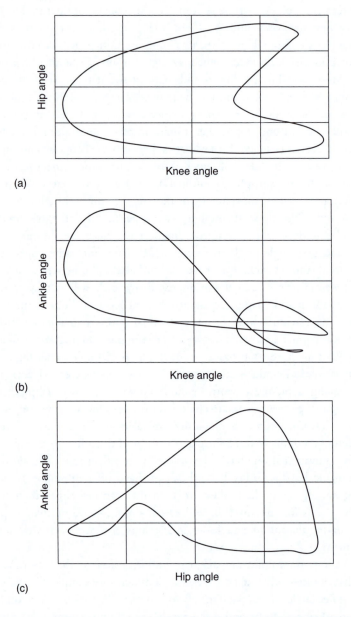

(a)

(b)

(c)

left and Figure 6.17(b) at top right. They are topologically equivalent but still different. The patterns for the two high performance rowers also differ. The rower represented by Figure 6.17(c) (high performance rower 1) has a single loop pattern, with the loop being broader at the start of the drive, whereas the rower in Figure 6.17(d) (high performance rower 2) has the broader part of the loop at the finish of the drive. The two patterns are

Figure 6.17 Hip–knee angle–angle diagrams for four rowers early in a five minute race trial on a rowing ergometer, one 'stroke' only shown on each: (a) and (b) club standard rowers; (c) and (d) high performance rowers. The angles are all normalised to the range –1 to +1.

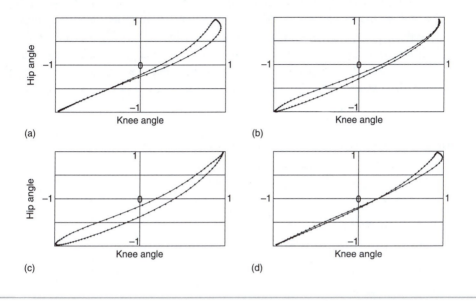

(a)

(b)

(c)

(d)

also not topologically equivalent, with high performance rower 2 having a clear two-loop pattern in contrast to the single-loop pattern of high performance rower 1. If we compare across performance standards, we note the general shapes of the hip–knee angle–angle diagrams for club rower 1 and high performance rower 2 are similar; they are also topologically equivalent, as both have two loops. The general shapes of club rower 1 and high performance rower 2 are also similar in having the broader part of the loop at the start of the drive; however, they are not topologically equivalent. Each of these four rowers has evolved a hip–knee coordination pattern that 'matches' their organismic constraints to those of the task and environment; none of these patterns is inherently 'right' or 'wrong'. Coordination profiling, over multiple trials, has been proposed as a comprehensive way of highlighting coordination differences or similarities between individuals (see, for example, Button et al., 2006).

Disadvantages of angle–angle diagrams include their unfamiliarity compared to time series. Also, it is not obvious from the diagram which way round the figure proceeds – clockwise or anticlockwise – or where key events, such as toe-off and touchdown in gait, occur; the latter is also true to some extent for time series. Some criticism can be made of the loss of 'time' as a variable, although marking the data, or time, points (similarly to that for the phase planes in Figure 6.20 in the next sub-section) would add some indication of how the angles change with time. We do, however, lose access to time-series shape patterns, that is slope = velocity and curvature = acceleration; such relationships do not apply to angle–angle diagrams.

Phase planes

Perhaps the main criticism of angle–angle diagrams is that they do not show coordination changes very clearly without painstaking analysis of the patterns, as for the hip–knee coupling above. Only the ankle–knee coupling of the three joint couplings that we compared between walking and running was qualitatively different topologically between the two modes of gait. Phase planes, a totally different approach, are based on the notion that any system, such as a body segment, can be graphed as diagrams of two variables; for the phase planes used in human movement analysis, these variables are usually joint angle

Figure 6.18 Phase planes for one treadmill running stride: (a) hip joint; (b) knee joint.

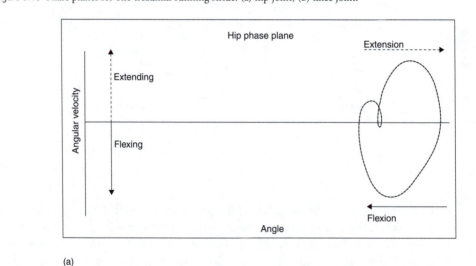

(a)

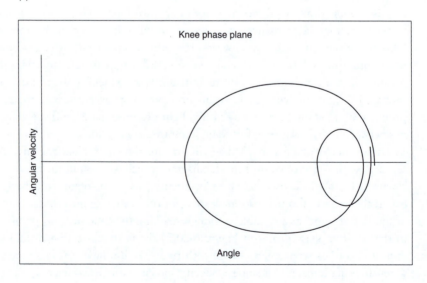

(b)

and angular velocity. Although the relevance of a phase plane for a single joint to coordination between joints may seem hard to fathom, phase planes turn out to be pivotal for our understanding of movement coordination, as will be evident later in this section.

Example phase planes, for the hip (Figure 6.18(a)) and the knee (Figure 6.18(b)) joints in a treadmill running stride, are shown in Figure 6.18. Their description – although not their analysis – is 'child's play' compared to both angle time-series and angle–angle diagrams. First, let us ask whether the phase plane progresses clockwise or anticlockwise with time around its loop – it must do one or the other. Because in sports biomechanics for two-dimensional analysis, we define flexion as a decrease in joint angle and extension as an increase, then flexion must be from left to right and extension from right to left in Figure 6.18. Similarly, as we saw in a previous sub-section on time series, a flexion velocity is negative and an extension velocity is positive; so, flexion must be below the horizontal zero line in Figure 6.18 and extension above it. The phase planes of

Figure 6.19 Phase planes for one treadmill walking stride: (a) hip joint.

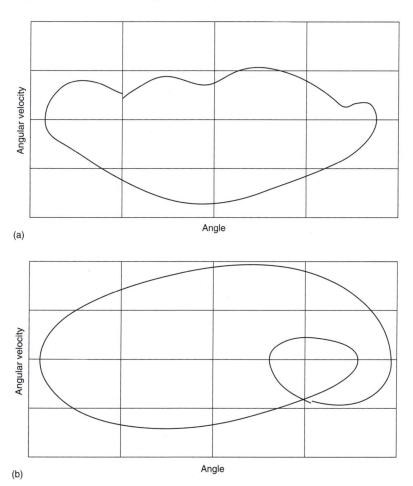

(a)

(b)

Figure 6.18 must, therefore, progress clockwise with time. Why? Well, let us assume the opposite – they progress anticlockwise with time. In this case, in Figure 6.18(a), the hip joint would be flexing – from right to left – while its angular velocity was positive (above the zero line) indicating extension. We have proved a contradiction: the phase plane cannot progress anticlockwise with time; therefore, it must progress clockwise with time.

It is also worth noting that phase planes for the hip angle in these examples of treadmill walking and running are not topologically equivalent (compare Figure 6.19(a) with Figure 6.18(a)); the phase plane for running has two loops while that for walking has only one. However, the example knee phase planes for treadmill running and walking are topologically equivalent as they both have two loops, as seen in Figures 6.19(b) and 6.18(b).

Continuous relative phase

The value of phase planes starts to become more evident when we define the so-called 'phase angle' as shown for the example of treadmill running in Figure 6.20. I have changed the graph so that it is 'centred' on its mean value, for reasons that need not concern us in this book. If we now subtract the phase angle – defined anticlockwise from the right horizontal – for one joint from that for a second joint at the same instant, we define a variable known as relative phase. Here, we subtract the knee phase angle from that for the hip, rp = pah – pak. We can do this for every time instant in the cycle to arrive at values of this relative phase as a function of time, which is known as 'continuous relative phase'.

A graph of continuous relative phase as a function of time for this example of treadmill running by a particular individual at the preferred running speed is shown in Figure 6.21. Continuous relative phase is simply another coordination 'pattern', although more difficult to interpret than angle–angle diagrams. In Figure 6.21, for example, we

Figure 6.20 Superimposed phase planes for the hip (dashed curve) and knee (continuous curve) joints in one treadmill running stride plus definition of their phase angles (pah and pak) and the relative phase angle (rp).

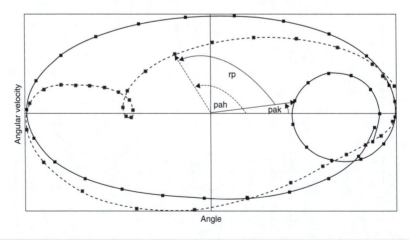

Figure 6.21 Continuous relative phase for the hip–knee angle coupling for one treadmill running stride, derived from Figure 6.20. The dashed vertical line indicates toe-off and the continuous vertical line indicates touchdown.

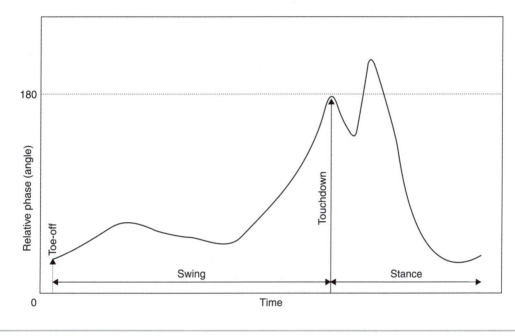

see that the knee 'lags' the hip in 'phase space' (rp<180°) except just after touchdown: the relative phase angle is around 30 to 60° for much of the swing phase (after toe-off) and changes to around 180° at touchdown, fluctuates about that value at the start of the stance phase before returning to around 30 to 60° before toe-off. The change from 30–60° to 180° or vice versa precedes the change from swing to stance or vice versa, which can be interpreted as a preparatory or anticipatory change.

The limitations of continuous relative phase (CRP) are, first, that phase angles can cross the 0–360° discontinuity, because the angle is plotted as a linear variable yet it is a circular one (i.e. 0° = 360° = 720° ...). This can lead to discontinuities in the CRP graph, unless plotted on the surface of a cylinder, not an easy task in a textbook. This leads to the possible need for the use of circular statistics to analyse data. The use of CRP assumes, for any statistical tests, that the datasets are sinusoidal – or very nearly so (mostly fairly close for cyclic movements) and 'stationary' – that is, the statistical description of the dataset is invariant with time, which will not be true, for example, if impacts are involved. However, CRP is a continuous, rich measure, which shows up as a pattern that can be qualitatively compared with others.

So what (you might be tempted to say)? Well, relative phase has been found to be the variable (the 'order parameter' or 'collective variable') that best expresses coordination changes in a wide range of biological phenomenon, including human movement. Examples in human movement include the transitions between walking and running, and bimanual coordination changes. For a further discussion of these and other biological examples of the use of relative phase (such as firefly synchronised flashing and lamprey swimming) see Kelso (1995) in the 'Further reading' section below. So, relative phase is very important in understanding coordination!

Cross-correlation functions

Here, we will consider another graphical representation of coordination between joints – cross-correlation functions – and look at the strengths and weaknesses of this approach. We will begin by revising (or introducing, if you have not comes across them before) Pearson product moment correlations, the basis of cross-correlation functions. Correlation tests are used when we suspect (hopefully from some theory) that two variables are meaningfully interrelated. A correlation is a statistical technique to help us ascertain the extent of such a relationship. Correlations (expressed by correlation coefficients, r) vary from +1 through 0 to –1 (the line, if there is one, associating the two variables is called the regression line). Plus 1 is a perfect positive correlation; minus 1 is a perfect negative (inverse) correlation; zero indicates that the two variables are uncorrelated. Most r values are not 1 or 0.

Cross-correlations are similar to Pearson product moment correlations, but involve correlating variables (often angles) from two time series. They can be easily implemented by the function PEARSON in Excel; e.g. = PEARSON(D2:102,E2:E102); where the data for one angle are in cells D2 to D102 and for the second angle in cells E2 to E102. The term 'cross' correlation is used to denote correlations between two different time series compared to 'auto-correlation' of one time series with itself. Cross-correlating two angle time series may obscure real relationships, if one angle 'leads' or 'lags' the other, in other words, if peaks and troughs are offset in time as below. If the time lag is removed, relationships may be revealed. As an example, consider simple cosine and sine series as in Figure 6.22(a) below ($r = 0$). The sine series lags the cosine series, here by 5 data points; for example, the cosine series reaches the value +1 five data points before the sine series does. If we now remove 1 lag (Figure 6.22(b)) $r = 0.32$; for –2 lags, $r = 0.61$; remove 3 lags (Figure 6.22(c)), $r = 0.82$: for –4 lags, $r = 0.96$; remove 5 lags and the two curves now overlie, so $r = 1$. If we now plot the correlation coefficients as a function of time lags for one time series against the other, showing the strength of the correlation at different lags, we obtain the cross correlation function (CCF, Figure 6.22(d)).

Now let us consider the hip and knee angle time series for treadmill walking, for which we looked at the angle–angle diagram in Figure 6.16 above, and plot correlation coefficients for various time lags for one angle time series against the other, showing the strength of the correlation at different lags. The resulting cross-correlation functions can show, for example, that joints can be coordinated but out of phase, as in this example (Figure 6.23). Here we have $r = 0.76$ at a lead of the hip over the knee of 17% of the stride time and $r = -0.75$ at 76%; by contrast, the original time series had $r \sim 0.2$, highly uncorrelated and, superficially, seemingly uncoordinated. Cross-correlations between suitable joint angles or angular velocities can also show proximal-to-distal joint sequencing in, for example, throwing.

Figure 6.22 Indication of change of correlation coefficient with time lag: (a) cosine and sine series; (b) cosine series and sine series with one time lag removed; (c) cosine series and sine series with three time lags removed; (d) resulting cross-correlation function plotted against removed time lag.

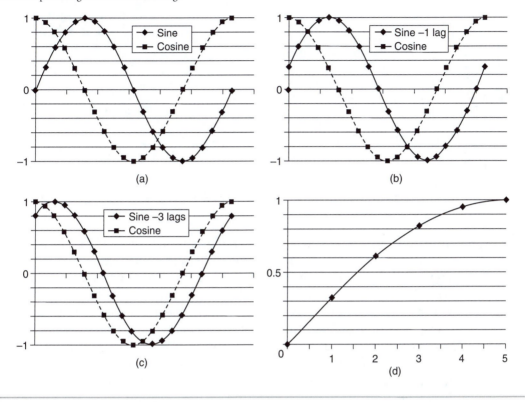

Figure 6.23 Cross-correlation function for the hip and knee angles in treadmill walking for a specific individual at preferred walking speed.

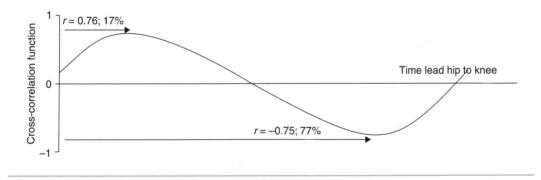

Conjugate cross-correlations consider coordination between three or more variables, such as the angles of the hip, knee and ankle in our example of treadmill walking (Figure 6.24), by plotting and analysing cross-correlation functions of the hip and knee, the knee and ankle, and the hip and ankle. Without going in to this in too much detail, it

Figure 6.24 Conjugate cross-correlation functions between the hip and knee, knee and ankle, and hip and ankle angles in treadmill walking for a specific individual at preferred walking speed.

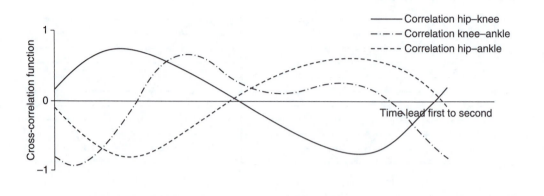

is clear that the cross-correlation functions of the hip and knee and the hip and ankle are inverted. The cross-correlation function of the knee and ankle is entirely different in shape and in time leads, or lags, to the largest positive and negative correlation coefficients.

Cross-correlation functions reveal aspects of coordination not apparent in other approaches. Although the calculation of cross-correlation functions might seem to be 'quantitative', their interpretation is essentially qualitative. The patterns are easy to interpret, although some people find the underlying concepts somewhat difficult. If we are only interested in calculating correlations, then the only underlying assumption is that the two variables are linearly related. It should be obvious that there must be a meaningful relationship between the two variables to be correlated, otherwise erroneous results will be obtained. Human movement dynamics are not, however, linear, but this is not an insurmountable difficulty as we can logarithmically transform the data. If we wish to test hypotheses, for example about the statistical significance of the correlation coefficient, the same assumptions must be met as for Pearson product moment correlations (see Howell, 2009); this would definitely take us into quantitative analysis.

QUALITATIVE MOVEMENT ANALYSIS PACKAGES

Most qualitative movement analysts will have access to a qualitative movement analysis software package, such as Dartfish (www.dartfish.com) or Siliconcoach (www.siliconcoach.com), which offer many options that can help the analyst to pinpoint weaknesses in performance. As I mainly use Siliconcoach – it was developed by graduates from the School of Physical Education at the University of Otago and is one of the best of these packages – the examples below will be based on that package.

It is worth noting that such software packages come at various prices, so it is important to ensure that you know what you need and what is on offer. All of them capture digital video recordings and allow still and slow motion replay and the capture of still images. All allow the viewing of at least two video sequences on the same screen, some up to four. Similarly, two or more still images can be displayed and saved on the same screen. These options are useful, for example, to look at two views of the same action, such as a golf shot (Figure 6.25) or of a successful and unsuccessful performance, such as a tennis serve (Figure 6.26). Some of these packages allow the viewing of two performances superimposed on one image, usually by matching the backgrounds, which can also allow the use of moving cameras. The use of any of these dual-screen or multiscreen options to compare different performers should be treated with great caution. Different individuals bring their own organismic constraints to a sports task, which interact with the constraints of the task and those of the environment to evolve unique solutions to the task. Seeking to copy others has not been proven to improve performance and can lead to an increased risk of injury. However, one justifiable use of such comparisons is when the view of one performer is used as an exemplar of one or more critical features of a deterministic model, such as the long jump take-off example of Figure 6.5; such exemplar images are used in the long jump 'wizard' below.

Figure 6.25 Simultaneous front and side views of the start of a golf swing. The ovals and lines highlight the viewing focus; the angle of 51° indicates the angle of the club shaft to the horizontal.

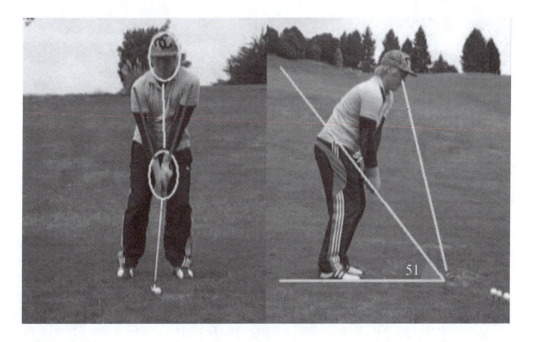

Figure 6.26 Views of the same instant in a successful and unsuccessful (the ball hit the net) tennis serve (the horizontal lines show the depth of knee flexion in each serve).

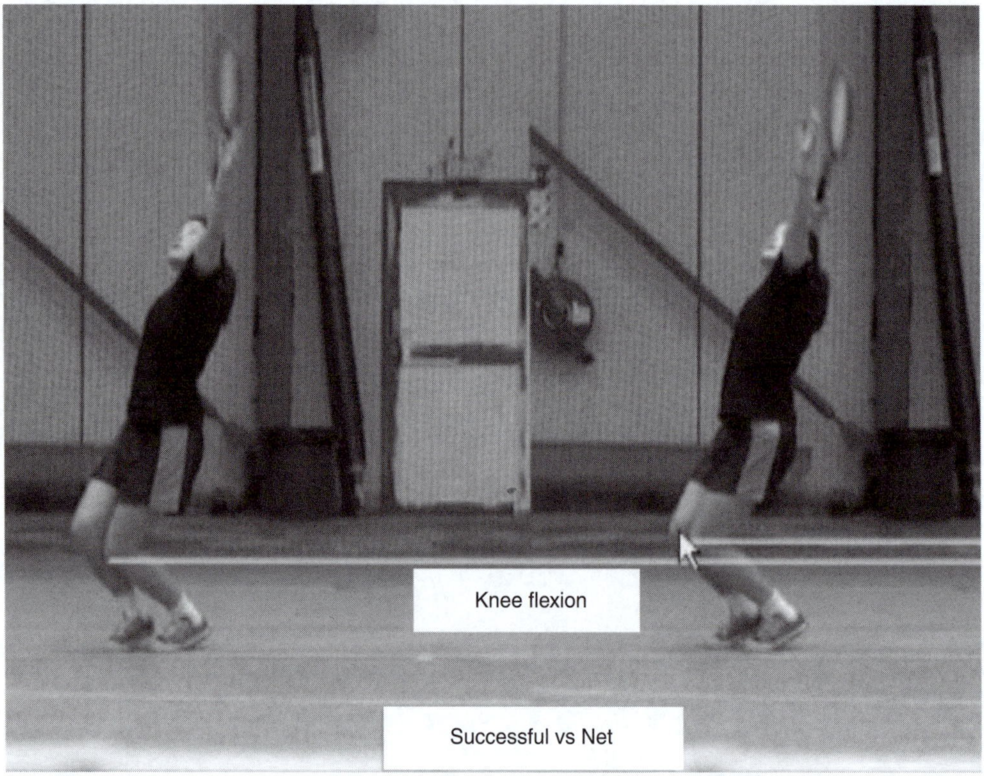

Most qualitative analysis software packages also allow simple line drawing to highlight, for example, body shape or viewing focus (the latter as in Figure 6.25) or another specific aspect of the movement (as in Figure 6.26). All of these packages provide simple measurement of angles (as in Figure 6.25) and lengths. Some also allow the calculation of speed and other derived variables; the sampling rate of the video footage or out of plane movements may compromise the accuracy of these calculations, however. Several video examples of the use of Siliconcoach in qualitative movement analysis are available on the book's website.

One of my favourite options in Siliconcoach was the ReportPak Wizard Editor, which allowed templates of correct movement technique to be developed and used, known as wizards. This option allowed the wizard editor easily to convert deterministic models, such as the one we developed earlier in this chapter for the long jump, into a wizard format, as in Figure 6.27, in which the 'aspects' of the model (dashed arrows) are key events or phases of the movement and the 'aspect details' (chain-dashed arrows), are the critical features of the movement. Once completed, the wizard could be put into a format to be used by a movement analyst (see Figure 6.28) and then put into a report for a coach (Figure 6.29). Although the wizard option is now being phased out by Siliconcoach for a more text-based approach, it is probably as near as anyone has come so far to developing an 'expert system' for performance diagnostics (see Chapter 7).

Figure 6.27 Siliconcoach wizard of long jump, based on the deterministic model developed in this chapter. The first level of indentation (continuous arrow) contains the title the wizard. The second level of indentation (dashed arrows) contains the 'aspects' of the jump – either phases of the movement (such as run-up) or key events (such as take-off). The third level of indentation (chain-dashed arrows) contains the 'details' of the jump – the 11 critical features.

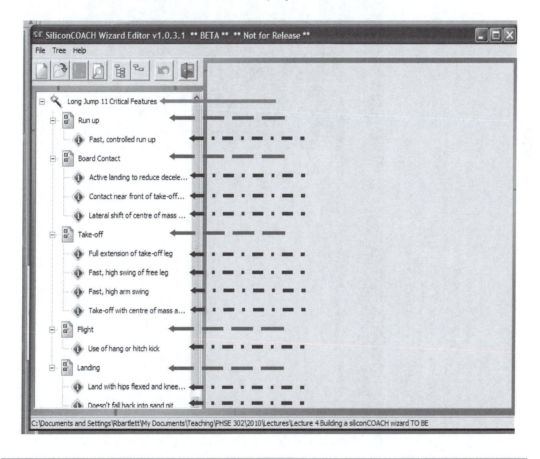

Figure 6.28 Long jump wizard as it appears to an analyst. The 'Value' (column 2) is based on one of several options. Yes (or no) is fairly self-explanatory – it is correct, hence the tick in the next ('Movement') column for 'Fast, controlled run up'. A second option for the value column involves the use of 'look-up tables'. Here, the critical feature (or detail) 'Contact near front of the board' has been highlighted, hence the exemplar image of board contact, to which the analyst has added his or her client image, and the aspect notes about board contact. In the value column, 'Too far back' is deemed 'insufficient' for 'Contact near front of the board', hence the minus sign in the next column, indicating a critical feature that needs attention. The 'Priority' column would be completed by the movement analyst to prioritise the order in which the critical features that need attention for the 'client' athlete should be addressed in the intervention stage of the analysis process.

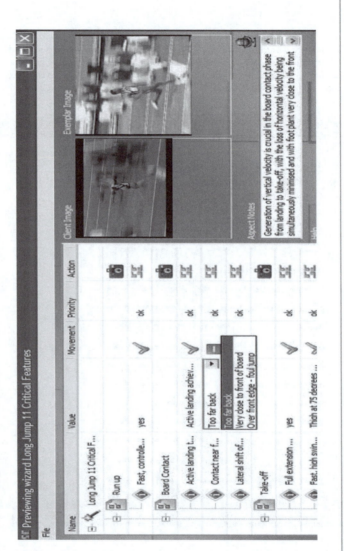

Figure 6.29 The same wizard as in Figure 6.28 as it would appear in ReportPak for a coach; the analyst has added his or her (client) images to compare with the exemplar images. Note that the exemplar images are being used only to highlight good (or not so good in the case of 'contact near the front of the take-off board' for the Board Contact aspect) examples of one or more critical features. The critical features provide the technique model for the jump, not the jump technique of another athlete.

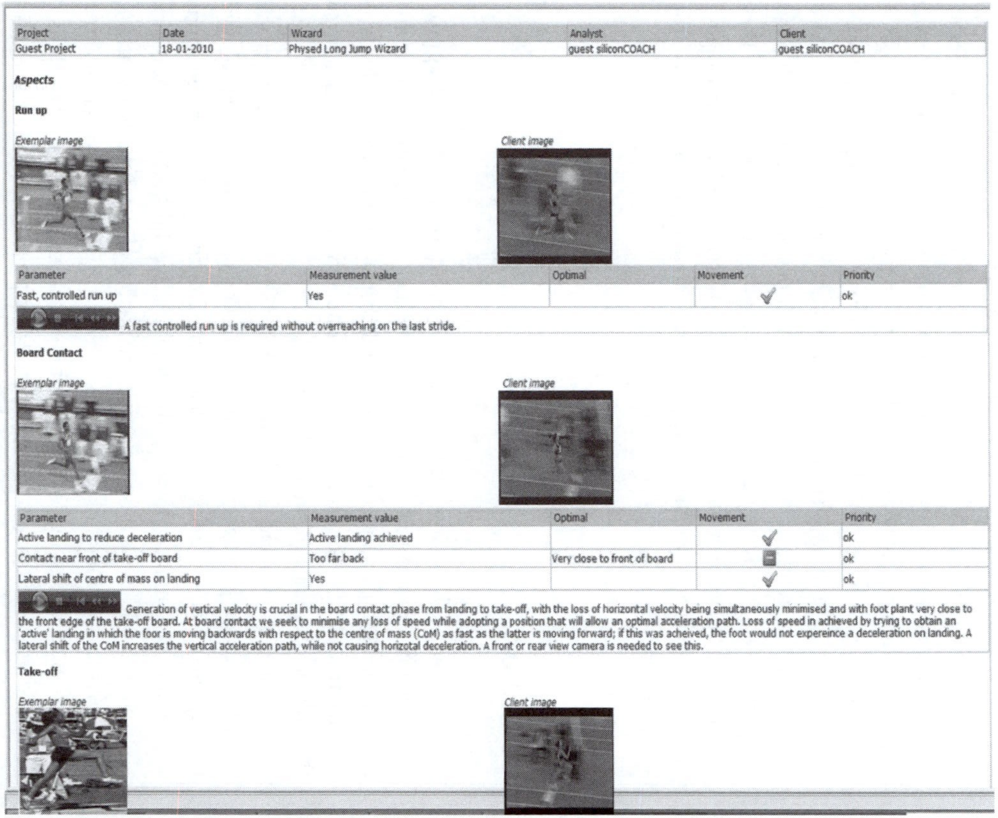

Project	Date	Wizard	Analyst	Client	
Guest Project	18-01-2010	Physed Long Jump Wizard	guest siliconCOACH	guest siliconCOACH	

Aspects

Run up

Exemplar image

Client image

Parameter	Measurement value	Optimal	Movement	Priority
Fast, controlled run up	Yes		✓	ok

A fast controlled run up is required without overreaching on the last stride.

Board Contact

Exemplar image

Client image

Parameter	Measurement value	Optimal	Movement	Priority
Active landing to reduce deceleration	Active landing achieved		✓	ok
Contact near front of take-off board	Too far back	Very close to front of board	!	ok
Lateral shift of centre of mass on landing	Yes		✓	ok

Generation of vertical velocity is crucial in the board contact phase from landing to take-off, with the loss of horizontal velocity being simultaneously minimised and with foot plant very close to the front edge of the take-off board. At board contact we seek to minimise any loss of speed while adopting a position that will allow an optimal acceleration path. Loss of speed is achieved by trying to obtain an 'active' landing in which the foot is moving backwards with respect to the centre of mass (CoM) as fast as the latter is moving forward; if this was achieved, the foot would not experience a deceleration on landing. A lateral shift of the CoM increases the vertical acceleration path, while not causing horizontal deceleration. A front or rear view camera is needed to see this.

Take-off

Exemplar image

Client image

SUMMARY

In this chapter, we identified four stages in a structured approach to movement analysis, considered the main aspects of the first three stages and noted that the value of each stage depends on how well the previous stages have been implemented. We saw that the most crucial step in the whole approach is how to identify the critical features of a movement, and we looked at several ways of doing this, but found that none is foolproof. We worked through a detailed example of the best approach, using deterministic models, and considered the use of 'movement principles'. Another focus of this chapter was movement and coordination patterns and their qualitative interpretation. The importance of being able to interpret graphical patterns of angular displacement and to infer from these the geometry of the angular velocity and angular acceleration patterns was stressed. We looked at how to assess joint coordination using angle–angle diagrams and cross-correlation functions, and, through phase planes, relative phase; we briefly touched on the strengths and weaknesses of these approaches. Finally, we looked at some of the options provided in software packages for qualitative movement analysis, which can help the qualitative analyst to improve the performance of an athlete.

STUDY TASKS

1 For one of the following sports activities, a movement phase approach to each of which is outlined in Chapter 5, identify the most important phase from a performance perspective and then derive, and display diagrammatically, levels 1 to 3 of a deterministic model for that phase. The activities are stroking in swimming, the volleyball spike and the javelin throw.

2 Use a deterministic model to identify about six observable critical features for performance of a sports activity of your choice. You will need to develop fully, and represent diagrammatically, levels 1 and 2 of the model, but you should not need to follow every branch down further levels (as we did in the long jump example above) – you should focus on developing the boxes in level 2 that most affect performance.

3 Devise a systematic observation strategy for your chosen activity in Study Task 2, including recording location, number of cameras, their positions, any auxiliary lighting, camera shutter speed, performer preparation, and the required number of trials. Set out an instruction sheet for conducting an initial pilot study. Outline, briefly, how you might assure validity, reliability and objectivity while minimising observer bias.

4 Describe the biomechanical, physiological, perceptual-motor and psychological errors that could contribute to a run-out in cricket.

5 Download a knee angle–time graph for walking from the book's website. From this, and using the relationships between the gradients and curvatures of the graph, sketch the appropriate angular velocity and acceleration graphs. Remember that you

move along the graph from left to right, going uphill and downhill noting the changes in gradient and curvature. Repeat the above exercise for the hip angle in walking, which you can download from the book's website. Keep repeating this for other datasets, until you are able to sketch the angular velocity and acceleration graphs without reference to either the figures in this chapter or the answers on the website. An ability to analyse such movement patterns is essential for all good movement analysts.

6   Describe the coordination sequences of the ankle–knee and ankle–hip joint couplings in Figures 6.15(b and c). Indicate the points on the figures that correspond to coordination changes (similar to points 'a–g' in Figure 6.15(a)). Indicate also whether the joints are in-phase or anti-phase in each region of the diagram (as, for example, for regions 'a–b' and 'g–a' in Figure 6.15(a)) – assume for this purpose that ankle plantar flexion is in-phase with knee and hip extension. Note that the points in Figures 6.15(b and c) at which coordination changes will not necessarily be the same as those in Figure 6.15(a); however, point 'a' and an anticlockwise progression with time are common to all three figures.

7   For this Study Task, download and save one of the walking and one of the running Excel files from the walking-to-running folder on the book's website (for one runner). Successful completion of this study task is absolutely crucial if you want to become a competent qualitative movement analyst, so do persevere.

   (a) By selecting the relevant columns from the Excel file, plot time series graphs for the hip, knee and ankle angles for both walking and running. Comment on any observable differences between the movement patterns for walking and running.

   (b) By selecting the relevant columns, plot angle–angle diagrams for the hip–knee and ankle–knee couplings for each activity. Again, comment on any observable differences between the coordination patterns for walking and running.

   (c) Again, by selecting the relevant columns, plot phase planes (angular velocity versus angle) for the hip, knee and ankle for each activity. Yet again, comment on any observable differences between the coordination patterns for walking and running.

   (d) Finally, by selecting the relevant columns, plot the cross-correlation functions between the hip and knee, hip and ankle, and knee and ankle (three curves) for each activity. Yet again, comment on any observable differences between the coordination patterns for walking and running.

8   Based on the differences you have noted in Study Task 7, explain whether each of the three types of coordination pattern help you to identify any qualitative differences between walking and running.

GLOSSARY OF IMPORTANT TERMS

Analyst bias An unconscious tendency that can arise in the evaluation and diagnosis stage of qualitative analysis for various reasons. Prior knowledge of a performer or a performer's age can be factors. Good definitions of, and correctness criteria for,

critical features and thorough training of the observational analysts can help to reduce analyst bias.

Anticipatory change Some change in body geometry or function that precedes, or anticipates, a particular movement change. In the context of this chapter, this means the change in continuous relative phase that occurs before the change from the stance to swing phase, or vice versa, in running.

Collective variable Simplistically, a variable that incorporates two or more other variables. Relative phase is a collective variable as it incorporates two angles and two angular velocities. In the context of this book, the collective variable should characterise coordination patterns or changes in coordination, which relative phase usually does. A collective variable is also known, in the coordination context, as an **order parameter**.

Conjugate cross correlations An extension of **cross-correlation functions** to cover more than two joints. Rules of compatibility between the time lags and between the signs of the correlation peaks for the various cross-correlation functions involved can be specified.

Coordination dynamics In essence, the science of coordination, which aims to describe, explain and predict how patterns of coordination form, adapt and change in living organisms. In the context of this book, the term can be applied to a single joint through to the entire human movement system.

Coordination patterns Whereas movement patterns express how a movement variable – for example, an angle, angular velocity, or angular acceleration – evolves or varies with time, coordination patterns look at how meaningful combinations of these variables co-vary. Coordination patterns include angle–angle diagrams, phase planes, continuous relative phase (itself a function of time) and cross-correlation functions.

Coordinative structures These are considered to be functional relationships between important anatomical parts of the body to perform a specific activity, such as when groups of muscles and joints temporarily function as coherent units to achieve a specific goal, such as hitting a ball.

Correlation coefficients These express the strength of the statistical relationship between two variables.

Critical features Those key features of a movement that are required for the movement to be performed optimally. The term is used mostly in qualitative biomechanical analysis, in which case the critical features need to be observable. The identification of the critical features of a movement is the most important task of the preparation stage of qualitative biomechanical analysis.

Cross-correlation functions These are obtained by calculating the **correlation coefficient** between two time series, then introducing various time lags between the two time series and recalculating the **correlation coefficient** for each time lag. Finally, the cross-correlation function is the graph of the correlation coefficient as a function of the time lag.

Impulse–momentum relationship An expression of Newton's Second Law of Motion, which states that the impulse of a force (the mean force multiplied by the time during which the force acts) is equal to the change in momentum of the body on which the force acts.

Individual specificity Term used to express the fact that any individual will find a specific solution (or set of solutions) to a movement task that fits his or her **organismic constraints** as well as the task and environmental constraints. The movement analyst has to be continually aware of the requirement for individual specificity when seeking to identify and correct movement faults. What works for one sports performer may not work for another.

In-phase and anti-phase coordination In-phase coordination involves two joints (or segments) moving in an anatomically similar way. Examples would be the knee and hip flexing together in the downward movement of a standing vertical jump or the index fingers on both hands abducting. Anti-phase, or out of phase, coordination occurs when the movements are antagonistic, as when the index finger on one hand adducts while that on the other hand abducts, or when the hip flexes while the knee extends. In this context, ankle plantar flexion is considered to be in-phase with hip and knee extension.

Intra- and inter-analyst reliability Intra-analyst (also called intra-rater or intra-operator) reliability is the consistency of the analyses carried out by one analyst on several occasions. Inter-analyst reliability (also called objectivity) is the consistency of the analyses of several analysts. Intra-analyst reliability is usually better than inter-analyst reliability. Neither is easy to determine accurately for qualitative movement analysis.

Joint angle conventions For two-dimensional analysis in the sagittal plane, the normal sports biomechanics convention is for a fully extended knee or elbow, for example, to be designated as 180°. Flexion then involves the joint angle decreasing and extension involves the joint angle increasing. This convention is used throughout this book. The angle conventions used by clinical biomechanists and in three-dimensional analysis are completely different. Movement analysts need to check carefully what joint angle convention is being used.

Needs analysis In the context of this book, a needs analysis is usually a semi-formal meeting or interview, led by the movement analyst, to ascertain what the 'clients' need from the movement analysis.

Optimal performance model A somewhat discredited concept of a universal optimal set of movement patterns to perform a given movement task – such as a javelin throw – that applies to all individuals. This concept led to the idea of copying the movements of the current world champion in that task (the so-called 'elite performer template'), completely ignoring the principle of **individual specificity**.

Order parameter See **collective variable** above.

Organismic constraints The set of characteristics, or constraints, that an individual possesses; these constraints influence the movement solutions that individual will adopt for a particular task and environment. These are internal to the individual and include anatomical–anthropometric characteristics, strength, flexibility and fitness.

Pearson product moment correlation This is the most common way of assessing the strength of a linear relationship between two variables. The strength of the relationship is expressed as the Pearson product moment **correlation coefficient**.

Sinusoidal A function having the form of a sine or cosine wave or a combination of these.

Subjective performance criterion A performance criteria (or result) that is judged subjectively, as in gymnastics, figure skating and diving.

Systematic observation strategy The development of a systematic 'observation' strategy pays attention to all matters that are relevant to good observation, and subsequent analysis, of movement.

Topological equivalence Two shapes (such as angle–angle diagrams) are said to be topologically equivalent if one can be deformed into the other without folding or cutting. For our purposes, two shapes can be said to be topologically equivalent if they contain the same number of loops. [In the branch of mathematics called topology, topological equivalence is a bit more complicated than these simple statements might imply.]

REFERENCES

Bartlett, R.M. (2007) *Introduction to Sports Biomechanics: Analysing Human Movement Patterns*, London: Routledge.

Bartlett, R.M., Bussey, M. and Flyger, N. (2006) Movement variability cannot be determined reliably from no-marker conditions. *Journal of Biomechanics, 39*, 3076–3079.

Bartlett, R.M., Wheat, J. and Robbins, M. (2007) Is movement variability important for sports biomechanists? *Sports Biomechanics, 6*, 224–243.

Button, C., Davids, K. and Schöllhorn, W. (2006) 'Coordination profiling of movement systems', in K. Davids, S. Bennett and K. Newell (eds) *Movement System Variability*, Champaign, IL: Human Kinetics, pp. 133–152.

Davids, K., Button, C. and Bennett, S. (2008) *Dynamics of Skill Acquisition: A Constraints-led Approach*, Champaign, IL: Human Kinetics.

Hay, J.G. and Reid, J.G. (1982) *Anatomy, Mechanics, and Human Motion*, Englewood Cliffs, NJ: Prentice Hall.

Howell, D.C. (2009) *Statistical Methods for Psychology*, Belmont, CA: Cengage Wadsworth.

Kelso, J.A.S. (1995) *Dynamic Patterns: The Self-Organization of Brain and Behavior*, Cambridge, MA: MIT Press.

Knudson, D.V. (2007) Qualitative biomechanical principles for application in coaching. *Sports Biomechanics, 6*, 109–118.

Knudson, D.V. and Morrison, C.S. (2002) *Qualitative Analysis of Human Movement*, Champaign, IL: Human Kinetics.

FURTHER READING

Bartlett, R.M. (2007) *Introduction to Sports Biomechanics: Analysing Human Movement Patterns*, London: Routledge. Chapter 3 looks in more basic detail at the qualitative analysis of movement patterns and at basic coordination patterns.

Kelso, J.A.S. (1995) *Dynamic Patterns: The Self-Organization of Brain and Behavior*, Cambridge, MA: MIT Press (Chapter 1: How Nature Handles Complexity). Most of you will not find this plain sailing, but not because of any mathematics – there are no equations in this chapter – but because of the novelty of much of the material. Stick with it; you too might be inspired by Scott Kelso's approach.

Knudson, D.V. and Morrison, C.S. (2002) *Qualitative Analysis of Human Movement*, Champaign, IL: Human Kinetics. The first edition of this book was for many years one of the few real gems in the Human Kinetics list of sports science texts; the second edition continues that tradition. However, the authors have not yet welcomed a wider interpretation of qualitative movement analysis and a crucial (perhaps the crucial) 'critical feature' of skilled human movement – coordination – receives only one page reference in the index. The structured approach to movement analysis outlined in this chapter is covered in far more detail in Part II, while Part I sets the scene nicely and Part III outlines applications of their approach, with many diagrammatic examples. Highly recommended and well written.

APPENDIX 6.1 MOVEMENT AND COORDINATION VARIABILITY

Introduction

As we mentioned several times in this chapter, differences occur in movements both between individuals performing the same task (inter-individual variability) and within the same individual (intra-individual variability). Inter-individual variability arises mainly because of different people finding solutions to a particular sports task, such as a long jump, a dart throw or a netball chest pass, that reflect not only the task and environmental constraints but their own organismic constraints. All biological systems are self-organising, within such sets of constraints. This means that no general 'optimal movement pattern' exists for different individuals performing the same task, as you can see from Figure 6.17 earlier in the chapter. We need models of performance that can be adapted to specific individuals, which we can obtain from qualitative deterministic models, the focus of the first half of this chapter.

Intra-individual variability arises from the observation that one person will not perform an identical movement from one trial to the next, for example over six throws in a javelin competition or several free throws in basketball (see Bartlett *et al.* (2007) for a review). Even in what appear to be stereotyped activities, such as treadmill running, movement patterns will vary from stride to stride, as shown in Figure 6.30. The person here, a 65-year-old male, was walking (Figure 6.30(a)), running fairly slowly (Figure 6.30(c)) and jogging at an intermediate speed between the two, known as the transition region, in which neither walking nor running felt normal (Figure 6.30(b)). In all three conditions, you can clearly observe differences between strides. The movements are not replicated exactly from stride to stride or, for example, in a throw or jump, from one trial to another. This casts considerable doubt on the concept of a 'representative trial' and is the main reason we analyse multiple trials in both qualitative and quantitative movement analysis.

Various functional roles have been proposed – although not necessarily proved – for movement variability. Among these are: facilitating a change in coordination, such as from walking to running; enabling adaptations to the environment, as in running on a treadmill or an asphalt road or sand; and reducing the possibility that the same tissues will be maximally loaded from stride to stride or trial to trial, thereby reducing the risk of overuse injury.

Figure 6.30 Movement variability in knee time series for a recreational walker: (a) walking at 5.5 km/h; (b) transition zone at 7.5 km/h; (c) slow running at 10 km/h; (d) walking showing mean and mean ±1 standard deviation lines.

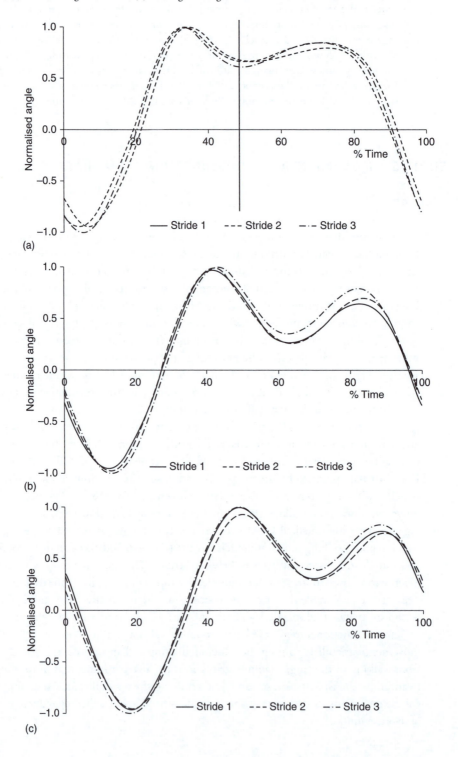

Figure 6.30 (*continued*)

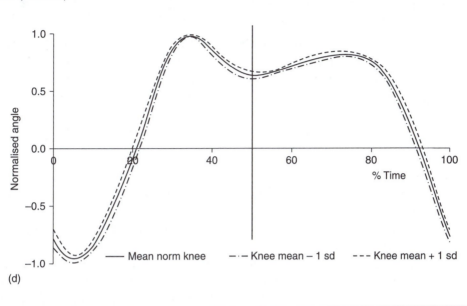

(d)

Movement variability

Variability in movement patterns, such as angle time series as in Figure 6.30, is referred to as 'movement variability'. We must admit here that we have to be able to measure the angles or any other variables used to produce these movement patterns accurately, which usually requires the use of joint markers and a quantitative analysis package such as SIMI rather than a qualitative one, such as Siliconcoach. However, these patterns can be analysed, in part, qualitatively. First, you can easily see the variability between the three strides in each condition in Figure 6.30. Second, with careful observation, you can see that the walking condition (Figure 6.30(a)) is slightly more variable than the other two; it has no regions, unlike those for transition and running, in which the variability is very small. The fact that the variability is greatest for walking for this individual can be explained through the idea that movements that are practised many times allow the individual to relax the degrees of freedom involved to find more flexible solutions to the task (degrees of freedom can approximately be considered to be the total number of degrees of rotational freedom in all the joints involved in the movement). Less familiar movements might lead to a freezing of the degrees of freedom in the chain of body segments. This individual is a very keen recreational walker, regularly walking at an average speed of 6 km/h for periods of 2–3 hours; he no longer runs, however, after a back injury when he was 60; so walking is well-practiced for him, running and the transition region are not.

If we wish to quantify, or measure, movement variability, we have a simple task. We need only a measure of dispersion. Standard deviation is a robust measure of dispersion and, for the purpose of this book, we will accept it as a good measure of variability, although many biomechanists use more complicated measures. We simply take the

Table 6.3 Movement variabilities in hip and knee time series and coordination variabilities in hip–knee angle–angle diagram (AAD)

CONDITION	WALKING 5.5 KM/H	TRANSITION 7.5 KM/H	RUNNING 10 KM/H
Hip angle	0.71°	0.65°	0.70°
Knee angle	1.28°	1.00°	1.02°
Normalised hip angle	0.042	0.041	0.038
Normalised knee angle	0.045	0.038	0.041
Normalised hip–knee AAD	0.064	0.058	0.057

standard deviation between the angles recorded at the same per cent time for each stride (t_i), represented by the vertical line at mid stride (50% time) in Figure 6.30(a). That enables us to plot the mean and ±1 standard deviation lines in Figure 6.30(d), for the same strides as in Figure 6.30(a). We can also obtain a measure of the average standard deviation over the whole 0–100 per cent times for the whole stride by adding the standard deviations at each per cent time interval (sd_{ti}) and dividing by 101, the number of time 'points', mean $sd = \Sigma(sd_{ti})/101$. This mean value is sometimes called the 'ensemble mean' or 'mean ensemble' variability and we can obviously compare values between conditions as in Table 6.3. In this case the mean ensemble value is greatest, by over 25%, for the knee angle in walking: walking = 1.28°; transition = 1.00°; running = 1.02°; it is also greatest for the hip angle in walking, but less so than for the knee. These values add to, and support, our qualitative observation that, for this individual (and such findings are individual-specific), walking is the most variable of the three conditions. The calculation is made simple because we have removed any variability in the time between strides by normalising the stride time to 100%. We can also account for the differences in the range of movement between conditions by normalising the angle in each condition to the range of movement at each joint, by fitting the values to the range ±1 (I did this when plotting all of the graphs in this appendix). This has little effect here on which joint is most variable, as you can see from Table 6.3; walking is still the most variable for both joints. The order of the other two has changed for the hip joint.

Coordination variability

If we assess variability in coordination patterns – angle–angle diagrams (Figure 6.31), phase planes, continuous relative phase (CRP) and cross-correlation functions – then we obtain coordination variability. Again in Figures 6.31(a–c) we can observe the variability in all three conditions. Less obvious than for Figure 6.30(a–c) is that the coordination variability of this male recreational walker is greatest for his familiar activity of walking. Table 6.3, however, clearly shows that the variability for walking is 10% greater than for the other two conditions. The reason this is visually less obvious is due to the dispersion of the data points for the same per cent stride time on an angle–angle diagram that we touch on in the next paragraph.

If we wish to calculate the coordination variability, then, for CRP and cross-correlation functions, it is similar to the calculation above for angle time series as the variable plotted on the horizontal axis – time for CRP and time lag for cross-correlation functions – is not subject to variability as plotted. Please note that cross-correlation functions are automatically normalised, as the range of the correlation coefficient is ±1, but this is not true for CRP, for which the range is usually ±180° or 0–360°.

Calculations of variability in angle–angle diagrams and phase planes are somewhat more complicated than for time series. Both variables – the two angles in an angle–angle diagram

Figure 6.31 Coordination variability in hip–knee angle–angle diagrams for a recreational walker: (a) walking at 5.5 km/h; (b) transition zone at 7.5 km/h;

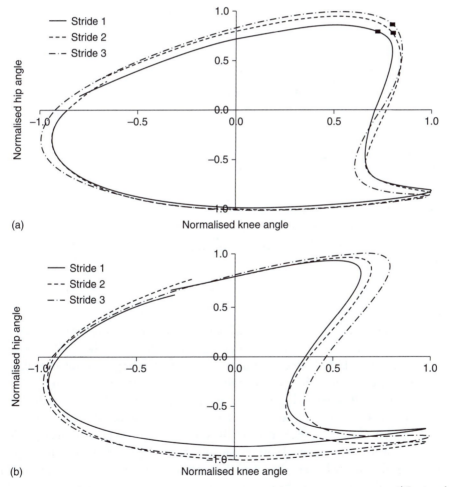

(a)

(b)

(*Continued Overleaf*)

Figure 6.31 *continued* (c) slow running at 10 km/h; (d) walking showing mean and mean ±1 standard deviation lines. The three rectangles at the top right of figure 6.31(a) are for 80% stride time for each of the three strides.

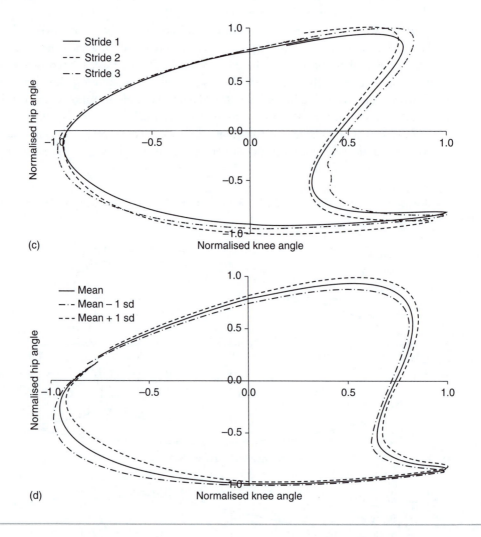

(c)

(d)

(Figure 6.31(a–c)) and the joint angle and angular velocity in a phase plane – contain variability. This affects the presentation of the mean ±1 standard deviation lines as in Figure 6.31(d), in which the lines cross over, which would be impossible for an angle time series. Again, we can normalise these diagrams to the range of movement for angles (and for phase planes to the largest positive or negative angular velocity). Different researchers have preferences as to whether or not to do this; I always do, as can be seen in Figure 6.31. In calculating the mean ensemble variability, we cannot simply add the standard deviations for the two angles – one is plotted horizontally and one vertically, effectively becoming vectors. We therefore use Pythagoras's theorem 'the square on the hypotenuse of a right angled triangle is equal to the sum of the squares on the two adjacent sides'. As the square of standard deviations is called the variance, we simply add the variances and then take the square root to arrive back at a standard deviation at each time point. In other words, $sd_{ri} = \sqrt{(sd_{ki}^2 + sd_{hi}^2)}$, where sd_{ki} and sd_{hi} are the standard deviations of the knee and hip angles, respectively, at time point t_i, where $i = 0$ to 100. We then sum the standard deviations across the 101 per cent times and divide by 101 as for movement variability. You can see the ensemble mean coordination variabilities for the normalised angle–angle diagrams of Figures 6.31(a–c) for the recreational walker in Table 6.3. The coordination variability for this person's familiar walking pattern is the most variable of the three conditions by about 10%, confirming the finding for movement variability above. Please note that the time points are not so obvious on an angle–angle diagram or phase plane as on a time series (however, these data are obvious in the tables of data from which the values are taken to plot the angle–angle diagrams) – the data points for each of the three strides for 80% stride time are shown by small rectangles at the top right of Figure 6.31(a) – and they are not vertically aligned as on an angle time series. This makes the variability between the strides on angle–angle diagrams (and phase planes) less easy to observe than on angle time series: many people would intuitively see Figure 6.31(b) as the most variable of the three conditions, which is disproved by Table 6.3.

Some final thoughts on movement and coordination variability

It is worth repeating that movement and coordination variability are ubiquitous in all animal movements, including humans in sport; they cannot and must not be ignored even by qualitative movement analysts in their day-to-day work. As a closure to this Appendix, you might like to reflect on how the presence of team members would affect movement and coordination variability in, say, a netball chest pass or a throw-in in soccer. Furthermore, reflect at your leisure, on how the presence of opponents would affect movement and coordination variability in, say, a rugby line-out throw or the two activities in the previous sentence. Movement and coordination variability are all around us, so embrace them and rejoice in them.

A warning is also appropriate here, however. If we sought to measure variability in the activities in the previous paragraph during competitions, then we would certainly not be able to use joint or other markers on the body. We would have to estimate joint positions by eye and manually digitise the assumed positions. We then have a far greater problem with errors in measurements contributing to variability between trials or strides than when using joint markers. Bartlett *et al.* (2006) found that it is not possible to measure variability either reliably (within one operator) or objectively (between operators) when no joint markers are used (for abridged details of this study, see Bartlett, 2007). This remains a considerable challenge to the assessment of movement and coordination variability in sports competitions.

7 Performance improvement through quantitative biomechanical models

Roger Bartlett

Knowledge assumed
Understanding of the basics
of performance analysis
(Chapter 5)
Familiarity with the use
of deterministic models
(Chapter 6)
Knowledge of basic statistical
tests

▊ INTRODUCTION

BOX 7.1 LEARNING OUTCOMES

After reading this chapter you should be able to:

- sketch and explain the relationships that can exist between a performance criterion and various performance variables
- describe and compare the: cross-sectional and longitudinal; contrast and correlational; and single-individual and group approaches to statistical modelling
- evaluate critically the limitations of statistical modelling in sports biomechanics
- understand the uses of deterministic modelling in quantitative analysis
- appreciate the advantages and limitations of computer simulation modelling when seeking to evaluate and improve sports performance
- define and distinguish between modelling, simulation, simulation evaluation and optimisation and explain the differences between static and dynamic optimisation and global and local optimums
- interpret graphical representations of optimisation and use contour maps to identify likely ways to improve performance
- understand some of the existing models of human skeletal muscle that are used in computer simulation models of the sports performer
- appreciate the various approaches from artificial intelligence that have been used in the context of the biomechanical improvement of sports performance.

In the previous chapter, we discussed the use of deterministic models of performance in the context of the four-stage qualitative analysis process. We noted that to improve performance we need a model against which to compare an athlete's current movement technique: deterministic models generally serve that purpose for the qualitative analyst. In this chapter we will look at the fundamentals underlying the optimisation of sports movements through the use of quantitative biomechanical models of performance. The emphasis is on theory-driven statistical modelling, computer simulation modelling and optimisation, and various approaches from artificial intelligence. Although these methods may help to improve performance directly, they are more often used to carry out research to obtain an in-depth understanding of the performance of a specific sports task, upon which strategies for performance improvement can then be built. All three of these approaches need quantitative data: these will generally be obtained from an automatic marker-tracking system, such as Vicon (www.vicon.com) or videography, for example, SIMI (www.simi.com). These quantitative approaches benefit from the use of a structured approach, such as that in Chapter 6; the emphasis, however, will be on measurement not observation. As the methods of quantitative biomechanical analysis are well-covered elsewhere (see, in particular, Payton and Bartlett, 2008), they will not be discussed further in this chapter. Most research in quantitative biomechanical modelling uses automatic marker-tracking systems; these systems require athletes to wear reflective markers and are, therefore, generally not useable in competition. Such laboratory-based data has good research (internal) validity but often lacks the ecological validity that is so important in the context of performance improvement; sports performances are not laboratory-based events. You should, however, note the warning of Bartlett *et al.* (2006) about the unreliability of data from the manual coordinate digitising of video records, which often provide the only way that we can obtain data from performances in top competitions.

STATISTICAL MODELS OF SPORTS PERFORMANCE

Underlying performance relationships

The characteristics of a sports movement technique that contribute to the successful execution of that technique are obviously of interest to sports biomechanists seeking to improve performance. The relationship between the desired outcome of the movement technique, called the performance criterion (p), and the various independent (performance) variables (v) are of vital interest (see Figure 7.1). Note here that the term 'performance variables' (or 'performance parameters') is essentially the quantitative analyst's equivalent to the qualitative analyst's 'critical features' (Chapter 6). For example, the performance criterion in the shot-put is the throw distance; the performance parameters include release speed, release angle and release height.

If a linear relationship exists between the performance criterion and a performance variable (Figure 7.1(a)), then improvements in performance should result from improvements in that variable at any standard of performance, providing that a logical cause–effect relationship exists, which can be established through the use of deterministic models. If the relationship is curvilinear – the two variables are related by a curved line – (Figure 7.1(b and c)) then we should seek to improve that variable at the standard of performance at which it is most relevant, i.e. where the slope of the curve is steepest. The nature of the relationship between performance variables and the performance criterion may be that of an 'inverted-U' such that, for any given athlete, there is an optimum value (v_0) for that performance variable (Figure 7.1(d)). There will also be performance variables that have no correlation to the performance criterion (Figure 7.1(e)). In practice, as we shall see in the next section, performance variables often interact to influence the performance criterion even when they are independent of one another. The relationships of Figure 7.1 are then replaced by n-dimensional surfaces; in the simplest case $n=2$ and they resemble contour maps (see, for example, Figure 7.6 later in this chapter).

Figure 7.1 Different functional relationships between performance criterion (p) and independent (performance) variable (v): (a) is linear; (b) is quadratic, but can be linearised by $x = \log v$; (c) is also non-linear, but can be linearised by $y = \log p$; (d) is an inverted-U relationship, typical of an optimal one, and can possibly be linearised by using $x = |v - v_0|$ and seeking a function to linearise p against x; (e) shows no relationship between the variables.

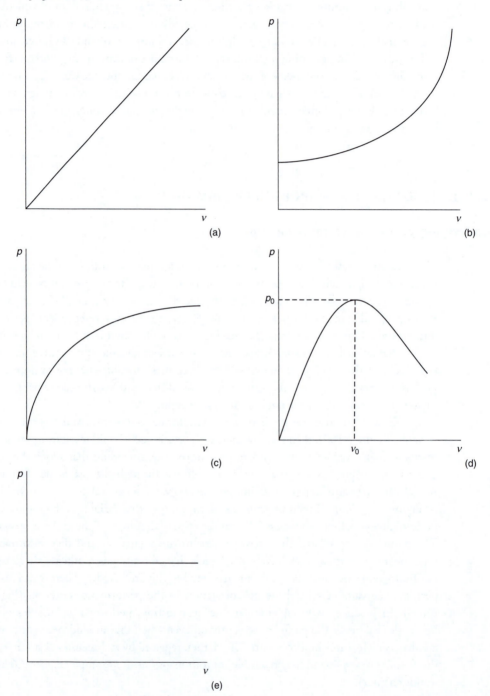

Types of statistical model

Several different approaches have been used to identify the features of a sports performer's movement technique that influence the success achieved. These approaches generally involve the collection and analysis of data from the performances of many performers of a wide range of ability. This is essentially an experimental approach, generally using image-based motion analysis (Payton and Bartlett, 2008). The data analysis will vary with the experimental design, but we can identify the correlation and contrast methods.

In the correlation method a single group of performers, or multiples trials by one performer, is generally used. Correlations between the performance criterion and various performance variables, and inter-correlations among variables are established in a correlation matrix. The correlation coefficients are then used to deduce which performance variables have an important influence on the performance criterion. Failure to select a sufficiently broad range of performances can lead to the omission of important causal variables. The correlation method essentially uses correlational statistics (see, for example, Howell, 2009) to ascertain relationships between selected independent variables and the performance criterion. This type of modelling can be performed as part of, or as an adjunct to, the provision of useful information to the athlete and coach through, for example, sports science support to elite sport.

Two approaches are used for correlational analysis, sometimes categorised as the cross-sectional and the longitudinal. The cross-sectional approach has often involved the analysis of a 'representative trial' by each performer within a single group (a 'group design'), usually, but not always, taken as a 'snapshot' in time, for example at a track and field athletics event. Often far too few trials or performers are analysed to allow conclusive results. Furthermore, the concept of 'representative trials' has been discredited by the recognition of the ubiquity of intra-individual (inter-trial) movement variability; however, the idea of a most successful trial – the one with the best outcome – can still be defended. The cross-sectional approach, which should involve a sufficiently large sample for the results to be generalised, is used to identify variables that are significantly related to performance for a population of athletes represented by that given sample. This may identify both the variables that are important and their best values for that sample.

The longitudinal approach generally uses multiple trials by the same performer (a 'single-individual' or 'within-individual' study). The term longitudinal can be somewhat misleading as it has been used to describe the study of multiple trials by the same performer on one occasion, such as a training session, or over a longer period of time, such as a competition season. The study of multiple trials by the same performer seeks to identify significant variables for a population of trials for the same athlete represented by the given sample of trials.

Comparing the longitudinal single-individual approach and the cross-sectional group approach, and providing that only causal variables are considered, the latter approach seeks to establish the important determinants of performance for athletes in general, while the former seeks to do the same for a particular performer. The two can yield different results. A certain factor may appear to be an important determinant in a group design but not in single-individual one. The results of a group study cannot be generalised to a specific performer, neither can the results from single-individual studies be generalised to other individuals. It should also be noted that a cross-sectional group design will not always identify as important all those biomechanical factors of a technique that a deterministic biomechanical model would contain; this is particularly true if the range of skills within the group is relatively narrow, as in an elite competition. There are many examples of cross-sectional group designs reported in sports science journals (see, for example, Leigh and Yu, 2007). However, single-individual studies are far less common, although there is now agreement that such studies are crucial for the improvement of an individual athlete's technique (see Salter *et al.*, 2007 for a comparison of within- and between-individual approaches). This is particularly emphasised by the constraints-led approach, which recognises that individuals find solutions to the constraints of a sports task that relate to their own organismic constraints.

It is also possible to conduct multiple single-individual studies using several individuals and multiple trials for each individual (for further details, see, for example, Bates *et al.*, 2004). Such studies could, in principle, be carried out at a competition. For example, in the Olympic men's shot-put, we could, theoretically, study nine throws by each of the eight throwers who progressed to the last three throws of the final – their three preliminary throws and six finals throws; unfortunately, not all of these throwers would probably take all three permitted preliminary throws. In multiple single-individual designs, it has been recommended that, to obtain good statistical power, 20 trials for each of a group of five performers should be analysed, or ten trials by each of ten performers, or five trials by each of 20 performers. Nine throws by each of eight throwers would seem to come acceptably close to these recommendations, although with some loss of statistical power.

An alternative to the correlation method is to divide the population into selected groups and use variational statistics to investigate the differences between the groups, but this method is less frequently used. In this contrast method, the participants are usually divided into groups of contrasting ability. Examples include the study of Leskinen *et al.* (2009) of elite and national-standard 1500-m runners, and that of Ho *et al.* (2009) of elite and sub-elite dragon boat paddlers. The means of the various performance variables are then computed for each group and the significance of the observed differences between the means are tested, using *t*-tests, analysis of variance (ANOVA) or multivariate analysis of variance (MANOVA). From the results obtained, conclusions are reached about the important determinants of the performance criterion. A more useful contrast approach, given the uniqueness of individual performers, is to divide multiple trials by the same performer into successful or unsuccessful trials, for example, successful or unsuccessful free throws in basketball. Variational statistics can then be used to analyse differences between the two groups of trials: this approach has not often been used.

Several limitations to the correlation and contrast approaches to statistical modelling have been identified. The arbitrariness, subjectivity and non-systematic nature of some contrast and correlational designs are not an inherent feature of statistical modelling, but rather of its inappropriate, or incorrect, use. The following limitations are worth highlighting. In the first place, relationships between variables will occasionally be revealed that are, in fact, random (Type I errors). These errors often arise when performance variables are not objectively prioritised or, simply, that there are too many of them. This problem can be minimised, if not avoided, by using statistical techniques not as an end in themselves but for theory verification and refinement. A second limitation relates to misidentification of the underlying relationships between independent and dependent variables, as, for example, seeking correlations between projection speed and distance thrown or jumped. However, the relationship between these two variables, from simple projectile motion theory, is essentially quadratic so that projection speed squared should be correlated with the distance thrown or jumped. Correlation statistics should never be used without first looking at a scattergram of the variables to ascertain the type of relationship between them (as in Figure 7.1). Furthermore, the most powerful statistical techniques are often not used; for example, a correlation matrix might be reported but the relative importance of the variable contributions might not be assessed.

A third limitation is that the effects of an uncontrolled physiological or anthropometric variable can mask or inflate the importance of one or more independent variables. A study of a single athlete has experimental control of the constitutional variables that distinguish individuals; a study of multiple athletes exercises no such control. Judicious use of partial correlations can provide some statistical control – such as partialling out the performer's mass if this appears to be a confounding variable (or covariate). However, there are limits to, and dangers in, the use of this statistical control. Each variable partialled out drastically reduces the population to which the results can be generalised.

A fourth limitation is that insufficient attention is often paid to the underlying assumptions of the statistical tests used. This can lead to large overall Type I error rates. Problems arise here, for example, when: parametric statistical tests are used with small, unequal groups; no checks are made with ANOVA designs for normality and homogeneity of variance; or multiple regression designs incorporate too few participants (or trials) for the number of predictor variables used. For a thorough discussion of these and related points, see Howell (2009) and Mullineaux *et al.* (2001). In multiple regression designs, it is generally accepted that for p predictor variables, the number of participants, or trials, n, should be at least $10p$ (preferably $20p$); few studies have used such large ratios of n/p. In multiple single-individual designs, it is often tempting to increase the ratio of n to p by combining participants and trials; this is permissible only under certain conditions – violations of those conditions can invalidate such a design (Donner and Cunningham, 1984).

Investigators also frequently fail to report the power of their statistical tests or the meaningfulness of the effects that they find, such as effect size, and concentrate only on statistical significance (for a further discussion, see Mullineaux *et al.*, 2001). Finally, if changes to a movement technique appear desirable from statistical modelling, the participation of the athlete is still needed to implement the changes and check whether they really are beneficial. This considerably limits the scope for investigating the 'what if?' questions that can provide great insight into sports movements.

Theory-based statistical modelling

The following three-stage approach helps to avoid the weaknesses that are too often apparent in the correlation and contrast approaches and ensures that the appropriate variables are measured and statistically analysed. First, we need to develop a theoretical model (usually as a deterministic model) of the relationships between the performance criterion and the various performance variables. This must be done 'up front' before any data collection takes place. Such deterministic models were considered in-depth in Chapter 6 in the context of qualitative biomechanical analysis. They identify the factors that should influence the performance outcome and relate them to the theoretical laws of biomechanics that underpin the movement (see also Bartlett, 2007). For a quantitative analysis, the second stage is the collection and analysis of data. Depending on the approach used, this may involve a large range of performers or many trials from the same performer. The latter approach – single-individual designs – is now recognised as more useful in seeking to improve an individual's sports performance, given that adaptations to the task, environmental and organismic constraints are individual-specific (see Chapter 5). The former approach – group designs – can be useful in trying to understand the underlying movement in general. Finally, we need to evaluate the results quantitatively with respect to the theoretical deterministic model (this will share many similarities with the evaluation and diagnosis stage of the qualitative analysis process in Chapter 6).

COMPUTER SIMULATION MODELS

Modelling

In computer simulation modelling, the models that are used to evaluate sports movements are based on physical laws, unlike statistical models that fit relationships to data. Two related concepts are simulation (or computer simulation) and optimisation. Modelling, simulation and optimisation encapsulate, in a unified structure (Figure 7.2), the processes involved in seeking the values of a set of variables or functional relationships that will optimise a performance. This can allow for the determination of optimal values of variables within a movement technique or, in principle, the optimal technique. Computer simulation modelling makes the link between the performer, or sports object, and its motions. It involves representing one or more of the characteristics of a system or object using mathematical equations. Every model is an approximation that neglects certain features of the system or object. The art of modelling is often described as putting only enough complexity into the model to allow its effective and meaningful use. All other things being equal, the simpler the model the better, as it is easier to understand the behaviour of the model and its implications. The difficulty of interpreting the results, particularly for feedback to coaches and athletes, increases rapidly with model

Figure 7.2 The relationship between modelling, simulation, simulation evaluation and optimisation.

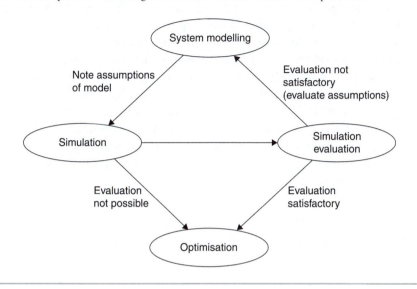

complexity. Thus, the modeller should always start with the simplest model possible that captures the essential features of the movement being studied. Only after a full understanding of this simple model has been gained, should the model be made more complex, and then only if this is necessary.

Simulation

Experiments measure what happens in the real world to real objects: a simulation model forms a similar basis for computer experiments. In fact, simulation can be defined as the carrying out of experiments under carefully controlled conditions on the real world system that has been modelled. It is much easier to control external variables in a computer simulation model than in the real world. The modelling process transforms the real system into a set of equations; simulation involves the performance of numerical experiments on these equations, after which we transform the results back to the real system to understand reality.

The necessity of adding complexity to an existing model should be revealed by continuously relating the results of the simulations to physical measurements. This tests the model to see if it is an adequate approximation and what new features might need to be added. This aspect of the process, termed simulation evaluation, will be considered further in a later sub-section. In many computer simulations, these evaluations are not carried out; in some, they are not even feasible. One approach to simulation evaluation, which has been reported for simulation models, particularly of airborne activities, has been to combine modelling and experimental studies so that the model results can be compared directly with the movements they model (e.g. Figure 7.3, from Yeadon and King, 2008). This approach could be adopted in many more cases and would help both in relating the model to the real world and in communicating the simulation results to coaches and athletes; we will return to the latter issue in Chapter 8.

Computer simulation clearly offers an inexpensive and harmless way of addressing the 'what if?' questions about how systematic changes affect important variables in sports movements. There are many unresolved issues in simulation modelling. These include model complexity, simulation evaluation, sensitivity analysis, what muscle models are needed for sport-specific models, and the adequacy of the rigid body model of human body segments. The problem of model validation remains by far the most serious limitation.

Figure 7.3 Simulation evaluation by the comparison of the performance (top) and simulation (bottom) for tumbling (adapted from Yeadon and King, 2008).

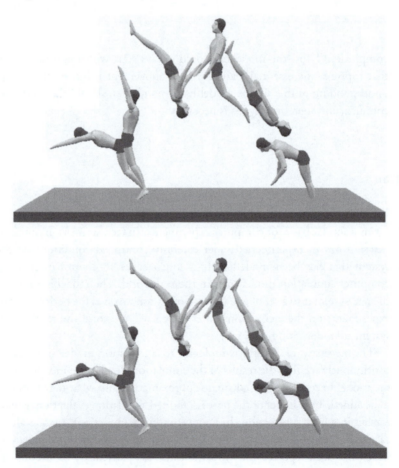

Optimisation

Formally, the process of optimisation is expressed as the method for finding the optimum value (maximum or minimum) of a function $f(x1, x2, \ldots xn)$ of n variables. Finding the maximum for the function f is identical to finding the minimum for $-f$. Because of this, optimisation normally seeks the minimum value of the function to be optimised. Biomechanically, this can be considered as an operation on the mathematical model (the equations of motion) to give the best possible motion, for example the longest jump, subject to the limitations of the model. Optimisation can be carried out by running many simulations covering a wide, but realistic, range of the initial conditions. This is a computationally inefficient way to search for the optimal solution to the problem and is now rarely used. We can distinguish between static and dynamic optimisation. Static optimisation (used for the javelin study below) computes the optimum values of a finite set of quantities of interest, such as a small set of input parameters. Dynamic optimisation (also known as optimal control theory), on the other hand, seeks to compute optimum input functions of time.

An important issue in optimisation is the choice of the performance criterion that is being optimised (compare with Chapter 6). In most running and swimming events this is time minimisation, which presents no problem. In the shot-put, javelin throw, long jump and downhill skiing, there is a simple performance criterion, which can be optimised. However, it may also be necessary to consider the rules of the event; it is possible to incorporate these rules as constraints on the optimisation. The points for judging aesthetic form could be included as constraints on permitted body configurations in, for example, a ski jump model. In sports such as gymnastics, ice-skating, tennis and hockey, the specification of an overall performance criterion is more complicated and may, indeed, not be possible. A further problem, to which we will return in the next subsection, relates to the possible existence of local and global optimums (Figure 7.4). The optimisation process may return a local, rather than the global, optimum. Furthermore, different starting points may give different answers for the local optimum while still missing the global one. For example, we may find A rather than C in Figure 7.4 but not arrive at B. This may reflect the fact that, for a particular sport, a range of different movements is possible, related perhaps to anthropometric factors, each of which has an associated local optimum. It is tempting to speculate that the process of evolutionary adaptation has led to the selection of the global optimum from the set of local ones, for a given athlete. This selection could be based on some fundamental principle of human movement (Chapter 5), probably that of minimisation of metabolic energy consumption. Evidence to support the minimal energy principle includes the existence of the stretch–shortening cycle of muscular contraction and the commonality of two-joint muscles. It is not necessarily the case that this minimum energy principle is always valid. Explosive sports events will not have a minimal energy criterion as their optimising principle, but it might still be involved in the selection of a global optimum from a set of local ones. In many sports, it could be postulated that the optimisation process may be extremely complex, requiring a 'trade off' between information processing capacity and muscle power.

Figure 7.4 Global optimum (minimum) at B and two local optimums at A and B.

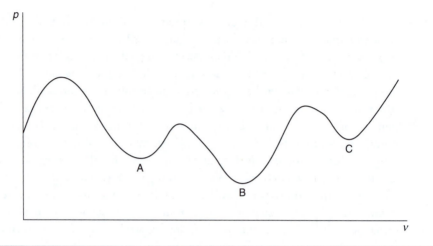

Optimal javelin release as an example of computer simulation modelling

The javelin flight model

Although the research to be discussed here was done in the last century of the second millennium, I use it as an example of computer simulation modelling as it is simple, illustrates the points I wish to make, and I was involved in the research. Throwing events can be considered to consist of two distinct stages: the thrust and the flight. The second of these is characterised by only gravitational and aerodynamic forces acting on the implement, the flight path of which is beyond the control of the thrower. This forms a relatively simple problem in comparison with the thrust stage, in which the implement is acted upon by the thrower. The flight phase of the throw is a classic initial condition problem in optimisation (Best *et al.*, 1995). The javelin flight is, in most respects, the most interesting of the four throwing events. The initial conditions for such an event are the set of release parameter values, which are specific to a given thrower; the optimisation problem is to find the optimal values of these to produce the maximum range (the performance criterion). This is a static optimisation, since only a finite set of instantaneous (parameter) values is involved.

In javelin throwing, the initial conditions needed to solve the equations of motion for the flight of the javelin include the initial linear position and velocity vectors and the initial angles and angular velocities. These initial conditions are the rates of pitch, spin and yaw at release (Figure 7.5(a)), the release height, the distance from the foul line, the speed of the javelin's mass centre (the magnitude of its velocity vector), the angle of the javelin's velocity vector to the ground (the release angle), and the angle of the javelin to the relative wind (the angle of attack) (Figure 7.5(b)). The vibration characteristics of the javelin at release can also be important, although they are not considered here. In addition to these initial

Figure 7.5 Javelin release parameters: (a) rotational, (b) translational.

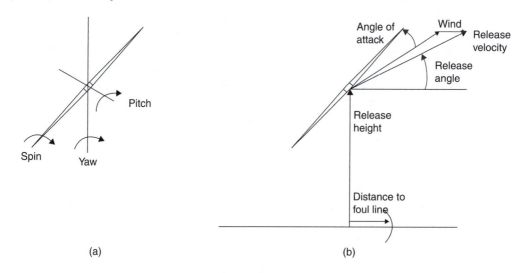

(a) (b)

conditions, the model requires the specification of the javelin's mass and principal moments of inertia and the aerodynamic forces and moments acting on the javelin in flight. Additionally, the model might need to incorporate the effects of wind speed and direction, although these are beyond the control of the thrower. A three-dimensional model of javelin release and flight would require aerodynamic force and moment data from a spinning and vibrating javelin at various speeds and aerodynamic angles. This would present a far from trivial wind tunnel experimental problem. Best *et al.* (1995), therefore, used a two-dimensional model of javelin release. They noted that an optimal release for an elite thrower is hardly likely to involve javelin yaw and will probably minimise vibration.

The equations of motion for this simplified, two-dimensional model include the moment of inertia of the javelin about its short (pitching) axis, and the lift and drag forces and pitching moments acting on the implement. Best *et al.* (1995) used a trifilar suspension method for accurately measuring the moment of inertia. They noted that accurate specification of the aerodynamic forces and moments acting on the javelin was essential to simulate and optimise the flight successfully, and that defects in these measurements were a feature of many previous studies. These defects were primarily the use of single sample data and a failure to account for interactions (or crosstalk) between the force balances used to measure the component forces and moments. Their identification of these as major errors was somewhat speculative, because most previous studies had reported insufficient experimental information even to enable error sources to be identified. Nevertheless, they took great pains to avoid such errors in their results, and they reported the methods for obtaining these data in considerable detail. However, it is not known what the discrepancies are between these results (from two-dimensional, laminar flow wind tunnel tests on non-spinning javelins), and the true aerodynamic characteristics of a spinning, pitching, yawing and vibrating javelin within a region of the turbulent atmosphere in which the air speed varies considerably with height.

Simulation

From the above modelling considerations and the two-dimensional equations of motion, the throw distance (the performance criterion) can be expressed in terms of the release parameters. This allows model simulation by varying the values of the release parameters, within realistic limits, and studying their effects. The range now depends solely upon: release speed $v(0)$; release height $z(0)$; release angle $\gamma(0)$; release angle of attack $\alpha(0)$; release pitch rate $q(0)$; and wind speed V^W (see Figure 7.5). The distance to the foul line (Figure 7.5(b)) is not included as it does not affect flight and relates to the thrust stage; different movement techniques in this stage might affect the required distance to the foul line to avoid making a foul throw. The wind speed is not a release parameter and is beyond a thrower's control. There is little evidence in the literature to assess the interdependence or otherwise of the five release parameters. The two for which there is a known interrelationship are release speed and angle. Two pairs of investigators have investigated this relationship, one using a 1 kg ball and the other using an instrumented javelin. Surprisingly, they obtained very similar relationships over the relevant range, expressed by the equation: release speed = nominal release speed (v_N) – 0.13 × (release angle – 35), where the angles must be in degrees and the speed in m/s. The nominal release speed is defined as the maximum at which a thrower is capable, at his or her current strength and fitness, of throwing for a release angle of 35° and replaces release speed in the set of release parameters. The numerical techniques used to perform the simulations are beyond the scope of this chapter (see Best *et al.*, 1995).

Optimisation

An optimisation can now be performed. Of the five remaining independent variables, after introducing the relationship between release speed and release angle, and neglecting wind speed, the nominal release speed is non-variable at a thrower's current strength and fitness. The release height is, in principle, an optimisable parameter. However, in normal javelin throwing it varies only slightly for a given thrower, and small changes beyond these limits detrimentally affect other, more important release parameters. If the remaining three parameters – release angle ($\gamma(0)$), release angle of attack ($\alpha(0)$), and release pitch rate ($q(0)$) – are allowed to vary independently, then an optimal set can be found at a global maximum where (with R as range): $dR/d\gamma(0) = dR/d\alpha(0) = dR/dq(0) = 0$. The solution to this optimisation equation involves, at least conceptually, a mathematical procedure to find a peak on a hill of n-dimensions (where n is the number of dependent plus independent variables, four in this case).

Sensitivity analysis

Best *et al.* (1995) carried out a sensitivity analysis – a detailed evaluation of the system's behaviour to changes in the release parameters – using contour maps. This fulfils two roles. First, the optimisation equation is true for all local optimums as well as the global optimum, so that all optimisation techniques find a local optimum that may, or may not, be global. Furthermore, different local optimums may be found from different starting points (as in Figure 7.4). This is important as it may relate to distinct identifiable throwing techniques. The only way to check on the number of peaks is to look at the full solution – a three-dimensional surface: $R=f(\gamma(0),\alpha(0),q(0))$. This is not usually possible as only two independent variables can be viewed at one time using contour maps (see below) while the remaining independent variables have to be kept constant. The second aspect of sensitivity analysis was a detailed evaluation of the contour maps to establish, for example, whether the optimum is a plateau or a sharp peak. This provides insight into the best way to reach the peak, helping to define positive directions for training regimes (Best et al., 1995). This is not possible using optimisation alone. An example of a contour map for this problem is shown in Figure 7.6, where only one

Figure 7.6 Full contour map showing range (R) as a function of release angle and release angle of attack for N86 javelin; remaining release parameters constant at nominal release speed 30 m/s, wind speed zero, release height 1.8 m and release pitch rate zero.

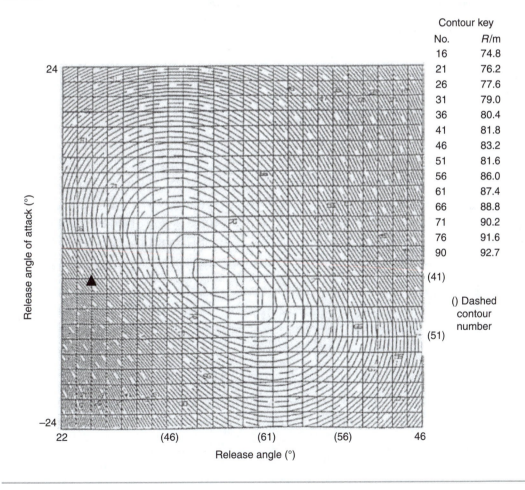

| Contour key | |
No.	R/m
16	74.8
21	76.2
26	77.6
31	79.0
36	80.4
41	81.8
46	83.2
51	81.6
56	86.0
61	87.4
66	88.8
71	90.2
76	91.6
90	92.7

(41)

() Dashed contour number

(51)

optimum is apparent. This solution was verified by zooming in on the global peak. For all javelins this showed a double peak to exist for a small (less than 3 m/s) range of nominal release speeds (Figure 7.7). The reality of the peaks – that they were not an artefact of the contour plotting algorithm – was verified by a plot of optimal release angle of attack as a function of nominal release speed (Figure 7.8). This figure shows a discontinuity where one peak 'overtook' the other. The peaks were so close together that the optimisation algorithm usually 'jumped over' the local optimum along the ridge approaching the global peak (shown by the black circle in Figure 7.7), except where the starting position for the search was at the other, local, optimum.

Best *et al.* (1995) reported that different optimal release conditions were found for throwers with differing nominal release speeds and for different javelins. For a given thrower and javelin, as the nominal release speed increased from 26 m/s (see Figure 7.8),

Figure 7.7 Contour map highlighting dual peak phenomenon for range (*R*) as a function of release angle and release angle of attack for N86 javelin; remaining release parameters constant at nominal release speed 30 m/s, wind speed zero, release height 1.8 m and release pitch rate zero.

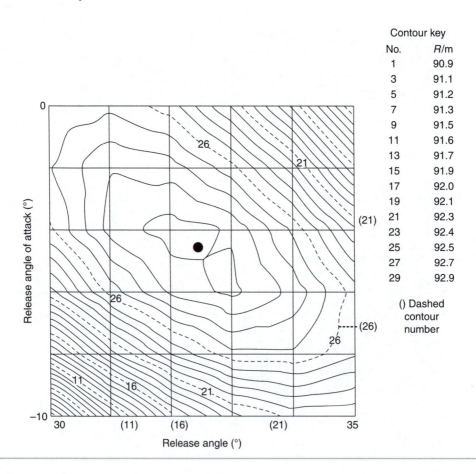

Figure 7.8 Optimal release angle of attack as a function of nominal release speed for three men's javelins: N86 – Nemeth New Rules (now illegal); A86 – Apollo Gold New Rules; A85 – Apollo Gold Old (pre-1986) Rules; and two women's javelins: A90 – Apollo Laser Old (pre-1991) Rules; A91 Apollo Gold New Rules.

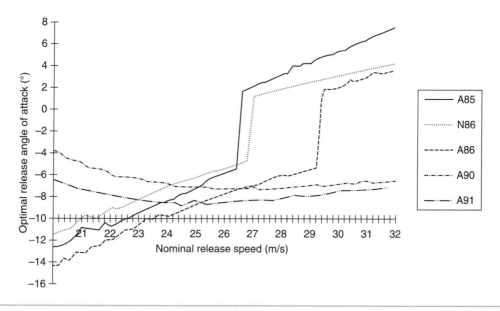

the optimal release angle and optimal release angle of attack increased and optimal pitch rate decreased. As Figures 7.6 and 7.7 demonstrate, the shape of the hill was simple and tended to a plateau as the optimal solution was reached. The shape of the hill provides insight into the complexity of coaching. Because of the plateau near the optimal solution, a thrower with near optimal values finds that the range is insensitive to small changes in release parameter values. Away from the optimum, however, the range will be very sensitive to at least one of the release parameters. Confusion could arise for a thrower with an optimal release angle of attack but a non-optimal release angle (see the black triangle on Figure 7.6), for whom changes in both angles have relatively large effects on the range. For this thrower, only a study of the contour map could reveal that it was the release angle that was non-optimal, and, therefore, required to be changed to improve performance. For further consideration of these issues, see Study Task 4. Furthermore, a wide range of non-optimal release conditions can produce the same range – indeed, any combination of release parameters around a particular contour. Also, throwers with different nominal release speeds can, in some circumstances, throw the same distance.

Simulation evaluation

Best *et al.* (1995) considered their findings to show the inadvisability of a 'trial and error' approach, seeking to change a movement technique without knowing the performer's current 'position' in the overall 'solution' – for example, where the thrower's release conditions are located on the contour maps. This might be considered as a caution that should be borne in mind by qualitative biomechanical analysts, who lack such knowledge. Furthermore, little is known about the interactions between independent variables and any physical or injury constraints that may be relevant. Only sensitivity analysis can define positive, relevant directions to improving performance.

Errors or uncertainties may be introduced in any one, or more, of the three stages of optimisation because of assumptions that have been made, perhaps necessarily. Simulation evaluation should always be at least considered, as the results of such a computer simulation should provide an accurate representation of the real world. In practice, the sheer complexity of such an evaluation may make it, in many cases, unfeasible. The release parameters from a 1991 World Student Games study were used to calculate the theoretical flight distances for three throws using javelins for which the inertia and aerodynamic characteristics had been measured. These distances were then compared with the measured throw distances. The discrepancy was not systematic, as might be expected if there were errors in the simulation model, and it was small, with an average discrepancy modulus of only 1.4 m (for throws over 81 m). This provided limited evidence of the accuracy of this simulation model of javelin flight.

Models of the human performer

The previous example dealt with the optimisation of the motion of a javelin. Computer simulation models of the sports performer are, necessarily, more complex. Among other things, they need to take into account how to model the inertia (and other parameters) of body segments and the behaviour of the muscles that drive the movement. We give the latter topic some consideration in the next sub-section; for other aspects, the reader is referred to the overview of Yeadon and King (2008). The problems that models of body segments have to address include the following: the number of segments required to model the particular sports motion; how the three-dimensional geometry of body segments is to be treated; how the degrees of freedom at each joint are to be represented or simplified; if, and how, variable densities within segments are to be accommodated; how personalised the model will be; and whether the rigid body representation of a segment is adequate (see also Bartlett, 1999).

Models of human skeletal muscle

Skeletal muscle models range from the deceptively simple to the incredibly complicated. Essentially, however, almost all of them are derived from the simple schematic model of Figure 7.9, in which skeletal muscle has a contractile component and series elastic and parallel elastic elements. The contractile component is made up of the actin and myosin filaments and their associated cross-bridge coupling mechanism. The series elastic

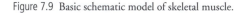

Figure 7.9 Basic schematic model of skeletal muscle.

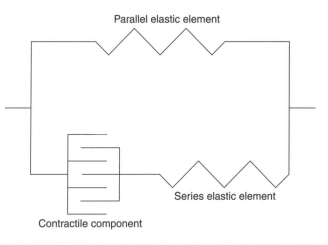

element lies in series with the contractile component and transmits the tension produced by the contractile component to the attachment points of the muscle. The tendons account for by far the major part of this series elasticity, with elastic structures within the cross-bridges and the Z-line of the sarcomere contributing the remainder. The parallel elastic element comprises the connective tissues around the whole muscle (epimysium), around groups of muscle fibres (perimysium), and around each muscle fibre (endomysium), as well as the sarcolemma (the membrane enclosing each muscle fibre). The elastic elements store elastic energy when they are stretched and release this energy when the muscle recoils. The series elastic elements are more important than the parallel ones in the production of tension. Biomechanically and physiologically, the elastic elements are important as they keep the muscle ready for contraction and ensure the smooth production and transmission of tension during contraction. They also ensure the return of the contractile component to its resting position after contraction. They may also help to prevent the passive overstretching of the contractile component when relaxed, reducing the risk of injury. The series and parallel elements are viscoelastic rather than simply elastic. This viscous property enables them to absorb energy at a rate proportional to that at which force is applied and to dissipate energy at a rate that is time-dependent (see also Chapter 1).

The muscle models used in computer simulations of sports movements vary in the number of elements they contain. Many of these models are relatively complex, although none of them exactly reflects the physiological and biomechanical behaviour of skeletal muscle. Their major restriction, however, lies in the modelling of their control. In many muscle models, the control is discontinuous ('bang–bang'), such that the muscles are either active or inactive – essentially this is a feature not of skeletal muscle but of a single muscle fibre. The behaviour of a whole muscle is, fortunately, more subtle.

The models of skeletal muscle developed by the late Herbert Hatze are widely reported in the biomechanics literature and are of interest as an example of trying to model complex behaviour through a complex model; their main points are summarised in Hatze (1981). The elastic elements in Hatze's models did not depart radically from those of Figure 7.9, other than in the introduction of damping to make them reflect viscoelastic reality. Essentially therefore, the series elastic elements were characterised by an exponential load–extension relationship; this also applied to the parallel elastic element but with length as the dependent variable. The greatest departure from earlier models lay in Hatze's treatment of the contractile component. Instead of seeking simply to incorporate the length–tension and force–velocity relationships, Hatze developed a mathematical model of a muscle fibre in which the force was a product of the state of the muscle before and during contraction (its 'active state'), the degree of actin–myosin filamentary overlap and the velocity of movement between the actin and myosin filaments. This model was based on a hypothesis that incorporated both the sliding filament theory and an assumption that the energy transformations in the muscle proceeded in a chain from chemical to electrical to heat and work (Hatze, 1981). The active state model also incorporated the decrease in the relative concentration of calcium ions as the muscle fibre diameter changed, and accounted for the occurrence of non-linearities, such as myosin filament and Z-line collisions at short fibre lengths. The response of this model to various nerve impulse trains was presented in, for example, Hatze (1981) and was claimed by the author to be confirmed by previous experimental results. This could be considered to be a form of simulation evaluation. The remainder of the fibre contractile element model was simple in comparison. The length–tension relationship followed an exponential–sinusoidal relationship. Hatze (1981) also noted the need for a statistical (Gaussian) spread of fibre lengths to be incorporated in the whole muscle model. The force–velocity relationship was non-linear, and the model also had to account for the internal resistance caused by deformation of the sarcolemma. The whole muscle model was considerably more complex. It allowed for a varying average stimulation rate and treated a varying number of stimulated motor units which are recruited sequentially according to their size. Further details of this model are beyond the scope of this chapter. Interestingly, the model's behaviour was controlled by variations in the motor unit recruitment rate and the stimulation rate, as happens physiologically. However, in reality these variables are discontinuous, although they generate a smooth muscle response. This discontinuity was represented in the model by continuous normalised values for simplicity.

In an attempt to investigate and validate his model of skeletal muscle, Hatze (1981) reported a series of experiments carried out in relation to a model of the triceps brachii (Figure 7.10). The author noted that the model needed the values of a set of parameters to be estimated. This required a series of observations of constant maximum isometric torques (moments of force) at various muscle lengths, of quasi-stationary torque outputs at various activation levels, and of linearly increasing torque outputs. On the basis of these experiments, with known moment arm and muscle length functions, and assuming tendon resting lengths and minimum and maximum fibre pennation angles, several important parameters were estimated. These included the maximum isometric force,

Figure 7.10 Triceps brachii model: BE represents the cross-bridge series elastic element; CE the contractile component; PS the sarcolemma parallel elasticity; SE the tendon series elastic element. The parallel elastic element, PE, is represented by a visco-elastic spring-dashpot. In addition, θ is the muscle fibre pennation angle, maximum θ_{max}, mean θ_{av}, minimum θ_{min}; subscripts 1–3 denote the three heads of the muscle (after Hatze, 1981).

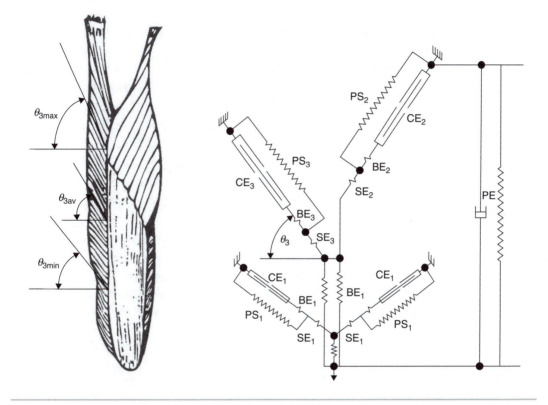

the 'spreads' (widths) of the length–tension curves, and the optimal muscle lengths. The experimental details are faithfully reproduced in Hatze (1981) and considerable trouble was obviously taken to obtain these parameter values. However, it is arguable whether this constitutes a model or simulation evaluation and it is difficult to dispute the criticism often made of this model that it is over-parameterised. The use of such muscle models in optimisations of sports motions and their evaluation have been limited, although the study of Hatze (1976) has become a classic of both the sports biomechanics and the motor control literature.

ARTIFICIAL INTELLIGENCE IN PERFORMANCE MODELLING

In this section, we will look at recent developments in the use of artificial intelligence (AI) in sports biomechanics. The section outlines possible uses of expert systems as diagnostic tools for evaluating faults in sports movements ('techniques') and presents some example knowledge rules for such an expert system. It then compares the analysis of sports techniques, in which expert systems have found little place to date, with gait analysis, in which they are routinely used. I also present an example of the use of evolutionary computation in movement optimisation in the soccer throw-in, which predicted an optimal technique close to that in the coaching literature. Consideration is then given to the use of artificial neural networks (ANNs) in sports biomechanics, focusing on Kohonen self-organising maps, which have been the most widely used in the analysis of sports movements; some examples of the use of Kohonen self-organising maps in sports biomechanics are presented.

Expert systems in sports biomechanics – or, rather, the lack of them

Lapham and Bartlett (1995) published a review of the use of AI in sports biomechanics, in which they reported no evidence of the use of AI in sports biomechanics, although expert systems and ANNs were being used in gait analysis. They did, however, predict a bright future for the use, in particular, of expert systems in sports biomechanics. So what has happened in the 15 years since?

Expert systems are, effectively, a database combined with a knowledge base, 'reasoning' and a user interface. The knowledge base contains specific knowledge, or facts, for the 'domain'. The knowledge rules can also include logic operations, managed by probability theory, as in this example from a hypothetical expert system for the analysis of fast bowling in cricket: "IF 'shoulder-axis counter-rotation' is high, THEN 'technique' is mixed ($p=0.8$)". This example of a knowledge rule illustrates that much information is vague – 'high' in the above example has varied from 10° to 20° to 30° to 40° in the scientific literature on fast bowling, showing that much information is 'fuzzy'. These fuzzy overlaps are supported by the division of the mixed technique into side-on-mixed and front-on-mixed.

Expert systems are good diagnostic tools and system 'shells' are available; it is, therefore, rather surprising that they are rare in sports biomechanics. As we noted in passing in Chapter 6, the closest approach to expert systems in sports biomechanics so far is found within qualitative video analysis packages, such as Siliconcoach's 'wizards'. Although not, strictly speaking, expert systems, these wizards do provide a formula engine that could be used by wizard developers to arrive at decisions by taking into account one or more responses to other data entered into the wizard; whether this provision is used is up to the wizard developer. This reality conflicts with the positive view of the utility of expert systems by Lapham and Bartlett (1995).

The use of expert systems in gait analysis suggests an extension to the analysis of sports movements; both are branches of biomechanics. In gait analysis, however, there is a strong developmental motivation – patient health – which helps to attract funding. Clinicians are expensive, making investment in complex software development worthwhile financially. Gait analysis is a confined expert domain, gait and its variants, with many experts. It is laboratory-based, so automatic marker tracking systems are common-place and data are abundant. Analysis of sports movements is more complex than gait analysis and there is a weak developmental motivation: research into sports performance is not well funded. Coaches and sports scientists are not expensive; the analysis of sports movements is often field-based, preventing the automatic tracking of markers; and it is a broad expert domain, involving many sports. There is relatively little data for expert systems for specific sports movement techniques and there are fewer experts than for gait analysis.

Evolutionary computation in sports biomechanics

Evolutionary computation uses artificial, or numerical, 'chromosomes' to simulate evolution (Negnevitsky, 2002). Bächle (2003) used an evolutionary strategy to optimise the joint moments of force (torques) at the hip, shoulder and elbow to maximise distance thrown in a soccer throw-in. This study predicted an optimal throwing technique close to that described in the coaching literature, with the initially passive moment of the hip accelerating the trunk forwards while the negative elbow moment kept the forearm back.

Artificial neural networks in sports biomechanics

Artificial neural networks (ANNs) allow computers to learn from experience and by analogy. They are computer programs that try to create a mathematical model of neurons in the brain. An ANN is an interconnection of simple adaptable processing elements or nodes. They are non-linear programs that represent non-linear systems, such as the human movement system, and, from a notational analysis perspective, games. Artificial neural networks have nodes, which are simplified models of brain neurons, inputs, outputs and weights. The network stores experiential knowledge as a pattern of connected nodes and synaptic weights between them. Multi-layer ANNs have several 'hidden' layers and normally learn using the 'back-propagation learning law'. Kohonen self-organising maps have one hidden layer and use 'competitive learning' – only one neuron is selected for weight adjustment each iteration, based on the minimum 'distance' between the sums of its inputs and its weight. These networks can require lots of 'training' data and, once trained, can only be used for testing, not further learning.

Given their usefulness for classification, clustering and prediction, and that they are easily available, how widespread is the use of ANNs in sports biomechanics? Well, unlike expert systems, they have been used, as well as in other aspects of performance analysis. Pattern recognition using ANNs is an important feature; the patterns can be tactical ones from a game, performance patterns in training, or – the focus here – movement patterns of sports performers. In this last application, the ANN is normally used to transform a high-dimensional vector space of biomechanical time series into a low-dimensional output map.

Kohonen self-organising maps were used to analyse discus throws by Bauer and Schöllhorn (1997). They used 53 throws (45 of a decathlete, 8 of a specialist) recorded using semi-automated marker tracking over a one-year training period. Each throw had 34 kinematic time series, for 51 normalised times; these complex, multi-dimensional time series were mapped on to a simple 11×11 neuron output space (Figure 7.11). Each sequence was then expressed as the 'mean deviation' (d in Figure 7.11) of the output map – the continuous line – from that of one of the throws by the specialist thrower, shown by the dashed line. It should be noted that this mean deviation is not a truly meaningful Euclidean distance. The deviations for the eight specialist throws are shown on the right of the dashed vertical line in Figure 7.12, the decathlete's 45 throws on the left of that line. The 'distances' are less for the specialist thrower as the comparison throw was one of his throws. Note the clustering within groups of throws, between the continuous vertical lines, in training or competition sessions. There was more variability between than within sessions; for five groups of five trials, the authors computed inter- and intra-cluster variances, giving an inter-to-intra variance ratio of 3.3 ± 0.6. This shows that even elite throwers cannot reproduce invariant movement patterns between sessions. The supposed existence of such invariant patterns – which arises from the

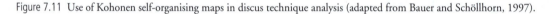

Figure 7.11 Use of Kohonen self-organising maps in discus technique analysis (adapted from Bauer and Schöllhorn, 1997).

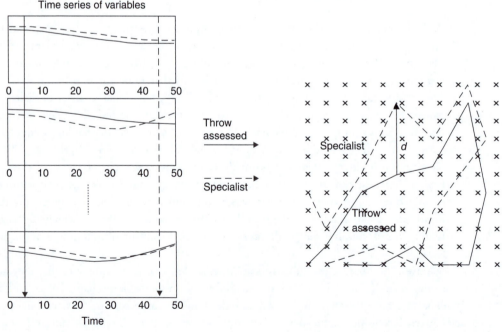

Figure 7.12 Grouping of throws within sessions, between continuous vertical lines (adapted from Bauer and Schöllhorn, 1997).

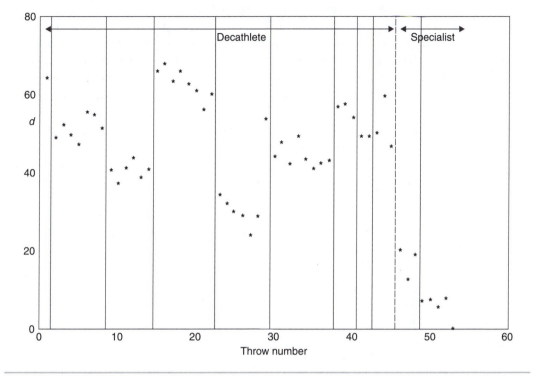

motor program concept of cognitive motor control – has often been used, explicitly or implicitly, to justify the use of a 'representative trial' in sports biomechanics. These results seem to disprove the existence of such invariant patterns. Schöllhorn and Bauer (1998) reported a similar approach to analyse 49 javelin throws from eight elite males, nine elite females and ten heptathletes. Clustering was found for the male throwers – as a group – and for the two females for whom multiple trials were recorded. Variations in the cluster for international male athletes were held to contradict any existence of an 'optimal movement pattern', another assumption once commonly made by sports biomechanists that is apparently overturned by this research.

Lees *et al.* (2003) reported the results of a study that used Kohonen maps to analyse instep kicks by two soccer players for distance or accuracy. Joint angles were obtained from the three-dimensional coordinates of automatically-tracked markers. These were then mapped on to a 12×8 node output matrix and showed differences between tasks and players; these output patterns were repeatable for the same task for one player.

Lamb *et al.* (2010) used Kohonen self-organising maps (SOMs) to classify the coordination patterns of four skilled basketball shooters performing the free throw, three-point shot and hook shot. They had hypothesised, based on the consideration that the free throw and three-point shot are modifications to the 'set shot' movement pattern, that these two shots would be more similar to each other than to the hook shot. Computer animations of the throws, which had been recorded using an automatic marker-tracking system, suggested that this hypothesis was true. However, for two of the four players, the coordination patterns, displayed on a 42×13 node output matrix, showed far more similarity between the three-point throw and the hook shot; both of these players used a jump hook shot. The graphical results of this study, which require multiple colours to be meaningful, and a detailed explanation of them, are available on the book's website. This study showed that movement analysts can be distracted by visual information in the movement, in this case by a focus on the arms, the distal segments in the proximal-to-distal shooting sequence. Furthermore, the results emphasised that different individuals find different coordination solutions to specific sports tasks, strongly supporting the need for single-individual studies if we wish to understand and improve the performance of an athlete.

In a study that aimed to explain changes in inter-limb coordination and to ascertain the validity of SOMs as an analysis technique for high-dimensional movement coordination, Lamb *et al.* (2011) looked at the golf chip shot. Four low-handicap golfers each performed ten chip shots to each of six target distances, from 4 m in 4 m steps to 24 m. Twenty four kinematic time series were used as the input for an SOM to produce a low-dimensional 24×16 or 25×15 output matrix (multiple-coloured graphical visualisations of these output maps are shown and explained on the book's website). The trajectories of the consecutive nodes on this output matrix were then used as a 'collective variable' and input into a second SOM, to create a visualisation of the stability of shot coordination. Similarly patterned trials 'drag' neighbouring nodes – depending on the Euclidean distance between them – into basins (Figure 7.13(a-c)); the deeper basins represent 'attractors' (see Kelso, 1995, for a full explanation and exploration of this concept).

One player (Figure 7.13(a)) showed clear bi-modal (two-basin) coordination at 4 m and 8 m – this is often referred to as multi-stability in coordination dynamics (Kelso, 1995). The two basins evolve to several at the middle distances but return to two for the longer distances; at no distance does this player show uni-modal coordination. A second player (Figure 7.13(b)) showed a clear non-linear phase transition from the uni-modal pattern (the left basin) at 4 m through the middle distances to a different uni-modal pattern (the right basin) at 20 m and 24 m; we might call these the short and long 'chipping' patterns respectively. The other two players (Figure 7.13(c) is for one of them) showed deep basins of attraction on the left side (short chipping pattern) for short shots, bi-modal coordination at 12 m and deep basins of attraction on the right side (long chipping pattern) of the diagram for longer shots. Instabilities at the middle distances are not as evident as for the player in Figure 7.13(b). As well as providing a novel insight into the non-linear dynamics of movement coordination, this study again emphasises (if further emphasis is needed) the uniqueness of the coordination patterns of each individual and, therefore, the need for intra-individual approaches to the improvement of sports performance.

Figure 7.13 Attractor layout diagram from second SOM for: (a) player showing bi-modal coordination; (b) player showing clear non-linear phase transition; (c) player showing clear uni-modal basins of attraction at short and long shots.

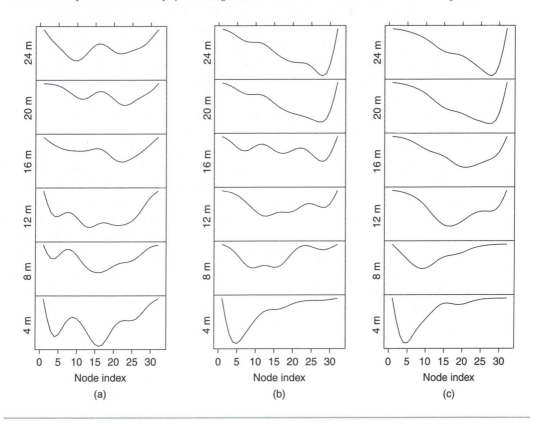

(a)

(b)

(c)

Artificial neural networks have been far more widely used than expert systems in sports biomechanics. In technique analysis, Kohonen self-organising maps have been claimed to reveal the 'forest' rather than the 'trees'. Simplification is undoubtedly an important feature of ANNs, although the ways in which we can best use the outputs of these mappings remain to be determined fully. Importantly, ANNs can transform multiple times series into a two-dimensional output map (as in Figure 7.11). This output could well be regarded as a 'collective variable', a crucial concept in the dynamical systems theory approach to movement coordination. It certainly combines far more variables (34 in the study of Bauer and Schöllhorn, 1997, and 24 in the study of Lamb *et al.*, 2011) than the four (two angles and two angular velocities) involved in relative phase (see Chapter 6). Artificial neural networks also represent an important link to non-linear dynamical systems theory; for example, Kelso (1995) reported the use of ANNs in studies of perception and noted that the networks model hysteresis, stimulus bias, and adaptation effects, all key tenets of non-linear dynamical systems theory. This link with what is becoming the strongest theoretical basis for sports biomechanics, indeed of performance analysis as a whole, is potentially of considerable importance.

SUMMARY

In this chapter, we considered the fundamentals underlying the biomechanical optimisation of sports movements, with an emphasis on theory-driven statistical modelling, computer simulation modelling and optimisation, and the approaches of artificial intelligence, particularly that of artificial neural networks. The relationships that can exist between a performance criterion and various performance variables were explained, the cross-sectional, longitudinal and contrast approaches to statistical modelling were described and the limitations of statistical modelling in sports biomechanics were evaluated. The use of computer simulation modelling, when seeking to evaluate and improve sports movements, were covered; brief explanations of modelling, simulation, simulation evaluation and optimisation were also provided. The differences between static and dynamic optimisation and global and local optimums were covered. We considered in detail the optimisation of javelin release as an example of computer simulation modelling of sports movements, and touched on the modelling of the human performer, with a couple of examples of models of skeletal muscle. Finally, we looked at the various approaches from artificial intelligence that have been used in the context of the biomechanical improvement of sports performance, focusing mainly on artificial neural networks and the links between this approach and the non-linear dynamical systems theory of movement coordination.

STUDY TASKS

1   Which of the following statistical tests would be appropriate for cross-sectional or longitudinal correlation studies and contrast research designs, respectively: analysis of variance (ANOVA), linear regression, or multiple linear regression? What difficulties might you face in satisfying the assumptions of these statistical tests in a field-based study of a specific sports technique?

2   Choose a sporting activity with which you are familiar and which, preferably, has a simple, objective performance criterion. Develop a deterministic model for this activity that identifies measurable performance variables (this is essentially similar to the critical features approach of Study Task 2 in Chapter 6, except that you need to identify measurable rather than observable features of the activity).

3   Distinguish between modelling, simulation and optimisation. Outline and evaluate the modelling, simulation, optimisation and simulation evaluation stages of the optimal javelin release study of Best *et al.* (1995). You should pay particular attention to the assumptions of the model and how these were evaluated.

4   Using Figures 7.6 and 7.7:

   (a) Specify four different pairs of release angle and release angle of attack that would produce the same range (e.g. 88.8 m, contour line 66); your set of values should include the maximum and minimum values of both angles (e.g. from

Figure 7.6, for 88.8 m, 22° release angle of attack (the minimum) and the corresponding release angle of 36°).

(b) For each of the four angle pairs, specify which angle should be changed, and in which direction, to increase the range; also what would be the maximum range that could be achieved simply by changing that angle? For the example above, the release angle of attack must be made more positive, and the greatest range (just over contour line 78, which is over 91.6 m) is obtained when the angle is about 28°.

(c) Outline three possible strategies to optimise the release conditions for a thrower currently throwing with a release angle of 36° and release angle of attack of 20°, and other release parameters as in Figures 7.6 and 7.7. Specify which of these strategies you would recommend to such a thrower, and give the reasons for your choice. You should bear in mind how easy the changes might be to implement and any likely effects on other release parameters.

5 After reading Yeadon and King (2008), undertake a critical evaluation of a computer simulation of an aerial sports movement of your choice. This should include consideration of the assumptions of the model, the range of simulations studied, and any optimisation performed. How might you perform a simulation evaluation for the example you chose?

6 Outline the main conclusions that you would draw from this chapter on the use of skeletal muscle models in a general simulation model of the sports performer.

7 Choose a sports activity in which you are interested. Run an on-line or library-based search to identify the ratio of the number of references that cover the use of artificial intelligence in modelling that activity to its total number of references. Are you surprised at the result? Try to explain why the ratio is so small (or large) in relation to what you might have perceived after reading this chapter to be the value of artificial intelligence in the study of sports movements.

8 After reading Bartlett (2006), critically evaluate the use of artificial intelligence in sports biomechanics, particularly with reference to how such approaches might help to identify ways to improve sports performance.

GLOSSARY OF IMPORTANT TERMS

Analysis of variance (ANOVA) In this statistical procedure, the observed variance in a particular variable is partitioned into components arising from different sources of variation. ANOVA provides a statistical test of the differences between the means of several groups. It is often used in the contrast approach to statistical modelling discussed in this chapter.

Artificial intelligence See glossary in Chapter 5.

Artificial neural networks These are computer programs that try to create a mathematical model of neurons in the brain. They allow computers to learn from experience and by analogy.

Automatic marker-tracking systems These are image-based motion analysis systems in which the system hardware and software automatically tracks, ideally without any user intervention, the trajectories of markers placed on the body.

Contractile component This is the component of models of skeletal muscle that incorporates the mechanisms of muscle contraction, essentially the actin and myosin filaments and their associated cross-bridge coupling mechanism.

Correlation matrix A correlation matrix is a square symmetrical $n \times n$ matrix that contains correlations among n variables, where n is a positive integer greater than 1. The ith row and jth column of the matrix contains the correlation coefficient between the ith and the jth variables. The leading diagonal elements are correlations of variables with themselves and are, therefore, equal to 1.

Elastic elements These are the components of models of skeletal muscle that store and release elastic energy. The series elastic element is in series with the contractile component and mainly consists of the tendons. The parallel elastic elements lie in parallel to the contractile component and consist mainly of the muscle's various connective tissues and sarcolemma.

Euclidean distance In the context of this chapter, this is used to describe a mathematically meaningful distance between two points on the output map of an artificial neural network.

Homogeneity of variance The assumption (in both ANOVA and t-tests, for example) that the variances of two or more datasets are equal.

Inverted-U A relationship between two variables that looks like an upside-down letter U.

Isometric force The tension (or force) developed in a muscle that is undergoing an isometric contraction – without change of length.

Local and global optimums A function may have a global optimum, defined over the whole range of the function, as well as several local optimums, which are optimal only within a limited (local) range of the function. A geographical analogy would be the many local peaks within the Himalayas, whereas the top of Mount Everest is the global Himalayan peak.

Multiple regression In multiple regression, more than one predictor variable is used to predict the value of the criterion variable. This contrasts with simple regression in which there is only one predictor variable.

Multivariate analysis of variance (MANOVA) is a generalisation of **ANOVA** to cases in which there are two or more dependent variables. It is sometimes used in the contrast approach to statistical modelling discussed in this chapter.

Normality The assumption (in both ANOVA and t-tests, for example) that a dataset conforms to a normal (or Gaussian) distribution (the bell-shaped curve).

Optimisation The mathematical process of finding the optimum value of a function of several variables. Static optimisation computes the optimum values of a finite set of quantities of interest, such as a small set of input parameters. Dynamic optimisation seeks to compute optimum input functions of time.

Parametric statistics assume that the data have come from a particular probability distribution; they involve assumptions about the parameters of that distribution, such as **normality** or **homogeneity of variance**. **ANOVA**, **MANOVA** and **t-tests**

are all parametric statistical tests, as are Pearson product moment correlations (see Chapter 6).

Performance criterion A formal term that means the factor by which a performance is assessed – the result or outcome. Examples are the distance jumped or thrown, the time of a race and the score of a dive or gymnastics vault.

Performance variables (or performance parameters) A term used mostly in quantitative biomechanical analysis for the factors that influence the performance criterion, or outcome. They are roughly comparable to the critical features in a qualitative biomechanical analysis or the performance indicators in performance analysis.

Self-organising maps are artificial neural networks that are trained using unsupervised learning to produce a low-dimensional output space representation (sometimes called a map) of the high-dimensional input space of the training data.

Simulation or computer simulation involves the carrying out of computer experiments on a set of equations (or a simulation model) that represent an aspect of the real world. Simulation models are based on physical laws not statistical relationships.

Simulation evaluation This is the process of seeking to evaluate whether the results of a computer simulation adequately represent the real-world system that was being modelled.

Statistical power The power of a statistical test is the probability that the test will reject a null hypothesis that is false, in other words, that it will not make a **Type II error**. The greater the power, the less is the chance of a Type II error.

t-tests provide a test of whether the means of two groups are statistically different from each other. They are often used in the contrast approach to statistical modelling discussed in this chapter.

Type I and Type II errors A Type I error occurs when a null hypothesis that is true is rejected, incorrectly. A Type II error occurs when a null hypothesis is not rejected although it is false.

Validity In the analysis of human movement in sport, there is often a conflict between internal, or research, validity and external, or ecological, validity. Laboratory studies generally have good research validity and field-based studies generally have good ecological validity. Ecological validity is of prime importance when seeking to improve sports performance.

Viscoelasticity This is a property of all biological materials, which exhibit both elastic and viscous behaviour when deformed. The stress-strain characteristics of viscoelastic materials are time-dependent (see also Chapter 1).

REFERENCES

Bächle, F. (2003) The optimisation of throwing movements with evolutionary algorithms on the basis of multi-body systems. *International Journal of Computer Science in Sport, Special Edition, 1*, 6–11.

Bartlett, R.M. (1999) *Sports Biomechanics: Reducing Injury and Improving Performance (First Edition)*, London: Routledge.

Bartlett, R.M. (2006) Artificial Intelligence in sports biomechanics: new dawn or false hope? *Journal of Sports Science and Medicine*, 5, 474–479.

Bartlett, R.M. (2007) *Introduction to Sports Biomechanics: Analysing Human Movement Patterns*, London: Routledge.

Bartlett, R.M., Bussey, M. and Flyger, N. (2006) Movement variability cannot be determined reliably from no-marker conditions. *Journal of Biomechanics*, 36, 3076–3079.

Bates, B.T., James, C.R. and Dufek, J.S. (2004) 'Single-subject analysis', in N. Stergiou (ed.) *Innovative Analysis of Human Movement: Analytical Tools for Human Movement Research*, Champaign, IL: Human Kinetics, pp. 3–28.

Bauer, H.U. and Schöllhorn, W.I. (1997) Self-organizing maps for the analysis of complex movement patterns. *Neural Processing Letters*, 5, 193–199.

Best, R.J., Bartlett, R.M. and Sawyer, R.A. (1995) Optimal javelin release. *Journal of Applied Biomechanics*, 12, 58–71.

Donner, A. and Cunningham, D.A. (1984) Regression analysis in physiological research: Some comments on the problem of repeated measurements. *Medicine and Science in Sports and Exercise*, 16, 422–425.

Hatze, H. (1976) The complete optimisation of a human motion. *Mathematical Biosciences*, 28, 99–135.

Hatze, H. (1981) *Myocybernetic Control Models of Skeletal Muscle: Characteristics and Applications*, Pretoria: University of South Africa Press.

Ho, S.R., Smith, R. and O'Meara, D. (2009) Biomechanical analysis of dragon boat paddling: a comparison of elite and sub-elite paddlers. *Journal of Sports Sciences*, 27, 37–47.

Howell, D.C. (2009) *Statistical Methods for Psychology*, Belmont, CA: Cengage Wadsworth.

Kelso, J.A.S. (1995) *Dynamic Patterns: The Self-Organization of Brain and Behavior*, Cambridge, MA: MIT Press.

Lamb, P.F., Bartlett, R.M. and Robins, A. (2010) Self-organising maps: an objective method for clustering complex human movement. *International Journal of Computer Science in Sport*, 9, 20–29.

Lamb, P.F., Bartlett, R.M. and Robins, A. (2011) Artificial neural networks for analysing inter-limb coordination: the golf chip shot. *Human Movement Science* (in press).

Lapham, A.C. and Bartlett, R.M. (1995) The use of artificial intelligence in the analysis of sports performance: a review of applications in human gait analysis and future directions for sports biomechanics. *Journal of Sports Sciences*, 13, 229–237.

Lees, A., Barton, G. and Kershaw, L. (2003). The use of Kohonen neural network analysis to qualitatively characterize technique in soccer kicking. *Journal of Sports Sciences*, 21, 243–244.

Leigh, S. and Yu, B. (2007) The associations of selected technical parameters with discus throwing performance: a cross-sectional study. *Sports Biomechanics*, 6, 269–284.

Leskinen, A., Häkkinen, K., Virmamirta, M., Isolehto, J. and Kyröläinen, H. (2009) Comparisons of running kinematics between elite and national standard 1500-m runners. *Sports Biomechanics*, 8, 1–9.

Mullineaux, D.R., Bartlett, R.M. and Bennett, S.J. (2001) Research methods and statistics in biomechanics and motor control. *Journal of Sports Sciences*, 19, 739–760.

Negnevitsky, M. (2002) *Artificial Intelligence: A Guide to Intelligent Systems*, Harlow: Addison-Wesley.

Payton, C.J. and Bartlett, R.M. (eds) (2008) *Biomechanical Evaluation of Movement in Sport and Exercise: The British Association of Sport and Exercise Sciences Guide*, London: Routledge.

Salter, C.W., Sinclair, P.J. and Portus, M.R. (2007) The associations between fast bowling technique and ball release speed: a pilot study of the within-bowler and between-bowler approaches. *Journal of Sports Sciences*, 25, 1279–1285.

Schöllhorn, W.I. and Bauer, H.U. (1998) 'Identifying individual movement styles in high performance sports by means of self-organizing Kohonen maps', in H.J. Riehle and M. Vieten (eds) *Proceedings of the XVI ISBS 98 Konstanz*, Konstanz: ISBS, pp. 574–577.

Yeadon, M.R and King, M.A. (2008) 'Computer simulation modelling in sport', in C.J. Payton and R.M. Bartlett (eds) *Biomechanical Evaluation of Movement in Sport and Exercise: The British Association of Sport and Exercise Sciences Guide*, London: Routledge, pp. 176–205.

FURTHER READING

Bartlett, R.M. (2006) Artificial Intelligence in sports biomechanics: New dawn or false hope? *Journal of Sports Science and Medicine*, 5, 474–479. This provides a general overview of the use of artificial intelligence in sports biomechanics up until 2006. It is necessary reading for Study Task 8. It does not, obviously, cover post-2006 research, from which the two references in the reference section to the work of Peter Lamb and his co-authors are highly recommended.

Payton, C.J. and Bartlett, R.M. (eds) (2008) *Biomechanical Evaluation of Movement in Sport and Exercise: The British Association of Sport and Exercise Sciences Guide*, London: Routledge. This book covers most aspects of the quantitative analysis of sports movements. Particularly recommended are Chapters 2 and 3 (by Carl Payton and Clare Milner, respectively) on 'Motion analysis using video' and 'Motion analysis using on-line systems', which have not been covered in this chapter. Chapter 8, by David Mullineaux, covers 'Research methods: sample size and variability effects on statistical power', much of which is relevant in the context of statistical modelling. Finally, 'Fred' Yeadon and Mark King provide a brief overview of 'Computer simulation modelling in sport'; this is necessary reading for Study Task 6. All of these chapters are highly recommended.

8 Intervention to improve performance

Roger Bartlett

Knowledge assumed
Understanding of the basics
of performance analysis
(Chapter 5)
Familiarity with the use of
models of sports performance
(Chapters 6 and 7)

INTRODUCTION – THE IMPORTANCE OF INFORMATION FEEDBACK

BOX 8.1 LEARNING OUTCOMES

After reading this chapter you should be able to:

- outline the fundamental points that must be satisfied for biomechanical feedback to the coach and athlete to be relevant
- describe the strengths and weaknesses of various biomechanical models of performance and their limitations in feedback
- appreciate the important roles played by technique training and skill acquisition in the process of modifying a sports technique
- understand some of the issues that must be addressed in seeking to optimise the provision of biomechanical information to the coach and athlete
- give examples of the use of computer-based feedback and consider likely developments in this mode of information provision
- critique several intervention case studies
- understand the limited amount of peer-reviewed evidence for the success of sports biomechanists in actually improving sports performance.

If, by using the methods described in Chapters 5 to 7, we have systematically identified a fault in an athlete's movement technique that is preventing him or her from achieving optimal performance, then we must communicate that information to the athlete and coach. This will require feeding back our results to show what the fault is, why it is a fault, and how it might be corrected. To do this successfully, we need: accurate and reproducible (reliable) results; results that provide information that is not directly observable by a skilled coach; and results that relate clearly to differences between good and poorer performance. These points clearly raise issues about fundamental research, some of which have been addressed in the last three chapters. They also raise issues about the feedback of results to coaches and athletes from performance analysis (Chapter 5), well-designed qualitative biomechanical studies (Chapter 6) or quantitative performance modelling (Chapter 7). These, in turn, point to some future research directions in which sports biomechanists should be involved within interdisciplinary teams (see also Cassidy *et al.*, 2006).

You should note that the intervention stage involves the movement analyst's administration of feedback, corrections or other changes in the environment to improve performance. Intervention is more comprehensive than just providing feedback, instruction or error correction. It can provide positive reinforcement, help in performance modelling, guide modifications to practise and prescriptions of training, and help to adjust equipment for optimal performance. You should also be aware that there is not enough documented evidence of successful interventions to improve performance over time.

Also related to the fundamental issue addressed in this chapter, are the topics of technique training – vital for a new movement technique to be refined – and skill acquisition – necessary for the relearning of a movement technique. These topics will be considered in later sections of this chapter.

AUGMENTED FEEDBACK

The information that we feed back augments that available to performers from their senses; it is referred to as augmented feedback. Augmented feedback can be in the form of knowledge of results (KR) – the outcome – or knowledge of performance (KP) – the movement process. The movement analyst must address what information is fed back, how this is done and when (this should have been partly addressed in the preparation stage of the movement analysis process, see Chapter 6). It should be self-evident that the feedback used should involve the right information at the right time and in an easily understood format; the speed of feedback and its presentation and interpretation are all important. However, there is often a great deal of information available, but it is not clear what should be provided, nor how. The frequent calls for rapid feedback and more feedback from both coaches and scientists often do not pay heed to the effects, if any, of feedback nor of how and when it should best be presented.

The main goal in providing feedback is to correct a 'fault' so as to improve performance (or, as we discuss later, to reduce the risk of injury). The intention of providing feedback to enhance performance is not to improve performance for the rest of the training session, or whenever feedback is provided (which immediate feedback can achieve), but to retain that performance improvement for the next competition. We need, therefore, to look critically at the retention phase of the overall feedback process, as we will do in a later section. The provision of feedback needs to address relevant motor learning theories. Although many of these theories have been developed for discrete laboratory tasks and have not been adequately tested on real world tasks, such as sport, they do provide some evidence to which sports biomechanists should attend.

Methods for providing augmented feedback include verbal feedback; use of verbal and other cues; visual models; manual or mechanical guidance; and modifying the task, practice or conditioning (see also, Knudson and Morrison, 2002). In a later section, we touch on the use of simple mechanical devices, such as cones and poles, to change cricket fast bowling technique. In giving verbal and other sensory feedback, we need to provide appropriate information – to translate critical features into intervention cues in behavioural terms, appropriate to the group with whom we are working. Cues can be verbal, visual, aural or kinaesthetic and we need to derive relevant cues for each critical feature that we intend to address in our intervention strategy. Verbal cues should be no more than six words and be figurative not literal. We must use analogies that are meaningful. The structure of a verbal cue should be: action; content (what does the action); qualification (how to gauge success); special conditions (if more information is needed). Examples would be: rotate hip and trunk; swing racket forwards relative to the ground. The latter example would seem preferable as it focuses externally (racket) rather than internally (hip and trunk) – see also Davids *et al.* (2008). Not all of these methods are equally effective in particular circumstances. For example, Guadagnoli *et al.* (2002) studied the effects of video, verbal and self-guided instruction on the distance and accuracy of fifteen 7-iron shots of 30 golfers with handicaps from 7 to 16. The golfers, who were randomly assigned to the three conditions, were tested before the first of four 90-minute practice sessions (one on each of four consecutive days), then immediately after the last session and, finally, two weeks later. The self-guided group were allowed to practise at a normal driving range with as many drives as they wished in 90 minutes but with no augmented feedback. The verbal feedback group were given verbal knowledge of results (KR) by a Professional Golfers' Association (PGA) teaching professional, while the video feedback group received both verbal and visual KR; both forms of feedback were provided throughout the practice session. On the immediate post-test, the only difference between the groups was that the self-guided group was less variable in the total distance the ball was hit than the other two groups. This finding was reversed in the two-week post-test, in which the two augmented feedback groups also had significantly better accuracy distances (the distance travelled towards the target minus any lateral deviation away from that line), with the video group outperforming the verbal group.

Video feedback is now routinely provided on competition performance or performance in training sessions. Unfortunately, much of this feedback is unstructured, often lacks a valid model against which to compare current performance, and rarely has an objective evaluation of its utility in improving performance. Sometimes video feedback is provided simply by replaying video footage to the athlete and his or her coach immediately after performance. The use of software packages for qualitative biomechanical analysis, such as Siliconcoach and Dartfish, allows video feedback of two or more performances simultaneously for comparison. As we noted in Chapter 6, this 'dual-screen' or 'multi-screen' option is very useful for comparing, for instance, successful and unsuccessful performances by one athlete. However, these options should be used very cautiously when comparing two different athletes, when one is often used as a 'model' of what the other should be doing. As we have previously noted, use of an inappropriate model of performance can be counterproductive and can increase injury risk. Video feedback works best when it is supported by a valid, underlying model of performance as discussed in the next section.

There are, of course, other reasons for providing biomechanical feedback to coaches and athletes other than to remedy movement deficiencies to improve performance, on which this chapter focuses. Feedback may be provided, for example, to fulfil an educational role. Some forms of feedback may be immediate (within seconds or minutes, usually after each trial), for example running speed measurements from photocells or simply replaying a video recording of a performance. Medium-term feedback, after several days or weeks, may be more appropriate when seeking to change a movement technique permanently, for example using detailed qualitative or quantitative video analysis and statistical modelling. Some aspects of modification of movements may require longer term research studies, carried out over months or even years, to provide the necessary scientific basis for a correct performance model; computer simulation modelling and artificial intelligence approaches would often fit here.

The implicit assumption, in many publications about the use of feedback, that any feedback is inherently good is not totally supported. It is important not to give too much feedback – providing more information does not always improve performance and may cause confusion, particularly if the information presented offers no clear solution to the problem identified; this may be true for complex kinetic variables, such as the forces on bicycle pedals or oars. Practitioners are not always receptive to feedback, particularly if it is not obviously relevant to improving performance. Despite these points, and the view that information feedback is the single most important variable (excluding practice) for skill learning and modification, too few studies have directly addressed the provision of augmented feedback to athletes and coaches of information from biomechanics research into sports movements.

There are many examples in which misleading or incorrect feedback has been provided to athletes and coaches. A classic example relates to how propulsive forces are generated in swimming. Before the research of 'Doc' Counsilman, Bob Schleihauf and others in the 1970s, the view of coaches had been that the hand acted as a paddle and that, in the front crawl, swimmers should pull their hands backwards in a straight line below the mid-line of the body using drag as the propulsive force (as in the straight line of Figure 8.1). This

Figure 8.1 Hand paths in swimming, showing a hypothetical straight line pull, the S-shaped path of the fingertip through the water, and the path of the fingertip relative to the rotating trunk.

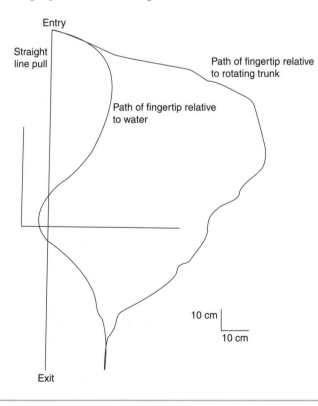

incorrect view was transformed by research based on cinematography that showed that swimmers' hands made an S-shaped pattern of an inward scull followed by an outward scull (Figure 8.1). From fluid dynamics testing, these sideways hand movements through the water were shown to maximise force production by using the hand as a hydrofoil, making use of lift and drag forces. The pitch of the hand (its orientation to the relative velocity vector with the water) plays an important role in this respect. Armed with this information, coaches switched to teaching a 'feel for the water', to optimise the pitch angle, emphasising the sideways sculling movements of the arm. Then studies in the 1990s, using simple models of the swimmer (Hay *et al.*, 1993; Payton *et al.*, 1997), showed that much of the sideways movement of the hand in the front crawl is attributable to body roll, which has a substantial influence on medial-lateral hand movements. The medial-lateral motion of the hand relative to the rotating trunk (the movement relative to the swimmer's body) involves the swimmer sweeping the hand away from the trunk in the first part of the pull and towards it in the second (Figure 8.1). This contradicted the previous research that had led to erroneous coaching beliefs about the relative motion of the hand.

MODELS OF PERFORMANCE AND THEIR USE IN PROVIDING FEEDBACK

To make meaningful statements about the movement technique of an athlete and how to improve it, we noted in Chapters 6 and 7 that a model is needed against which we can compare that movement technique and which will help in improving it. Important requirements for movement analysts are, therefore, to be able to construct and use 'performance models' of the sports activities we analyse and choose the most appropriate model for our purposes. The effectiveness of any feedback will depend not only on observing or measuring an athlete's current performance, but also on identifying that athlete's 'target, or model, performance'.

In Chapter 6, we discussed the use of deterministic models of performance in the context of the four-stage qualitative analysis process. We noted that to improve performance we need a model against which to compare an athlete's current movement technique: deterministic models generally serve that purpose for the qualitative analyst. In Chapter 7, we looked at the fundamentals underlying the biomechanical optimisation of sports movements through the use of quantitative models of performance. The emphasis was on theory-driven statistical modelling, computer simulation modelling and optimisation, and various approaches from artificial intelligence. We noted that, although these methods may help to improve performance directly, they are more often used to carry out research to obtain an in-depth understanding of the performance of a specific sports task, upon which strategies for performance improvement can then be built. An important question is how the results of these qualitative and quantitative models can best be used in the intervention stage of the movement analysis process to compare an athlete's model performance with his or her current performance.

If providing knowledge of performance, then we definitely need a 'model' against which we can assess current performance. There is no general agreement about how we establish a model performance or movement pattern. However, such models can function in comparing and improving movement techniques, developing training, and aiding communication. I emphasise that there is no such thing as a general optimal performance model, so any 'models' must be individual-specific. From a qualitative analysis viewpoint, the correct set of critical features, perhaps expressed in a 'wizard' or something similar, provides such a model.

Our 'model' performance could take the form of a live demonstration (for a full discussion of observational learning and the use of demonstrations, see Hodges and Williams, 2007). These have their use in the field, to show an athlete how to perform or modify their movements. However, they can be subjective, depending very much on the coach or whoever provides the demonstration. Furthermore, they require far deeper information about the movement technique to be known by the coach if this approach is not to degenerate into simply copying the movements of a more successful performer. Their lack of individual-specificity is their major drawback. Historically, the 'textbook' movement technique often served as the model against which others were evaluated. Such models are often hard to digest, particularly where complex movements are involved, and often contain too much information. Examples can be found in almost all coaching texts in which sports movement techniques are described in detail. These models have little practical use in the process of identifying and eradicating movement faults. Again, they lack individual-specificity.

To summarise, useful feedback to improve the performance of an athlete generally requires a target performance against which an athlete's current performance can be compared. The most appropriate performance model should be used (natural language is the least useful). The model should seek to manage detail and establish clarity. The structure of the model should be carefully considered. Some evidence supports the idea that the best feedback involves the presentation of the target and current movement techniques in the same form, for example both as computer graphic displays. Hierarchically structured graphical models have the potential for easy management and informative display of such complex information. Computer simulation and optimisation theoretically allow direct comparison of current and target movements. These modes of providing feedback are discussed in the section on computer-based feedback.

INFORMATION FEEDBACK AND MOTOR LEARNING

In a training context, it is now possible to feed back rapidly information relating to, for example, javelin release speed and angle and what these would have been for an optimal throw, and kinetic data from force pedals (Lieberman and Franks, 2004). The motor learning literature (e.g. Schmidt, 1991) provides evidence that summary feedback of results (after several practice trials) provides better results in the retention phase of learning than does immediate feedback provided after each trial (Figure 8.2). As we noted in the previous section, the retention phase of the feedback process is the important one in interventions to improve performance. If

Figure 8.2 Comparison of immediate and summary feedback (as knowledge of results) for a discrete task. Open circles: summary feedback; filled circles: immediate feedback; filled squares: both immediate and summary feedback (adapted from Schmidt, 1991).

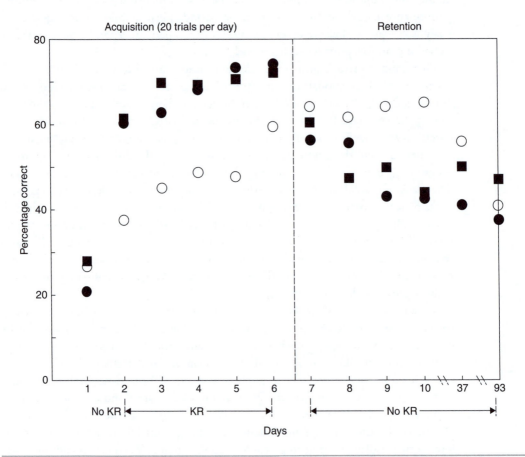

the results of Schmidt (1991) also apply to skilled sports movements (this has not been fully demonstrated), then sports biomechanists need to pay attention to these findings when structuring feedback to athletes and coaches, particularly during training sessions.

Although no difference between summary and immediate feedback was reported by Broker *et al.* (1993) for the learning of modifications to pedalling technique by inexperienced cyclists (Figure 8.3), there is insufficient evidence, at present, about whether this is general for sports tasks. Many studies of feedback during technique training, such as that of Broker *et al.* (1993), relate to early learning of skills; it is unclear whether they generalise to more skilful performers. Published results relating to video feedback and the sequence in which current and target performances are presented may not apply to more skilled performers. Although it has been hypothesised that the usefulness of feedback decays rapidly with time and, therefore, that feedback must be provided within

Figure 8.3 Comparison of immediate and summary feedback for a sports task (cycling). Open squares: summary feedback; filled diamonds: immediate feedback (adapted from Broker *et al.*, 1993).

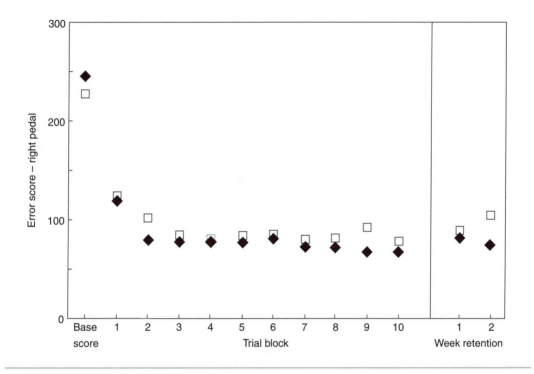

minutes, there is little empirical research to support this particularly in the context of a retained improvement in performance.

Mononen *et al.* (2003) studied the effect of augmented feedback of knowledge of performance (KP) about the aiming trajectory of the rifle barrel on target shooting performance – the shooting score and its variability. Forty participants, from the Finnish Air Force, were randomly assigned to control, no-KP, 50% KP and 100% KP groups and performed 40 shots in each of three training sessions per week during a four-week period. The no-KP, 50% and 100% KP groups received knowledge of results (KR); the no-KP group had only that feedback, the control group did not participate in the training sessions. The 100% KP group also received KP after each shot; the 50% KP group had KP after only the shots in the first and third blocks of ten (i.e. after shots 1–10 and 21–30). The shooters were also tested before the training began and at post-tests two and ten days into the retention period after the acquisition (training) period; the results are summarised in Figure 8.4. All experimental groups improved their shooting score throughout the acquisition period. In the two-day retention test, all experimental groups had significantly higher, and less variable, shooting scores than the control group; the 100% KP group had significantly better scores and variability than the other two experimental groups. In the 10-day retention test, however, no significant

Figure 8.4 Mean shooting scores during provision of knowledge of performance (KP) and in two retention tests. Open circles: control group; filled diamonds: no-KP; filled square: 50% KP; filled circle: 100% KP. The lines between the data points are added only for clarity not to imply linear trends (adapted from Mononen *et al.*, 2003).

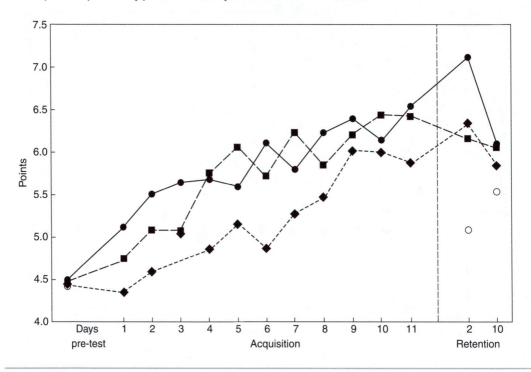

differences were found between any of the groups for shooting scores or their variability. Had the shooters been competing two weeks after the end of the training period, no improvement in performance would have been sustained. Unfortunately, the study did not include a group that received only summary feedback after several shots rather than after each shot (although the 50% KP group received KP after each of 20 shots but not after each of the other 20). This could have been accommodated by providing summary feedback in the rest interval the shooters were allowed after each block of 10 shots.

Anderson *et al.* (2005) looked at the provision of accelerometer-based feedback to 13 experienced rowers (performing on a rowing ergometer) and its effect on performance consistency (power-stroke dispersion) and kinematic consistency (based on acceleration patterns). Detailed visual feedback of acceleration and consistency patterns during the stroke (KP) was found to improve kinematic and performance consistency significantly more so than summary feedback (KR) of the kinematic consistency scores only after the completion of the stroke. Summary feedback was no better than a no-feedback condition in improving performance consistency but was significantly better in improving kinematic consistency. No improvements in performance-related parameters were found for any of the modes of feedback. The study did not examine whether any of the consistency improvements were retained over time, neither was it clear why kinematic consistency is important to rowing performance.

We might ask if the 'picture' about when to provide feedback, and how much to provide, changes if we accept the 'constraints-led' views of ecological motor control. That viewpoint sees augmented feedback as directing the performer's search for solutions to a specific sports task that satisfy the constraints imposed on him or her. Researchers from this paradigm have suggested that an external focus of attention, on movement effects, is better than an internal one, focusing on movement dynamics. An emphasis on task outcomes allows learners to search for a task solution and does not interfere with the self-organisational processes of movement dynamics. These views have been supported by research in slalom skiing and the forehand drive in tennis and in the golf pitch shot and basketball free throw (see also Davids *et al.*, 2008). There is evidence that 'less is more', in other words, that better performance is achieved with less frequent augmented feedback, for example, in learning the lofted pass in soccer. Again, it is, however, unclear if these results generalise to all stages of skill acquisition. If a focus of attention on movement effects is better than one on movement dynamics in correcting movement faults in skilled performers, we must be careful to tailor our feedback accordingly. This could be held to support the qualitative analysis approach, rather than the complexities of quantitative modelling of performance.

There are clearly many unresolved issues relating to optimal feedback to performers and coaches of sports biomechanics information. Biomechanists and motor skill experts can beneficially combine to research such topics and to establish whether motor learning paradigms for simple tasks do generalise to more complex ones. Such research would be valuable in helping athletes to learn and incorporate modifications to a movement pattern. More collaborative research between the sports science disciplines should also seek to identify if changes to the movement technique of a highly skilled performer can be made successfully, what the implications of this are for technique training (and other training), and whether the effects are beneficial to improving performance or reducing injury risk. We look at several case studies on this theme in a later section. It is often difficult to separate the direct effect of biomechanics feedback on the performance of sports movements from other effects. An example is shown by the study of Judge *et al.* (2008), in which video-based feedback was provided to the coach of the leading US female hammer thrower. After this feedback, substantial changes were made to her general training programme. The following season, her release speed had increased and, therefore, her throw distance. The available evidence suggested that the improvement was more likely to have been due to increases in muscular strength and power through training rather than the result of biomechanical feedback. Nevertheless, this is an issue worth revisiting for more thorough investigation by researchers in sports biomechanics and motor learning.

THE ROLE OF TECHNIQUE TRAINING

Many sports movements involve very complex motor skills, for example javelin or hammer throwing, gymnastics routines, racket sports, or the pole vault. It follows, therefore, that much of the training required to modify such movements will involve relearning of the required movement patterns to perform the skill and constant attempts to improve them. As noted in the previous section, for the feedback provided to be useful in improving movement technique in training, we require not only the presentation of the current performance but also instruction on the target movements that the training is seeking to achieve. It is possible to define the goal of technique training as being to develop the optimal movement pattern to achieve the performance goal within the organismic constraints of the athlete. Some organismic constraints, such as lever lengths or body height, are permanently, or for the growing athlete temporarily, unalterable. All intelligent coaches must be aware that the optimal motor pattern for their athletes will evolve within these constraints and may not, therefore, conform to those of an athlete with different organismic constraints but similar performance standard, let alone to athletes of different standards of performance. Other organismic constraints such as flexibility, strength, body weight, power, speed and endurance can be changed, usually by training, to allow better performance. This is the function of much training for the technique-dominated sports, such as gymnastics and the field events in athletics.

An important role of the coach is to guide the athlete in modification of his or her movement technique to eliminate faults. To do so correctly, the movement analyst needs to work with the coach in the intervention stage; to do this effectively requires attention to the following points. The analyst needs to be aware of the essential features of a particular movement technique to achieve a high standard of performance – this requires a theory-based performance model, as discussed in Chapters 6 and 7. He or she needs to recognise these features in performance, usually assisted by slow motion video replays and increasingly supplemented by computerised biomechanical analysis and modelling. It is essential to discriminate between a desirable movement technique and the highly individualised stylistic variations that are seen in performances of individual athletes, performing under their specific organismic constraints. The analyst and coach need to be aware of the current organismic constraints of the athlete and how these will affect what technique or other training should be prescribed to bring about improved performance. As an example, comparison of the movement techniques of two top female throwers might suggest that one is very powerful, but lacks mobility (especially in the lumbar–sacral region), while the other is very flexible but possibly lacks some strength or speed. The pronounced stylistic variations in their throwing movements (although using the same basic movement technique) follow quite logically from these organismic differences. Several issues need to be addressed when planning a technique training programme to remove perceived flaws. For further details, you should refer to a suitable text on motor learning (e.g. Davids *et al.*, 2008).

COMPUTER-BASED FEEDBACK

Computer graphics in feedback

The use of three-dimensional computer graphics has now become widespread in biomechanical feedback to sports practitioners. There has been little research to establish the most effective ways in which information should be presented to achieve the required outcome of improved performance even, for example, in terms of the best degree of abstraction of the graphic image. For example, some researchers have found an increase in performance retention with increased abstraction, while others have indicated the superiority of real representations. The former would support the use of, for example, computerised stick figure displays, while the latter would favour much more realistic solid body presentations.

When using computer graphics to provide feedback, we can represent the movement either serially or in parallel. Serial representations include videos of the performance and computer animations of the data from automatic marker-tracking systems (for examples, see the book's website) and from computer simulation models. They permit repeated study, but have to be studied serially, frame by frame or image by image. Video software analysis packages (such as Siliconcoach) allow two or more serial representations to be viewed simultaneously. These options are useful in providing feedback, for example, to look at a successful and an unsuccessful performance, such as a tennis serve (Figure 6.26). As we noted in Chapter 6, the use of any dual-screen or multi-screen options to compare different performers should be treated with great caution. Different individuals bring their own organismic constraints to a sports task, which interact with the constraints of the task and those of the environment to provide unique solutions to the task. Seeking to copy others has not been proven to improve performance and can lead to an increased risk of injury.

Parallel representation can be obtained from computer-generated images such as stick figures (Figure 8.5) or solid body models (see Figure 8.7 later in the chapter), as well as from biomechanical analysis packages, such as Siliconcoach and SIMI. As for serial representations, they presuppose a deeper model of performance. Examples of Siliconcoach presentations for use in the intervention stage of the four-stage qualitative

Figure 8.5 'Parallel' stick figure display of a javelin thrower.

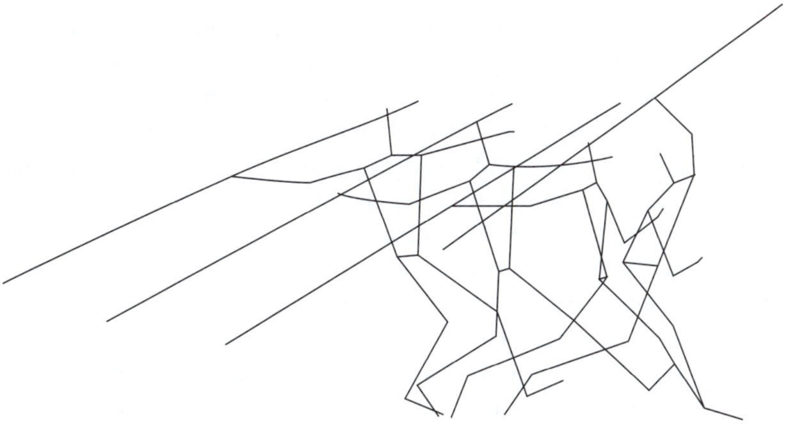

analysis process are shown on the book's website. Parallel representations also allow repeated study and they add a very useful concurrent representation of the movement. Again, their use to compare performers should be treated very cautiously.

Also useful in feedback to improve performance is the use of computerised three-dimensional image-based motion analysis (see Payton and Bartlett, 2008), in which the movement can be viewed from any chosen viewing direction. For example, hammer throwers and their coaches can see the throw viewed from above even if it was filmed using two horizontal cameras. By concentrating only on specific parts of the body, the computer software can also show aspects of the movement that would not have been revealed even by an appropriately placed camera. Many sports biomechanists have found these approaches to be very useful, if very time-consuming, in feeding back the results of quantitative analyses to athletes and coaches. Fundamentally, this approach still relies on the existence of an underlying performance model, if the data are to have some real meaning for the improvement of performance. For quantitative analyses, this would involve a statistical model (Chapter 7) or, better still, a computer simulation model (Chapter 7; see also the sub-section later on), so that simulated and actual performances could be compared.

Expert systems

In Chapter 6 we looked at how deterministic models can be developed into Siliconcoach wizards. These can then be used by the movement analyst or coach to compare an athlete's performance of the critical features incorporated in the wizard with a good execution of the performance, represented by optimal values of the critical features. An alternative approach would use graphical models to break the movement down into simpler elements. By doing so, such models would reduce complexity, possibly hiding information until it is needed while still maintaining the overall structure of the movement. One such approach would combine deterministic models with statistical modelling (Chapter 7). It could provide a strong theory-based graphical model to underpin other more field-based or computerised approaches. Deterministic models were discussed in detail in Chapter 6. They can produce far too much information on one diagram, particularly for those not familiar with the movement represented or the use of such models (see, for example, Figure 6.10). They do, however, allow hierarchical organisation; this could lead on to menu-based systems. One such system would be a logical and fully computerised extension of the hierarchical structure of deterministic models, in which information would be organised to enforce the use of a hierarchical structure and to hide information. The menus would ensure that only an 'easily digested' amount of information was presented, with the user dropping down to further levels of the model as required. However, they are, to date, largely non-existent, although Siliconcoach wizards capture some of this concept. A diagrammatic representation of part of a possible menu-driven system (it does not actually exist) is shown in Figure 8.6. This type of approach could form part of the structure of an 'expert system'.

Figure 8.6 Schematic representation of a menu-based system for a performance assessment model. The left-hand part of the diagram shows levels 2 and 3 of the 'landing distance' (Figure 6.12) branch of the deterministic model of the long jump that was developed in Chapter 6. Other levels of the model are hidden from the hypothetical user, who interacts with the model through the pointer, controlled by the mouse or touchpad. The right-hand part of the diagram represents the user-interaction menu. The 'Show previous level' function would allow the user to backtrack to level 1 of the model (see Figure 6.4). The user could choose to 'Go to model links for:' to access a sub-menu that, in this case, would explain why landing distance is the distance of the centre of mass behind the feet at landing minus the distance from the point of contact of the jumper's body closest to the take-off board to where the feet land (i.e. the links between the boxes are justified); if a statistical model had been developed, then statistical justification could be provided. In the illustration, the user has chosen (box shaded in light grey) to 'Show next level for:' in this case, either 'Land with CoM [centre of mass] behind feet' or 'Don't touch sand beyond landing point'. Selection of either would show the next level down (level 4) of the model and hide the previous level; selection of the former would reveal 'Hips flexed, knees extended', selection of the latter would reveal 'Control rotation off take-off board'. If 'Land with CoM behind feet' were to be chosen, the 'Show next level for:' option would now be disallowed, as 'Hips flexed, knees extended' is a lowest level box of the model.

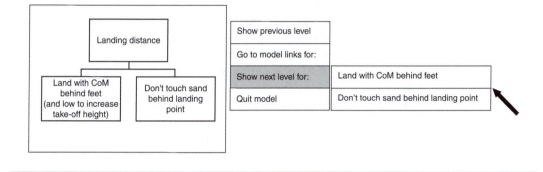

As we noted in Chapter 7, an expert system is a computer program that simulates the actions of a human expert. It consists of a great deal of specific knowledge (data and representations of the rules used by the expert), a way of matching that data to the expertise (an 'inference engine') and a user-friendly interface. There is little reason to doubt the value that such systems could have in providing biomechanical advice to coaches and athletes, and that they could have a profound effect in diagnosing faults in, and subsequently improving, sports performance. However, Lapham and Bartlett (1995) surprisingly found no reports of the development of an expert system to provide biomechanical advice to athletes and coaches on problems of movement technique; nothing much has changed in the intervening 15 years. An expert system in this context would involve a database of available quantitative information on a sports movement and on body characteristics and qualitative information about the movement technique. The system's inference engine would match these data with expertise – the rules and probabilities that emerge from analysis of how experts in that movement technique detect faults in performance. The development of such systems requires fundamental research, in which sports biomechanists should be involved. As we noted in the previous chapter, Siliconcoach wizards are about as close as we have come so far to such a diagnostic tool. It is tempting to speculate that expert systems will be developed in the near future as diagnostic tools for performance faults and injury risk factors. However, my experience over the last 15 years prevents me from being too optimistic.

The uses of computer simulation and optimisation in feedback

The computer simulation and optimisation of sports movements were discussed in Chapter 7, where the practical limitations of some simulation models were also addressed. The provision of information relating to javelin release speed and angle and what these would have been for an optimal throw was touched upon in that chapter (Best et al., 1995). We looked at how contour maps can provide guidelines to training by indicating where current performance lies on the map in relationship to the optimal performance. We noted, for example, that confusion could arise for a thrower with an optimal release angle of attack but a non-optimal release angle (see the black triangle on Figure 7.6), for whom changes in both angles have relatively large effects on the range. For this thrower, only a study of the contour map could reveal that it was the release angle that was non-optimal, and, therefore, required to be changed to improve performance. An approach based on that simulation model was used in the initial stages of a sports science support project for the UK's elite javelin throwers in which I was involved. At that time (the early to mid 1990s) the top British javelin throwers and their coaches found feedback of information derived from quantitative analysis of cine film, and later video, to be more valuable to them than the results of our computer simulations. I should add a note of caution here: the graphical display of computer simulations was very crude in those days and that, rather than the underlying model, might have been the reason for the throwers and coaches in our study not seeing the relevance of such feedback to improving performance. It is also worth noting that our computer simulation model was only for the flight stage of the javelin throw; at that time, it did not direct throwers to the aspects of their movements that needed attention to achieve an optimal throw.

Computer simulation models have been used both to teach and to correct movement patterns in several aerial sports; however, no systematic evaluation of the usefulness of the feedback given to coaches and performers has yet been reported. However, the ability to compare computer animations of an actual performance with one that has been found to be optimal using a computer simulation model for the same athlete is very powerful (for example, see Yeadon and King, 2008). In fact, it comes close to an ideal way of comparing current and optimal performance (see also Figure 7.3).

Kinetic feedback and virtual reality

It is now possible to feed back immediately kinetic information, such as the forces on the pedals in cycling, the forces on the oars in rowing (see, for example, Smith and Loschner, 2002), and force information from virtual reality simulations in bob-sled dynamics (for further examples, see Liebermann and Franks, 2004). The assumption is often made that immediate feedback of such information improves performance. There is little evidence-based research to support this assumption for the crucial retention phase of the learning process. Providing this information seems to conflict with ecological motor learning research touched on in an earlier section. Kinetic information just might not relate to the performer's immediate problem.

The evaluation of real-time computer simulators in skills training is not widely reported: indeed that developed by Huffman *et al.* (1993) for the bob-sled is a rare example. Even in that example, no attempt was made to ascertain whether the feedback provided by such a simulator resulted in improvements in performance, for example by comparing the results from a group of athletes trained on the simulator with a control group. However, such simulators do have great potential for providing relevant feedback of sports biomechanics information, particularly when combined with the use of virtual reality. Some examples of the use of virtual reality in feedback were reported by Liebermann *et al.* (2002), but while useful from a training perspective, the model performance against which to compare an athlete's current performance is somewhat lacking. The use of sophisticated computer technology to provide immediate information feedback to athletes should not be confused with feeding back information based on movement fault diagnosis to improve a specific aspect of performance in the retentive stage of the whole process.

INTERVENTION CASE STUDIES

As we noted in the introduction to this chapter, there is little documented evidence of successful interventions to improve performance over time – certainly few related to a clearly-established performance model. As Elliott and Bartlett (2006) noted, sports biomechanists, often with minimal evidence, claim that they can improve movement technique and reduce injury risk. A well-documented example is that of Blanksby *et al.* (2002), who looked at the effectiveness of a training session on grab, handle and track start techniques in elite swimmers. They reported that the training intervention significantly improved performance; however, the only evidence for their performance model was that it was 'based on mechanical factors considered to be important from the diving literature and on opinions from experienced coaches'. Somewhat more convincing attempts have been made to evaluate interventions to reduce injury risk. This concluding section, therefore, brings us full circle back to the theme of the first half of the book – reducing injury risk; a reduced susceptibility to injury generally leads, if not to an improved performance, then certainly to sustained good performance over time.

There are few sports movements in which strong links have been established with a specific injury. The one most often cited is the association between low back injury in cricket fast bowlers and the 'mixed' bowling technique. In this section, we will review evidence for the mixed fast bowling technique in cricket (Figure 8.7(a)) being a cause of low-back injury in cricket. We will then look at several intervention studies that have sought to reduce low back injuries to fast bowlers, by changing to another bowling style – mixed to front-on (Figure 8.7(b)) or side-on (Figure 8.7(c)) – among other factors.

Many studies, details of which can be found in the references cited in this section and in the review paper of Elliott (2000), have reported an association between low back

Figure 8.7 Side (top) and front (bottom) views of different fast bowling techniques in cricket: (a) mixed technique; (b) front-on technique; (c) side-on technique.

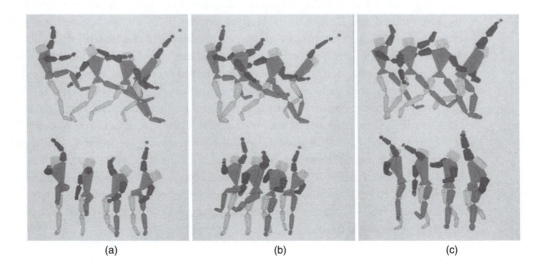

(a)	(b)	(c)

injury and the mixed fast bowling technique. Several studies have found fast bowlers to be prone to lumbar spine stress fractures of the neural arch (spondylolysis or spondy-lolisthesis) as in the following data: 50% of the bowlers in an Australian A grade club team over five years, age 20; 20% of a group of 72 bowlers, age 15–19; 11% of a group of 82 bowlers over one season, mean age 17; and 45% of 20 bowlers in an Australian state squad over one month. You should bear in mind that, for the normal population, the incidence of these stress fractures is only 4–6%, so the incidence in fast bowlers is very much more prevalent. In addition a widespread incidence of disc damage – degeneration and bulging – has been reported, with around 60% of fast bowlers being affected in one study.

The etiology of these injuries is multifaceted, involving several factors. The first is overuse – 59% of those affected have been found to bowl more than the average number of overs. Also implicated are poor physical preparation, poor footwear, and hard ground surfaces, both in play and in net practice sessions. Abnormal biomechanics is also a factor; for example, a statistically significant ($P < 0.05$) link has been established between these injuries and low foot arches. The final factor is the use of potentially injurious movement techniques. Two movement techniques are generally considered to be at fault here; one is the use of a straight front leg knee at landing in the delivery stride, which has been inadequately researched. The second, which has received much attention, is the association between the mixed fast bowling technique and low back injury.

The most common 'mixed technique', as should be evident from Figure 8.7(a), involves landing on the back foot at the start of the delivery stride with an open chest position, similar to that for the front-on technique (Figure 8.7(b)), but then counter-rotating the shoulders away from the bowling direction before front foot landing, so that they are in a more closed position, similar to that of the side-on technique (Figure 8.7(c)). Shoulder counter-rotation (with a mean value of 40°) has been found to be statistically significantly related to low back injury ($P < 0.05$) for a group of 17 mixed technique bowlers, six of whom had stress fractures of the lumbar spine and seven had soft tissue injury.

Three risk factors are present in the mixed technique – forced rotational stress, backward arching or lateral flexion, and high impact forces at front foot contact. Clearly the mixed technique is a risk factor. So, mixed technique fast bowlers are prone to lumbar spine stress fractures, but does the etiology of these injuries lend theoretical support to this assertion? Well, the mechanical etiology of this injury involves flexion overload, unbalanced shear forces, and forced rotational stress (remember that the normal lumbar spine allows very little rotation to take place about the longitudinal axis because of the disposition of the articular surfaces of the facet joints). Rotation is more important than hyperextension, as 80% of these stress fractures occur on the side of the non-bowling arm, whereas hyperextension is more marked on the side of the bowling arm. The neural arch has been shown to be vulnerable to damage from repeated flexion, hyperextension and rotation in cadavers and computer models. The mixed technique has far more forced torsional loading of the lumbar spine than the front-on or side-on techniques, often expressed, somewhat approximately, through shoulder counter-rotation and the shoulder alignment angle. So, the underlying etiology of neural arch stress fractures supports the injury risk of the mixed fast bowling technique.

There are some important limitations to this seemingly hard-and-fast association. First, the thorax–pelvis alignment – which gives a very close approximation to the movements of the lumbar spine – is well estimated by the three-dimensional shoulder alignment angle but not by the two-dimensional angle used in most studies before 2000. A second issue is that shoulder counter-rotation is a continuum, most fast bowlers counter-rotate to some extent; in one study, for example, the mean shoulder counter-rotation angle was reported as 17° for side-on bowlers, 20° for front-on bowlers and 46° for mixed technique bowlers. Another confounding factor is that variable shoulder counter-rotations have been used to classify mixed technique, from 10 to 40°: changing the cut-off value from 40° to 20° changes the classification of bowlers dramatically. Finally, front-on bowlers often tend to increase their shoulder counter-rotation late in a bowling spell, thereby becoming more 'mixed'.

A crucial issue, and the main point of this chapter, is whether anything can be done about the problem. It is one thing to identify an aspect of a movement technique that reduces performance or increases injury risk, another altogether to do something about it. Well first some anecdotal evidence. I was involved in such an intervention study in the late 1990s and early 2000s. This study is only considered here – it has not been published – to illustrate the value of using the structured four-stage approach to move-ment analysis. This study drew on the results of a seven-year project with the England and Wales Cricket Board (ECB) studying the fast bowling techniques of 27 test match cricketers from various nations, and on the research outlined above. It was a low-budget qualitative analysis project for Lancashire County Cricket Club and started with a needs analysis with the coach of the county's youth teams, whose requirement was the need to reduce the incidence of low back injury so that these players could continue to bowl fast as seniors. The main critical feature was, therefore, very straightforward to identify – was each bowler's technique side-on, front-on or mixed? This was based on previous research and was to be assessed observationally from video recordings. The young fast bowlers in the club's age-group squads were video recorded annually, using a single camera, by the county youth coach. At least six balls were recorded for each bowler in indoor nets (a slight challenge to ecological validity). The main limitations (owing to cost) were the frequency of assessment (only done annually) the number of video cameras and their quality, indoor lighting, and camera placement. The evaluation and diagnosis stage involved video analysis independently by the biomechanist and the county youth coach (to reduce analyst bias and improve objectivity). All balls for each bowler were analysed; one of these was analysed on different days by the biomechanist to check on and improve reliability. The biomechanist and coach then met to agree recommendations on changing mixed techniques (prioritising on the best chance of changing mixed to side-on or front-on), including input from physiotherapists working with the squads. This threefold approach provides a 'triangulation' of opinions common in some disciplines in sports science but rare in sports biomechanics. The intervention stage began with a meeting of the biomechanists and county youth coach with each bowler and his coach or parents to explain why and how changes were to be made. All recommendations had to be implemented by the bowler's coach or parents in practice sessions using cones (for the run-up) and simple verbal instructions (for the pre-bound and bound strides). As a result, many bowlers became far less mixed when evaluated the next year; those who had had low back pain mostly had reduced symptoms, based on feedback from the club's physiotherapist. One bowler, who had been very much 'mixed', had his technique successfully modified and went on to play senior international cricket. However, the annual observation–intervention process was insufficiently frequent to draw firm conclusions.

Elliott and Khangure (2002) used an initial half-day coaching course and six small-group coaching sessions over a three- to four-year period in an attempt to reduce the incidence of the mixed fast bowling technique among the young Australian bowlers involved in their study (mean age 13 years). The session emphasised the characteristics and safety of side-on and front-on techniques. Their intervention reduced shoulder counter-rotation during the delivery stride and the number of mixed bowlers but not, in their view, to a sufficient extent. Also, there was no reduction in disc degeneration. Ranson et al. (2009) used a two-year coaching intervention with a group of 14 elite UK fast bowlers (mean age 18.5 years). The intervention was based on movement data collected indoors with an automatic marker-tracking system. Suggested movement technique modifications, and ways to achieve them, were agreed with the bowler and county fast bowling coach. The intervention used verbal feedback, visual feedback and correction drills using poles. The outcome was a significantly more side-on shoulder alignment at back-foot strike and decreased shoulder counter-rotation. There was no change in back or front knee flexion or trunk lateral flexion. Unfortunately, no injury data or changes in injury occurrence were reported.

Wallis *et al.* (2002) used a completely different approach from the two studies reported in the previous paragraph. They assessed the effectiveness of a bowling harness on selected characteristics of the fast bowling technique. Their intervention featured an eight-week coaching programme with two 15-minute sessions each week, with harness and control groups (13 and 20 Australian bowlers respectively; mean age 13 years). The harness group also received visual and verbal feedback. The study found that the harness helped align the hips and shoulders better at back foot contact, thereby improving this aspect of the mixed technique, when worn. It also increased the negative shoulder separation angle at front foot strike and did not significantly affect shoulder counter-rotation, or trunk extension or lateral flexion to the left (for right-handed bowlers). More crucially, the group of bowlers that wore the harness did not retain any desirable changes to their movement technique even after the harness was removed. The success of all three of the published intervention studies that we have touched on in this and the previous paragraph in reducing the injury risk of the mixed fast bowling technique has, therefore, been limited.

SUMMARY

In this chapter, consideration was given to how the results of biomechanical studies of sports movements can be communicated and fed back to the athlete and coach to improve performance (or reduce injury risk). The fundamental points that must be satisfied for biomechanical feedback to the coach and athlete to be relevant were covered. The strengths and weaknesses of various performance models and their limitations in feedback were described. An appreciation was provided of the important roles played by technique training in the process of modifying a sports movement. The issues that must be addressed in seeking to optimise the provision of biomechanical information to the coach and athlete were considered, including input from a motor learning perspective. We looked at the use of computer-based feedback and outlined some recent developments in this mode of information provision. The chapter concluded with consideration of case studies that have evaluated the success of intervention strategies, particularly involving the reduction of injury risk to fast bowlers in cricket.

STUDY TASKS

1 List and briefly discuss three points that must be satisfied for biomechanical feedback to be relevant to the sports practitioner.
2 With reference to the example of propulsive force generation in swimming (Figure 8.1), assess which of the three points that you discussed in Study Task 1 were violated in providing information to swimming coaches about the S-shaped pull pattern based on cinematography.

3   List and briefly explain how various models of performance have been, or could be, used in conjunction with biomechanical feedback. Illustrate the usefulness of each of these various approaches in the context of identifying and correcting a specific movement fault in a sporting activity of your choice, for example a low take-off angle in long jump or over-rotation in a high-board dive.

4   Produce a schematic diagram of a menu-based analysis system for all the levels of the hierarchical model of Figure 6.8.

5   Outline the points to which a coach should attend when seeking to eliminate faults in the movement technique of an athlete. Illustrate these points by reference to a possible movement fault for a club standard performer in a sport of your choice.

6   After consulting the appropriate further reading, compare and contrast the results of Schmidt (1991), Broker *et al.* (1993) and Mononen *et al.* (2003) on the value of immediate and summary feedback.

7   After consulting the appropriate further reading, outline the major developments in the computerised feedback of information from sports biomechanics that you think are most likely in the next five years.

8   After consulting the three references to intervention studies to reduce injury in cricket fast bowlers, critically assess the various approaches that have been reported in trying to change mixed technique fast bowlers in cricket to side-on or front-on bowlers.

GLOSSARY OF IMPORTANT TERMS

Accelerometers Devices that measure acceleration. They are sometimes used in providing **augmented feedback**. They provide accurate information when mounted on a rigid structure, such as an oar, but very inaccurate information when mounted on the skin, owing to soft tissue movements.

Artificial intelligence See glossary in Chapter 5.

Augmented feedback In the context of this chapter, information that we provide to sports performers that supplements (or augments) that already available to them through their senses. It can be in the form of knowledge of performance (KP) or knowledge of results (KR).

Computer-based feedback This term is used for feedback provided through a digital computer, usually in the form of computer graphics. Most **augmented feedback** to sports performers is provided in this way.

Constraints-led approach A key approach in ecological motor control, in which the solution to a motor, or sports, task for a given individual is determined not only by the constraints of the task itself and the environment but also by the individual's organismic constraints (see glossary in Chapter 6).

Dual-screen displays Used in the context of this chapter to refer to the viewing of two still images or video sequences, usually in a qualitative movement analysis package, from different camera views, performances or performers on the computer screen at the same time, either side by side or one above the other. This can be extended to more than two images in some packages – multi-screen displays.

Etiology (or aetiology) In the context of this book, etiology is the study of the causes of sports injuries.

Immediate and summary feedback These terms are normally used to distinguish between **augmented feedback** provided after each trial of a task (immediate feedback) or only after several trials (summary feedback).

Menu-driven systems In the context of this book, this is used to describe a system using drop-down menus, such as those used in many Windows user interfaces, to present the information contained in a possible expert system for the diagnosis and correction of movement errors.

Optimisation See glossary in Chapter 7.

Serial and parallel representations Used in the context of this book to refer to representations, or animations, of a movement presented sequentially, or frame by frame, as in a video recording, or as a series of images presented 'in parallel' on one 'picture', as in stick figure representations of a whole movement.

Simulation (or computer simulation) See glossary in Chapter 7.

Statistical modelling Modelling data using various statistical methods such as ANOVA, MANOVA, t-tests and multiple regression (see Glossary in Chapter 7).

REFERENCES

Anderson, R., Harrison, A. and Lyons, G.M. (2005) Accelerometry-based feedback – can it improve movement consistency and performance in rowing? *Sports Biomechanics*, *4*, 179–195.

Best, R.J., Bartlett, R.M. and Sawyer, R.A. (1995) Optimal javelin release. *Journal of Applied Biomechanics*, *12*, 58–71.

Blanksby, B., Nicholson, L. and Elliott, B. (2002) Biomechanical analysis of the grab, track and handle swimming starts: an intervention study. *Sports Biomechanics*, *1*, 11–24.

Broker, J.P., Gregor, R.J. and Schmidt, R.A. (1993) Extrinsic feedback and the learning of kinetic patterns in cycling. *Journal of Applied Biomechanics*, *9*, 111–123.

Cassidy, T., Stanley, S. and Bartlett, R.M. (2006) Reflecting on video feedback as a tool for learning skilled movement. *International Journal of Sports Science and Coaching*, *1*, 279–288.

Davids, K., Button, C. and Bennett, S. (2008) *Dynamics of Skill Acquisition: A Constraints-led Approach*, Champaign, IL: Human Kinetics.

Elliott, B. (2000) Back injuries and the fast bowler in cricket: a review. *Journal of Sports Sciences*, *18*, 983–991.

Elliott, B. and Bartlett, R.M. (2006) Sports biomechanics: does it have a role in coaching? *International Journal of Sports Science and Coaching*, *1*, 177–183.

Elliott, B. and Khangure, M. (2002) Disk degeneration and the young fast bowler in cricket: an intervention study. *Clinical Biomechanics*, *34*, 1714–1718.

Guadagnoli, M., Holcomb, W. and Davis, M. (2002) The efficacy of video feedback for learning the golf swing. *Journal of Sports Sciences*, *20*, 615–622.

Hay, J.G., Liu, Q. and Andrews, J.G. (1993) Body roll and handpath in free style swimming: a computer simulation study. *Journal of Applied Biomechanics*, 9, 227–237.

Hodges, N.J. and Williams, M.A. (eds) (2007) *Journal of Sports Sciences*, 25(5) Special Issue on Observational Learning.

Huffman, R.K., Hubbard, M. and Reus, J. (1993) 'Use of an interactive bobsled simulator in driver training', in *Advances in Bioengineering*, Vol. 26, New York: American Society of Mechanical Engineers, pp. 263–266.

Judge, L., Hunter, I. and Gilreath, E. (2008) Using sports science to improve coaching: a case study of the American record holder in the women's hammer throw. *International Journal of Sports Science and Coaching*, 3, 477–488.

Knudson, D.V. and Morrison, C.S. (2002) *Qualitative Analysis of Human Movement*, Champaign, IL: Human Kinetics.

Lapham, A.C. and Bartlett, R.M. (1995) The use of artificial intelligence in the analysis of sports performance: a review of applications in human gait analysis and future directions for sports biomechanics. *Journal of Sports Sciences*, 13, 229–237.

Liebermann, D.G. and Franks, I.M. (2004) 'The use of feedback-based technologies', in M.D. Hughes and I.M. Franks (eds) *Notational Analysis of Sport: Systems for Better Coaching and Performance in Sport*, London: Routledge, pp. 40–58.

Liebermann, D.G., Katz, L., Hughes, M.D., Bartlett, R.M., McClements, J. and Franks, I.M. (2002) Advances in the application of information technology to sport performance. *Journal of Sports Sciences*, 20, 755–769.

Mononen, K., Viitasalo, J.T., Konttinen, N. and Era, P. (2003) The effects of augmented kinematic feedback on motor skill learning in rifle shooting. *Journal of Sports Sciences*, 21, 867–876.

Payton, C.J. and Bartlett, R.M. (eds) (2008) *Biomechanical Evaluation of Movement in Sport and Exercise: The British Association of Sport and Exercise Sciences Guide*, London: Routledge.

Payton, C.J., Hay, J.G. and Mullineaux, D.R. (1997) The effect of body roll on hand speed and hand path in front crawl swimming: a simulation study. *Journal of Applied Biomechanics*, 13, 300–315.

Ranson, C., King, M., Burnett, A., Worthington, P. and Shine, K. (2009) The effect of a coaching intervention on elite fast bowling technique over a two year period. *Sports Biomechanics*, 8, 261–274.

Schmidt, R.A. (1991) *Motor Learning and Performance: From Principles to Practice*, Champaign, IL: Human Kinetics.

Smith, R.M. and Loschner, C. (2002) Biomechanics feedback for rowing. *Journal of Sports Sciences*, 20, 783–791.

Wallis, R., Elliott, B. and Koh, M. (2002) The effect of a fast bowling harness in cricket: an intervention study. *Journal of Sports Sciences*, 20, 495–506.

Yeadon, M.R. and King, M.A. (2008) 'Computer simulation modelling in sport', in C.J. Payton and R.M. Bartlett (eds) *Biomechanical Evaluation of Movement in Sport and Exercise: The British Association of Sport and Exercise Sciences Guide*, London: Routledge, pp. 176–205.

FURTHER READING

Broker, J.P., Gregor, R.J. and Schmidt, R.A. (1993) Extrinsic feedback and the learning of kinetic patterns in cycling, *Journal of Applied Biomechanics*, 9, 111–123. This presents the first example considered in this chapter comparing immediate and summary feedback.

Schmidt, R.A. (1991) *Motor Learning and Performance: From Principles to Practice*, Champaign, IL: Human Kinetics. This contains clear expositions of all issues relating to learning, and relearning, of motor skills. It also presents the second example considered in this chapter comparing immediate and summary feedback. Mononen, K., Viitasalo, J.T., Konttinen, N. and Era, P. (2003) The effects of augmented kinematic feedback on motor skill learning in rifle shooting. *Journal of Sports Sciences*, *21*, 867–876. This reading is necessary for you to undertake Study Task 6.

Davids, K., Button, C. and Bennett, S. (2008) *Dynamics of Skill Acquisition: A Constraints-led Approach*, Champaign, IL: Human Kinetics. This gives an excellent overview, from the constraints-led approach, to skill acquisition. Some of this material is relevant to the theme of this chapter: changing movement patterns to improve performance.

Elliott, B. and Khangure, M. (2002) Disk degeneration and the young fast bowler in cricket: an intervention study, *Clinical Biomechanics*, *34*, 1714–1718. Ranson, C., King, M., Burnett, A., Worthington, P. and Shine, K. (2009) The effect of a coaching intervention on elite fast bowling technique over a two year period. *Sports Biomechanics*, *8*, 261–274. Wallis, R., Elliott, B. and Koh, M. (2002) The effect of a fast bowling harness in cricket: an intervention study. *Journal of Sports Sciences*, *20*, 495–506. Three studies that sought to reduce the incidence of the mixed fast bowling technique in cricket; this reading is necessary for you to undertake Study Task 8.

Liebermann, D.G. and Franks, I.M. (2004) 'The use of feedback-based technologies', in M.D. Hughes and I.M. Franks (eds) *Notational Analysis of Sport: Systems for Better Coaching and Performance in Sport*, London: Routledge, pp. 40–58. Liebermann, D.G., Katz, L., Hughes, M.D., Bartlett, R.M., McClements, J. and Franks, I.M. (2002) Advances in the application of information technology to sport performance. *Journal of Sports Sciences*, *20*, 755–769. This reading is necessary for you to undertake Study Task 7.

Glossary

Abrasion (graze) Skin surface broken without a complete tear through the skin.

Accelerometers Devices that measure acceleration. An accelerometer measures the acceleration of the free-fall reference frame (inertial reference frame) relative to itself. They are sometimes used in providing **augmented feedback**. They provide accurate information when mounted on a rigid structure, such as an oar, but very inaccurate information when mounted on the skin, owing to soft tissue movements.

Adhesion Bands of fibrous tissue, usually caused by inflammation.

Analysis of variance (ANOVA) In this statistical procedure, the observed variance in a particular variable is partitioned into components arising from different sources of variation. ANOVA provides a statistical test of the differences between the means of several groups. It is often used in the contrast approach to statistical modelling.

Analyst bias An unconscious tendency that can arise in the evaluation and diagnosis stage of qualitative analysis for various reasons. Prior knowledge of a performer or a performer's age can be factors. Good definitions of, and correctness criteria for, **critical features** and thorough training of the observational analysts can help to reduce analyst bias.

Anticipatory change Some change in body geometry or function that precedes, or anticipates, a particular movement change. In the context of this chapter, this means the change in continuous relative phase that occurs before the change from the stance to swing phase, or vice versa, in running.

Apophysis The type of growth plate that occurs between a tubercle (e.g. tibial tuberosity) and parent bone (e.g. tibia).

Artificial intelligence The branch of computer science that deals, loosely speaking, with 'intelligent machines' – machines (computers) that do things that would require intelligence if done by a human. The two most important branches to date for performance analysts are expert systems and artificial neural networks.

Artificial neural networks These are computer programs that try to create a mathematical model of neurons in the brain. They allow computers to learn from experience and by analogy.

Augmented feedback In the context of this book, information that we provide to sports performers that supplements (or augments) that already available to them through their senses. It can be in the form of knowledge of performance (KP) or knowledge of results (KR).

Automatic marker-tracking systems These are image-based motion analysis systems in which the system hardware and software automatically tracks, ideally without any user intervention, the trajectories of markers placed on the body.

Avulsion fracture Fracture where the two halves of the bone are pulled apart.

Ballistic movements Movements that are initiated by muscle activity in one muscle group, continue with a period (sometimes called coasting) of no muscle activity, and end by deceleration by the antagonistic muscle group or by passive tissues, such as ligaments.

Bone mineral content The measure of the total mineral content in bone, measured in grams.

Bone mineral density (BMD) The measure of mineral content in a volume of bone, measured as area bone mineral density (g/cm^2) or volumetric bone mineral density (g/cm^3).

Bursitis Inflammation of the fluid-filled sac (bursa) that lies between a tendon and skin, or between a tendon and bone.

Calcification Deposit of insoluble mineral salts in tissue.

Callus Material that first joins broken bones, consisting largely of connective tissue and cartilage, which later calcifies.

Cancellous bone Internal material of long bone; appears trellis-like.

Capsulitis Inflammation of the joint capsule.

Centripetal force Force directed toward the centre of rotation in a rotating body.

Chondromalacia patellae The softening and breakdown of the cartilage that lines the underside of the patella.

Coefficient of restitution The measure of elasticity of an object is a fractional value representing the ratio of velocities after and before an impact.

Collateral ligament An accessory ligament that is not part of the joint capsule.

Collective variable Simplistically, a variable that incorporates two or more other variables. Relative phase is a collective variable as it incorporates two angles and two angular velocities. In the context of this book, the collective variable should characterise coordination patterns or changes in coordination, which relative phase usually does. A collective variable is also known, in the coordination context, as an order parameter.

Comminuted fracture One in which the bone is broken into more than two pieces.

Computer-based feedback This term is used for feedback provided through a digital computer, usually in the form of computer graphics. Most **augmented feedback** to sports performers is provided in this way.

Conjugate cross correlations An extension of **cross correlation functions** to cover more than two joints. Rules of compatibility between the time lags and between the signs of the correlation peaks for the various cross correlation functions involved can be specified.

Constraints-led approach A key approach in ecological motor control, in which the solution to a motor, or sports, task for a given individual is determined not only by the constraints of the task itself and the environment but also by the individual's **organismic constraints.**

Contractile component This is the component of models of skeletal muscle that incorporates the mechanisms of muscle contraction, essentially the actin and myosin filaments and their associated cross-bridge coupling mechanism.

Contusion Bruise, usually caused by an escape of blood from ruptured vessels after injury.

Coordination dynamics In essence, the science of coordination, which aims to describe, explain and predict how patterns of coordination form, adapt and change in living organisms. In the context of this book, the term can be applied to a single joint through to the entire human movement system.

Coordination patterns Whereas movement patterns express how a movement variable – for example, an angle, angular velocity, or angular acceleration – evolves (or varies) with time, coordination patterns look at how meaningful combinations of these variables co-vary. Coordination patterns include angle–angle diagrams, phase planes, continuous relative phase (itself a function of time) and cross-correlation functions.

Coordinative structures These are considered to be functional relationships between important anatomical parts of the body to perform a specific activity, such as when groups of muscles and joints temporarily function as coherent units to achieve a specific goal, such as hitting a ball.

Correlation coefficients These express the strength of the statistical relationship between two variables.

Correlation matrix A correlation matrix is a square symmetrical $n \times n$ matrix that contains correlations among n variables, where n is a positive integer greater than 1. The ith row and jth column of the matrix contains the correlation coefficient between the ith and the jth variables. The leading diagonal elements are correlations of variables with themselves and are, therefore, equal to 1.

Cortical bone Outer layer (cortex) of bone having a compact structure.

Cost function A function used to constrain the optimisation model; a feasible solution to the cost function that minimises or maximises, if that is the goal, the cost function is called an optimal solution. The minimisation of the cost functions is an attempt to imitate the body's criteria for deciding which muscles to recruit and the order of recruitment. We can also define the level of activation that will produce appropriate motion or posture for a specific task. The selection of the most appropriate criterion to use in the optimisation process resides upon several aspects such as the type of motion under analysis, the objectives to achieve or the presence of any type of pathology.

Critical features Those key features of a movement that are required for the movement to be performed optimally. The term is used mostly in qualitative biomechanical analysis, in which case the critical features need to be observable. The identification of the critical features of a movement is the most important task of the preparation stage of qualitative biomechanical analysis.

Cross correlation functions These are obtained by calculating the **correlation coefficient** between two time series, then introducing various time lags between the two time series and recalculating the **correlation coefficient** for each time lag. Finally, the cross correlation function is the graph of the correlation coefficient as a function of the time lag.

Cross-sectional designs The term is used to refer to research designs taken at a specific time (a 'snapshot'). As an example, one or more trials by each finalist in the javelin throw at an international championship would be studied.

Cumulative trauma Caused by accumulated microtrauma resulting in acute or overuse type of injury. It is assumed that the acumulated microtrauma is caused by repeated overloading and inadequate rest of the tissues involved.

Degeneration A gradual deterioration of specific tissues changing them to a lower or less functionally active form.

Deterministic (or hierarchical) performance models These are models of the factors that influence sports performance in which the factors in the lower levels of the model completely determine (hence, deterministic) those in the higher levels. The top level is the factor by which performance is assessed, called the performance criterion – such as the time of a race or distance of a throw or jump. They resemble hierarchical models, for example in Microsoft Word, hence the alternative name.

Diaphysis The central ossification region of long bones (adjective: diaphyseal).

Dislocation Complete separation of articulating bones consequent on forcing of joint beyond its maximum passive range.

Dual-screen displays Used in the context of this book to refer to the viewing of two still images or video sequences, usually in a qualitative movement analysis package, from different camera views, performances or performers on the computer screen at the same time, either side by side or one above the other. This can be extended to more than two images in some packages – multi-screen displays.

Ductile To be drawn out, to become thinner or narrower before breaking.

Elastic elements These are the components of models of skeletal muscle that store and release elastic energy. The series elastic element is in series with the contractile component and mainly consists of the tendons. The parallel elastic elements lie in parallel to the contractile component and consist mainly of the muscle's various connective tissues and sarcolemma.

Empirical modelling This involves devising mathematical models, usually statistical ones, using experimental data. It is used widely in sports biomechanics and notational analysis.

Epiphysis The separately ossified ends of growing bones separated from the shaft by a cartilaginous (epiphyseal) plate.

Epiphysitis Inflammation of the epiphysis.

Etiology (or aetiology) In the context of this book, etiology is the study of the causes of sports injuries.

Euclidean distance In the context of this book, this is used to describe a mathematically meaningful distance between two points on the output map of an artificial neural network.

Exposure A method of quantifying injury risk due to participation in sport. Injury rates are reported as per athlete-exposures (number of practices or games where the athlete might be exposed to injury risk) or time-exposures (amount of time spent practising or participating in risk activity). If an athlete participated in 100 practices per season lasting 60 minutes each, and sustains one injury during practice, the exposure risk is said to be 1 per 100 or 1 per 1000 hours.

Finite element modelling Used to visualise stresses and strains in a structure. It uses a numerical technique called 'finite element analysis' for finding approximate solutions of partial differential equations as well as of integral equations.

Fracture A disruption to tissue (normally bone) integrity. In traumatic fracture a break will occur, whereas in a stress fracture the disruption is microscopic.

Golgi tendon organs These are small stretch receptors located at the junction of a muscle and its tendon. Their discharge causes inhibition of the muscle in which they are located (which helps to protect the muscle) and facilitation of the antagonist muscle.

Haemarthrosis Effusion of blood into a joint cavity.

Headform An instrumented system for testing head impacts.

Hemarthosis Bleeding or extravasation of blood into the joint spaces.

Hematoma An extravasation of blood outside the blood vessels, usually in liquid form within the tissue and generally the result of a haemorrhage.

Homogeneity of variance The assumption (in both ANOVA and *t*-tests, for example) that the variances of two or more datasets are equal.

Hooke's Law Within the elastic limit of a solid material, the deformation or strain produced by a stress of any kind is proportional to the force. If the elastic limit is not exceeded, the material returns to its original shape and size after the force is removed. If the elastic limit is exceeded, the material remains deformed or stretched. The force at which the material exceeds its elastic limit is called the 'limit of proportionality'.

Immediate and summary feedback These terms are normally used to distinguish between **augmented feedback** provided after each trial of a task (immediate feedback) or only after several trials (summary feedback).

Impulse–momentum relationship An expression of Newton's Second Law of Motion, which states that the impulse of a force (the mean force multiplied by the time during which the force acts) is equal to the change in momentum of the body on which the force acts.

Indeterminate system A system of simultaneous equations that has infinitely many solutions or no solutions at all. If there are fewer unique equations than variables, then the system must be indeterminate.

Individual specificity Term used to express the fact that any individual will find a specific solution (or set of solutions) to a movement task that fits his or her **organismic constraints** as well as the task and environmental constraints. The movement analyst has to be continually aware of the requirement for individual specificity when seeking to identify and correct movement faults. What works for one sports performer may not work for another.

Inequality constraints A restriction that limits the value of a dependent or independent variable. An inequality constraint is used to apply a limitation to a feature that may vary, such as joint movement, speed and torque.

Inertial reference frame A 'frame of reference' is a standard relative to which motion and rest may be measured. An inertial reference frame is relative to motions that have distinguished dynamical properties. An inertial frame is a spatial reference frame together with some means of measuring time, so that uniform motions can be distinguished from accelerated motions. In Newtonian dynamics, an inertial frame is a reference frame with a timescale, relative to which the motion of a body (disregarding external forces) is always rectilinear and uniform, accelerations are always proportional to and in the direction of applied forces, and applied forces are always met with equal and opposite reactions.

Inflammation Defensive response of tissue to injury indicated by redness, swelling, pain, loss of function and warmth.

Injury incidence The number of new cases of an injury within a specified time period divided by the size of the population initially at risk.

Injury prevalence Defined as the total number of cases of the injury in the population at a given time, or the total number of cases in the population, divided by the number of individuals in the population.

Injury rate May be defined as case rates or athlete rates. Athlete rates are determined by dividing the total number of athletes injured by the total number of athletes participating. Case rates are determined by dividing the total number of reported cases occurring during the study period by the total number of population exposed to the possibility of injury.

Innervation ratio The number of muscle fibres that are stimulated, or innervated, by a single motor neuron; the number of muscle fibres in a particular motor unit. This ratio varies from as few as 10 for muscles requiring very fine control to over 1000 for the weight-bearing muscles of the lower extremities.

In-phase and anti-phase coordination In-phase coordination involves two joints (or segments) moving in an anatomically similar way. Examples would be the knee and hip flexing together in the downward movement of a standing vertical jump or the index fingers on both hands abducting. Anti-phase, or out of phase, coordination occurs when the movements are antagonistic, as when the index finger on one hand adducts while that on the other hand abducts, or when the hip flexes while the knee extends. In this context, ankle plantar flexion is considered to be in-phase with hip and knee extension.

Intra- and inter-analyst reliability Intra-analyst (also called intra-rater or intra-operator) reliability is the consistency of the analyses carried out by one analyst on several occasions. Inter-analyst reliability (also called objectivity) is the consistency of the analyses of several analysts. Intra-analyst reliability is usually better than inter-analyst reliability. Neither is easy to determine accurately for qualitative movement analysis.

Inverse dynamics Inverse rigid-body dynamics is a method for computing forces and moments of force (torques) based on the kinematics of a body and the body's inertial properties (mass and moment of inertia).

Inverse optimisation An optimisation technique in which the ideal solution or outcome (i.e. movement) is known. We use the technique to optimise the muscle recruitment or muscle forces involved so as to simulate the known movement criteria.

Inverted-U A relationship between two variables that looks like an upside-down letter U.

Isometric force The tension (or force) developed in a muscle that is undergoing an isometric contraction – without change of length.

Joint angle conventions For two-dimensional analysis in the sagittal plane, the normal sports biomechanics convention is for a fully extended knee or elbow, for example, to be designated as 180°. Flexion then involves the joint angle decreasing and extension involves the joint angle increasing. This convention is used throughout this book. The angle conventions used by clinical biomechanists and in three-dimensional analysis are completely different. Movement analysts need to check carefully what joint angle convention is being used.

Laceration An open wound or cut.

Local and global optimums A function may have a global optimum, defined over the whole range of the function, as well as several local optimums, which are optimal only within a limited (local) range of the function. A geographical analogy would be the many local peaks within the Himalayas, whereas the top of Mount Everest is the global Himalayan peak.

Markov chains Named after A. A. Markov, a Markov chain is a random process in which one state depends only on the previous state. Markov chains are useful as tools for statistical modelling, particularly, in the context of this book, in modelling the outcomes of games, such as squash.

Mathematically indeterminate A problem that has an infinite number of solutions, or one in which there are fewer imposed conditions than there are unknowns.

Maximum tetanic force Maximum force produced by a muscle in a state of sustained maximal tension.

Maximum voluntary contraction A measure of strength that can be expressed as a maximal exertion of force, reported either as a force or as a moment (or torque) around a joint.

Menu-driven systems In the context of this book, this is used to describe a system using drop-down menus, such as those used in many Windows user interfaces, to present the information contained in a possible expert system for the diagnosis and correction of movement errors.

Metaphysis Region of long bone between the epiphysis and diaphysis.

Movement trajectory analysis A term normally used to refer to the analysis of the two-dimensional paths (or trajectories) taken by players over time across the surface of a sports pitch or court.

Multiple regression In multiple regression, more than one predictor variable is used to predict the value of the criterion variable. This contrasts with simple regression in which there is only one predictor variable.

Multivariate analysis of variance (MANOVA) A generalisation of ANOVA to cases in which there are two or more dependent variables. It is sometimes used in the contrast approach to statistical modelling discussed in this book.

Muscle latency period Refers to the lack of visible change that occurs in the muscle fibre during (and immediately after) the action potential.

Musculotendinous unit A muscle tendon unit functions as a single system, whose two components contribute to force production at different times. The force is produced by a combination of muscle actions and a release of elastic energy from the tendon component.

Needs analysis In the context of this book, a needs analysis is usually a semi-formal meeting or interview, led by the movement analyst, to ascertain what the 'clients' need from the movement analysis.

Net-wall games Games involving a net or a wall. Table tennis, tennis, badminton and volleyball are net games and squash and fives are wall games. One of the three common categories of formal games, the others being striking and fielding games (such as cricket and baseball) and invasion games (such as rugby, basketball, soccer and netball).

Normal force The force component that is perpendicular to the surface of contact.

Normality The assumption (in both ANOVA and *t*-tests, for example) that a dataset conforms to a normal (or Gaussian) distribution (the bell-shaped curve).

Optimal performance model A somewhat discredited concept of a universal optimal set of movement patterns to perform a given movement task – such as a javelin throw – that applies to all individuals. This concept led to the idea of copying the movements of the current world champion in that task (the so-called 'elite performer template'), completely ignoring the principle of **individual specificity**.

Optimisation The mathematical process of finding the optimum value of a function of several variables. A procedure or set of procedures that are used to make a system as functional as possible. Static optimisation computes the optimum values of a finite set of quantities of interest, such as a small set of input parameters. Dynamic optimisation seeks to compute optimum input functions of time.

Order parameter See **collective variable** above.

Organismic constraints The set of characteristics, or constraints, that an individual possesses; these constraints influence the movement solutions that individual will adopt for a particular task and environment. These are internal to the individual and include anatomical–anthropometric characteristics, strength, flexibility and fitness.

Orthogonal Two or more lines are said to be orthogonal if they are perpendicular or form right angles to each other.

Osteitis Inflammation of bone.

Osteochondrotic diseases Characterised by interruption of the blood supply of a bone, in particular to the epiphysis, followed by localised bony necrosis and, later, regrowth of the bone.

Parametric statistics assume that the data have come from a particular probability distribution; they involve assumptions about the parameters of that distribution, such as **normality** or **homogeneity of variance**. ANOVA, MANOVA and *t*-tests are all parametric statistical tests, as are **Pearson product moment correlations**.

Pearson product moment correlation This is the most common way of assessing the strength of a linear relationship between two variables. The strength of the relationship is expressed as the Pearson product moment **correlation coefficient**.

Pennate muscles The class of muscles, accounting for 75% of the body's musculature, with relatively short fibres angled away from the tendon. The arrangement allows more fibres to be recruited, which provides a stronger, more powerful movement at the expense of range and speed of movement. The class includes the tibialis anterior (a unipennate muscle), flexor hallucis longus (a bipennate muscle) and the deltoid (a multipennate muscle).

Performance criterion A formal term that means the factor by which a performance is assessed – the result or outcome. Examples are the distance jumped or thrown, the time of a race and the score of a dive or gymnastics vault.

Performance variables (or performance parameters) A term used mostly in quantitative biomechanical analysis for the factors that influence the performance criterion, or outcome. They are roughly comparable to the critical features in a qualitative biomechanical analysis or the performance indicators in performance analysis.

Peritendinitis Inflammation of the tissues around a tendon (the peritendon).

Perturbation analysis Used in notational analysis of sports (particularly, to date, squash) to refer to disruptions to steady rhythms of play, through critical incidents or perturbations. These perturbations may then lead to the end of a rally or be smoothed out, resulting in the establishment of a new steady rhythm of play. They can often be seen by experienced observers as well as measured.

Pes cavus Also known as a 'high arch' is a human foot type in which the sole of the foot is distinctly hollow when bearing weight.

Pes planus Also known as 'flat footed' is a condition in which the arch or instep of the foot collapses and comes in contact with the ground.

Phagocytosis A specific form of endocytosis involving the vesicular internalisation of solid particles, such as bacteria, and is the body's mechanism used to remove pathogens and cell debris after injury.

Physiological cross-sectional area The cross-sectional area of a muscle perpendicular to the muscle fibres.

Plantar fasciitis An irritation and swelling of the thick tissue (fascia) on the bottom of the foot.

Polar second moment of area is also known as the area moment of inertia, moment of inertia of plane area, or second moment of inertia. It is a property of a cross section that can be used to predict the resistance of beams to bending and deflection, around an axis that lies in the cross-sectional plane.

Polyethylene A type of polymer that is classified as a thermoplastic, meaning that it can be melted to a liquid and remoulded as it returns to a solid state. Polyethylene is chemically synthesised from molecules that contain long chains of ethylene, a monomer that provides the ability to double bond with other carbon-based monomers to form polymers.

Polypropylene A thermoplastic polymer used in a wide variety of applications. It is an addition polymer made from the monomer propylene and it can serve as both a plastic and a fibre.

Polyurethane Any polymer consisting of a chain of organic units joined by urethane links. It is an incredibly resilient, flexible, and durable manufactured material. It is made by combining a diisocyanate and a diol, two monomers, through a chemical reaction. This makes a basic material whose variations can be stretched, smashed, or scratched, and remain fairly indestructible.

Porous bound macadam The foundation layer of most artificial sports surfaces, the term macadam refers to the method of laying the stone and sand aggregates that are sprayed with the porous binding material.

Proprioceptive stretching Proprioceptive neuromuscular facilitation (PNF) is a more advanced form of flexibility training that involves both the stretching and contraction of the muscle group being targeted. Exercises are based on the stretch reflex which is caused by stimulation of the **Golgi tendon organs** and muscle spindles. This stimulation results in impulses being sent to the brain, which leads to the contraction and relaxation of muscles. After an injury, there is a delay in the stimulation of the muscle spindles and Golgi tendon organs resulting in weakness of the muscle. PNF exercises are used in rehabilitation programmes to re-educate the motor units that are lost due to the injury.

Right hand rule A procedure for identifying the direction of an angular motion vector.

Rotator cuff The group of muscles (supraspinatus, infraspinatus, teres minor and subscapularis) that act to stabilise the shoulder. The four muscles of the rotator cuff, along with the teres major and the deltoid, make up the six scapulohumeral muscles.

Rupture or tear Complete break in continuity of a soft tissue structure.

Self-organising maps are artificial neural networks that are trained using unsupervised learning to produce a low-dimensional output space representation (sometimes called a map) of the high-dimensional input space of the training data.

Serial and parallel representations Used in the context of this book to refer to representations, or animations, of a movement presented sequentially, or frame by frame, as in a video recording, or as a series of images presented 'in parallel' on one 'picture', as in stick figure representations of a whole movement.

Shin splints The more common term for 'medial tibial stress syndrome', which is a slow healing and painful condition in the anterior medial tibia.

Simulation (or computer simulation) involves the carrying out of computer experiments on a set of equations (or a simulation model) that represent an aspect of the real world. Simulation models used are based on physical laws not statistical relationships.

Simulation evaluation This is the process of seeking to evaluate whether the results of a computer simulation adequately represent the real-world system that was being modelled.

Sinusoidal A function having the form of a sine or cosine wave or a combination of these.

Sprain Damage to a joint and associated ligaments. The three degrees of sprain involve around 25%, 50% and 75% of the tissues, respectively. Grade I sprains are mild and involve no clinical instability; Grade II are moderate with some instability; and Grade III are severe with easily detectable instability. There may be effusion into the joint.

Statistical modelling Modelling data using various statistical methods such as **ANOVA, MANOVA, *t*-tests** and **multiple regression**.

Statistical power The power of a statistical test is the probability that the test will reject a null hypothesis that is false, in other words, that it will not make a **Type II error**. The greater the power, the less is the chance of a Type II error.

Strain Damage to muscle fibres. A Grade I strain involves only a few fibres, and strong but painful contractions are possible. A Grade II strain involves more fibres and a localised haematoma, and contractions are weak; as with Grade I, no fascia is damaged. Grade III strains involve a great many, or all, fibres, partial or complete fascia tearing, diffuse bleeding and disability.

Stretch reflex The contraction of a muscle in response to a sudden stretching of that muscle. It occurs in the stretch-shortening cycle.

Subjective performance criterion A performance criteria (or result) that is judged subjectively, as in gymnastics, figure skating and diving.

Subluxation Partial dislocation.

Superior labrum The labrum is a lip-like piece of cartilage that deepens the glenoid of the shoulder joint that aids in stabilising the shoulder joint. The labrum is divided into superior, inferior, anterior and posterior parts.

Systematic observation strategy The development of a systematic 'observation' strategy pays attention to all matters that are relevant to good observation, and subsequent analysis, of movement.

t-tests provide a test of whether the means of two groups are statistically different from each other. They are often used in the contrast approach to statistical modelling discussed in this book.

Tendinitis Painful tendon with histological signs of inflammation within the tendon.

Tendinopathy Disease of the tendon including tendinitis, tendinosis and tenosynovitis.

Tendinosis Degenerative condition of a tendon.

Tenosynovitis Inflammation of the synovial sheath surrounding a tendon.

Thermomoldable plastics A type of plastic that can be moulded using a heat source such as a heat gun or special oven.

Tibia varum A frontal plane deformity where the distal third of the tibia is angled closer to the mid-sagittal plane than the proximal end.

Topological equivalence Two shapes (such as angle–angle diagrams) are said to be topologically equivalent if one can be deformed into the other without folding or cutting. For our purposes, two shapes can be said to be topologically equivalent if they contain the same number of loops. [In the branch of mathematics called topology, topological equivalence is a bit more complicated than these simple statements might imply.]

Type I and Type II errors A Type I error occurs when a null hypothesis that is true is rejected, incorrectly. A Type II error occurs when a null hypothesis is not rejected although it is false.

Ultimate tensile stress The maximum stress that a material can withstand while being stretched or pulled before necking, which is when the injury occurs.

Valgus Abduction of the distal segment relative to the proximal one (as in genu valgum, knock-knees).

Validity In the analysis of human movement in sport, there is often a conflict between internal, or research, validity and external, or ecological, validity. Laboratory studies generally have good research validity and field-based studies generally have good ecological validity. Ecological validity is of prime importance when seeking to improve sports performance.

Varignon's theorem Is also called the 'principle of moments' and it states that the moment of any force is equal to the algebraic sum of the moments of the components of that force.

Varus Adduction of the distal segment relative to the proximal one (as in genu varum, bow-legs).

Viscoelasticity This is a property of all biological materials, which exhibit both elastic and viscous behaviour when deformed. The stress–strain characteristics of viscoelastic materials are time-dependent.

Wobbling mass model One of the assumptions of linear inverse dynamics is that the body being studied is a series of rigid segments. However, we can see from high-speed recordings of impacts, the soft parts of each segment of the human body are shifted relative to the bony parts and start to 'wobble' in a complex damped manner. Therefore, some researchers have developed ways of modelling the essential properties of the human body as 'wobbling masses', which are coupled quasi-elastically and strongly damped to each rigid bony part. The wobbling mass model allows the researcher to study the effects of the different mechanical behaviour of the soft tissues and the rigid bony parts of the human body.

Index

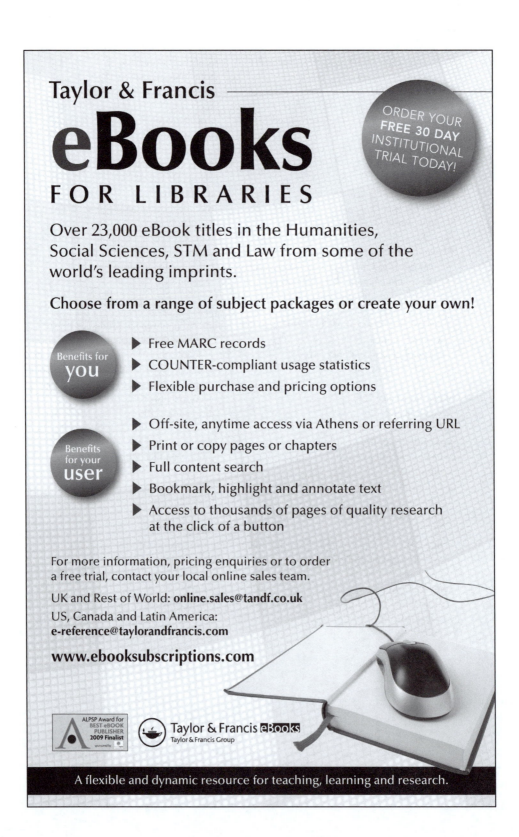